Comprehensive Manuals of Surgical Specialties

Richard H. Egdahl, editor

Edward W. Humphrey   Deanne Lawrence McKeown

Manual of Pulmonary Surgery

Includes 215 illustrations, 190 in full color

Springer-Verlag
New York Heidelberg Berlin

SERIES EDITOR
Richard H. Egdahl, M.D., Ph.D., Professor of Surgery, Boston University Medical Center, Boston, Massachusetts 02118

AUTHORS

Edward W. Humphrey, M.D., Ph.D., Professor of Surgery, University of Minnesota; Chief of Surgery, Minneapolis Veterans Administration Medical Center, Minneapolis, Minnesota 55417

Deanne Lawrence McKeown, Medical Illustrator, P.O. Box 1388, Sedona, Arizona 86336

CONTRIBUTORS

Richard L. Varco, M.D., Ph.D., Regents Professor of Surgery, Emeritus, University of Minnesota, Minneapolis, Minnesota 55417

Alan R. Shons, M.D., Ph.D., Associate Professor of Surgery, Director of Division of Plastic and Reconstructive Surgery, University of Minnesota, Minneapolis, Minnesota 55417

Sponsoring Editor: Marie D. Low
Production: Berta Steiner
Illustration Consultant: Fredric M. Harwin
Design: Caliber Design Planning, Inc.
Typeset by Kingsport Press, Kingsport, Tennessee
Printed and bound by R.R. Donnelley & Sons Company, Crawfordsville, Indiana

Library of Congress Cataloging in Publication Data
Humphrey, Edward W., 1926–
Manual of pulmonary surgery.

(Comprehensive manuals of surgical specialties)
Includes bibliographies and index.
1. Lungs—Surgery. I. McKeown, Deanne Lawrence.
II. Title. III. Series.
RD539.H85 1982 617'.542 82-16992

Printed in the United States of America.
9 8 7 6 5 4 3 2 1
ISBN 0-387-90732-7 Springer-Verlag New York Heidelberg Berlin
ISBN 3-540-90732-7 Springer-Verlag Berlin Heidelberg New York

This book is dedicated to
Dr. Richard L. Varco
from whom I have learned thoracic
surgery and much more.

E.W.H.

Contents

Editor's Note

Comprehensive Manuals of Surgical Specialties is a series of surgical manuals designed to present current operative techniques and to explore various aspects of diagnosis and treatment. The series features a unique format with emphasis on large, detailed, full-color illustrations, schematic charts, and photographs to demonstrate integral steps in surgical procedures.

Each manual focuses on a specific region or topic and describes surgical anatomy, physiology, pathology, diagnosis, and operative treatment. Operative techniques and stratagems for dealing with surgically correctable disorders are described in detail. Illustrations are primarily depicted from the surgeon's viewpoint to enhance clarity and comprehension.

Other volumes in the series:

Published:

Manual of Endocrine Surgery
Manual of Burns
Manual of Surgery of the Gallbladder, Bile Ducts, and Exocrine Pancreas
Manual of Gynecologic Surgery
Manual of Urologic Surgery
Manual of Lower Gastrointestinal Surgery
Manual of Vascular Surgery, Volume I
Manual of Cardiac Surgery, Volume I
Manual of Cardiac Surgery, Volume II
Manual of Liver Surgery
Manual of Ambulatory Surgery

In Preparation:

Manual of Vascular Surgery, Volume II
Manual of Soft Tissue Tumor Surgery
Manual of Orthopedic Surgery
Manual of Upper Gastrointestinal Surgery
Manual of Trauma Surgery
Manual of Sports Surgery
Manual of Aesthetic Plastic Surgery
Manual of Breast Surgery

Richard H. Egdahl

Preface

The *Manual of Pulmonary Surgery* has been designed primarily as a guide to the techniques of surgery on the lungs of adults and older children. The information included and the technical points stressed are those in which, in more than 20 years of teaching thoracic surgery, I have found residents to most commonly need instruction. An effort has been made to depict the usual anatomy of the lung and its more frequent variations, as it is encountered by the surgeon. This was necessary because a detailed description of pulmonary anatomy is not readily available. The excellent monograph on *Segmental Anatomy of the Lung* by Professor Edward Boyden, one of my teachers, is no longer in print.

The techniques illustrated are those preferred by the author; no attempt has been made to describe all of the possible variations. Deanne McKeown has illustrated the entire book. Her drawings of the procedures are based on sketches or photographs made in the operating room. The use of full color illustrations to emphasize important technical or anatomical detail adds to the ease of understanding the text.

A section on the indications for pulmonary resection that contains the information commonly used for surgical decision-making has been included. The reader is referred for more complete information on the pathophysiology and epidemiology of pulmonary disease to the several texts available on diseases of the chest. Because the lung cannot be considered in isolation from the rest of the respiratory mechanism, a discussion of the surgery of the major airways, of the chest wall and diaphragm, and of the mediastinum has also been included. Finally, since postoperative complications will occur in spite of the best efforts of the surgeon, and will provide some of the most difficult management problems encountered, the treatment of those complications unique to pulmonary surgery is discussed in the last chapter.

I am grateful to Dr. Richard Varco for writing the section on pectus excavatum, and to Dr. Alan Shons for writing the section on cutaneous and myocutaneous flaps for chest wall reconstruction. The secretarial and administrative staff of the surgery department worked diligently in the preparation of the manuscript, and my wife was very helpful in editing. The assistance and support of the publisher is gratefully acknowledged.

Edward W. Humphrey

Diagnostic Procedures 1

The goal of the initial workup is to determine therapy; therefore, the selection of diagnostic procedures should be based on their direct contribution to this decision. If the clinician's decision will not be affected by the result of a given examination, that examination is probably not worth the time, the discomfort, the risk, or the money it entails. The decision-making potential of any diagnostic test is a function of the risk of the therapy, the risk of the disease, and the error rate of the examination. A test used to screen for a particular abnormality should be chosen also on its probability of a significant yield in the affected population.

Understandably, a clinician may wish to spare a patient the discomfort of an invasive test, but noninvasive tests usually give only indirect evidence, which is often inaccurate. For example, in reviewing examinations of the mediastinal lymph nodes for metastasis from carcinoma of the lung, Fishman and Bronstein (8) reported that results of all indirect tests were negative in 38% of patients in whom mediastinoscopy showed metastasis; one or more indirect test was positive in 52% of the patients in whom mediastinoscopy did not show metastasis. This does not imply that invasive tests routinely have decision-making potential, but rather argues that the potential contribution of any test should be evaluated before it is ordered and that excessive importance should not be attached to a test on the basis of its being noninvasive.

Bronchoscopy

In the diagnosis and preoperative evaluation of patients with pulmonary disease, bronchoscopy is second in importance only to chest radiographic examinations. A bronchoscopic examination should probably be performed on most patients prior to pulmonary surgery. This test permits the inspection of the tracheobronchial tree for sites of ulceration, obstruction, laceration, or bleeding; of the intrabronchial extent for known or suspected tumors; and for the presence of previously undetected tumors. A histologic or cytologic diagnosis of a tumor may be made either by direct biopsy or by the use of intrabronchial brushing or biopsy under fluoroscopy. The histology of diffuse parenchymal disease can sometimes be determined by a transbronchial biopsy.

The examination can be performed either with a rigid Jackson bronchoscope or with a flexible fiberoptic bronchoscope. Although the rigid scope is still essential for the removal of many foreign bodies, and for certain more rare applications, such as the endoscopic resection of benign intrabronchial tumors, the fiberoptic scope has almost replaced the rigid scope for diagnostic purposes. The fiberoptic scope is easier to introduce, it is less uncomfortable for the patient, and it permits easy examination of segments of the bronchial tree that are accessible to the rigid scope only with difficulty. Although the fiberoptic scope is smaller and more prone to biopsy crush artifacts than is the rigid scope, biopsy specimens obtained through a fiberoptic scope are almost always adequate for the clinician's purposes.

Instruments

Rigid Bronchoscope

A 7-mm Jackson bronchoscope (Fig. 1-1) is the most useful size for adults. For children and for adults with tracheal stenosis, a series of smaller scopes with lumen diameters down to 3 mm must be available. With a rigid bronchoscope, the lobar and segmental bronchi are examined closely by using telescopic inserts that magnify and view at various angles to the long axis of the bronchoscope. Figure 1-2 shows two such inserts, a right angle and a fore-oblique telescope. The ventilating bronchoscope is used for patients who must have general anesthetic or who are on a ventilator. This scope couples to the ventilating equipment and may have an observation port that closes off the proximal end of the scope.

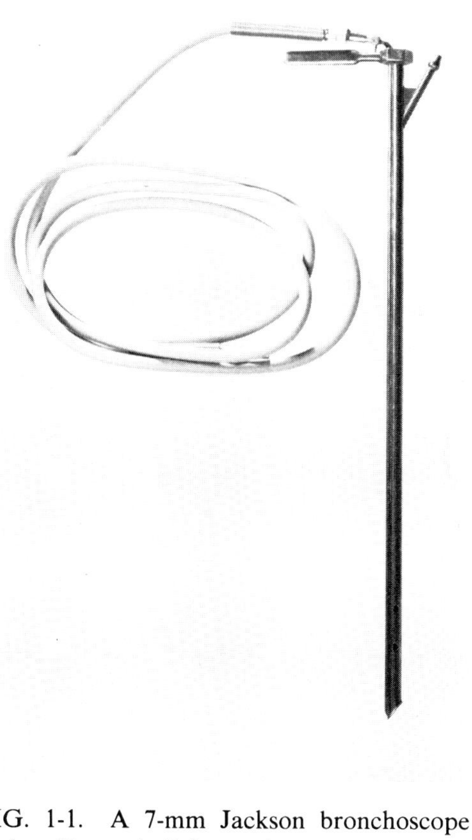

FIG. 1-1. A 7-mm Jackson bronchoscope with a fiberoptic light carrier.

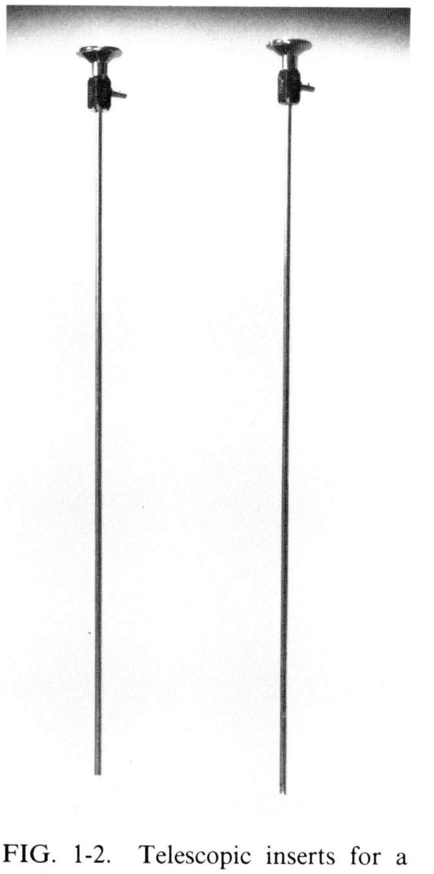

FIG. 1-2. Telescopic inserts for a Jackson bronchoscope. *Right,* a right angle telescope; *left,* a fore-oblique telescope.

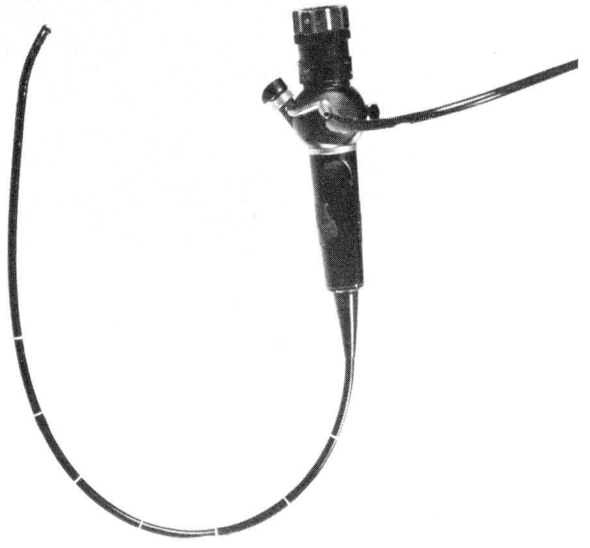

FIG. 1-3. An Olympus bronchofiberscope.

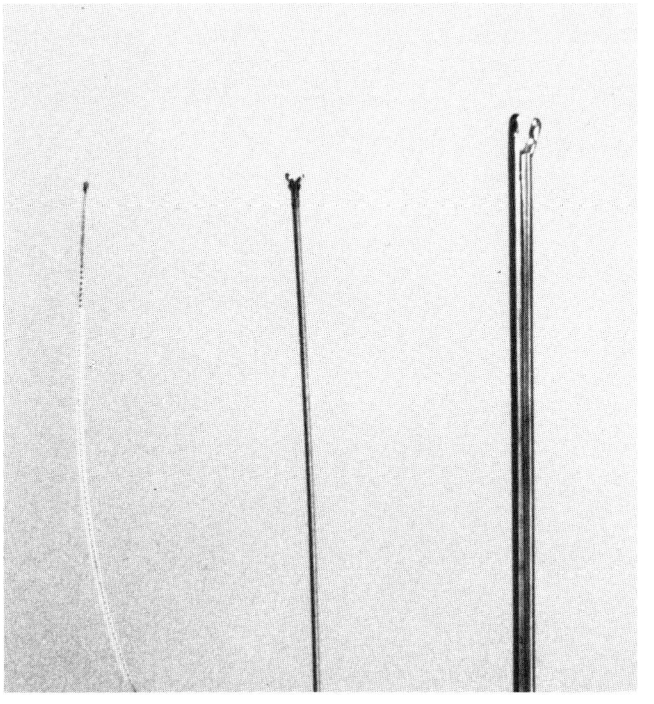

FIG. 1-4. *Right,* a biopsy forceps for a Jackson bronchoscope. *Center,* a biopsy forceps for a bronchofiberscope. *Left,* a cytology brush for the bronchofiberscope.

Fiberoptic Bronchoscope

The bronchofiberscope consists of three parts: an upper control unit, a flexible tube of optic fibers that is available in diameters from 3 to 6 mm, and a distal section that can be bent from 60° to 180° by a lever on the control unit (Fig. 1-3). An inner channel 2–2.6 mm in diameter is used for the insertion of biopsy forceps or brushes, for the instillation of liquids, and for aspiration. In addition to the lever for the bending section, the control unit has an ocular lens, attachments for the light source and for suction, and a port for the inner channel.

Accessories

A wide range of accessories is available for both rigid and fiberoptic bronchoscopes. In Figure 1-4, biopsy forceps for the rigid bronchoscope are shown on the right and for the bronchofiberscope in the center. Cytology brushes, such as that on the left in Figure 1-4, grasping forceps, and baskets are available also.

Anesthesia

An adequate anesthetic is essential for a satisfactory examination. Most bronchoscopic examinations are now performed with local anesthesia. The anesthetic technique and the preoperative preparation of the patient are the same for both rigid and fiberoptic bronchoscopy. The patient should be allowed nothing by mouth for six hours prior to the procedure. Premedication is usually 50–75 mg meperidine and 0.25 mg atropine by intramuscular injection 60 min before the procedure.

Several local anesthetic drugs may be used, but the most satisfactory at the present seems to be a 2% or 4% solution of lidocaine. With the patient in a sitting position, spray the nasopharynx and the oropharynx with a 4% solution of lidocaine. Using a laryngeal mirror, drop 1–2 ml of 4% lidocaine solution on the epiglottis and on the superior surface of the vocal cords. When anesthesia of this area is adequate, inject 2–3 ml of 2% or 4% lidocaine solution as a bolus past the vocal cords into the trachea as the patient is phonating. This injection may be made through the flexible bronchoscope or by using a syringe with a curved cannula, positioned using a laryngeal mirror. The intratracheal injection is usually sufficient to anesthetize the trachea and bronchi within a few minutes. It causes a cough that distributes the lidocaine onto the under surface of the vocal cords; if anesthesia of the bronchi is incomplete, an additional 1–2 ml of the lidocaine solution can be injected through the bronchoscope as it is being advanced into the bronchi. In an adult, the maximum total dose of lidocaine should not exceed 300 mg.

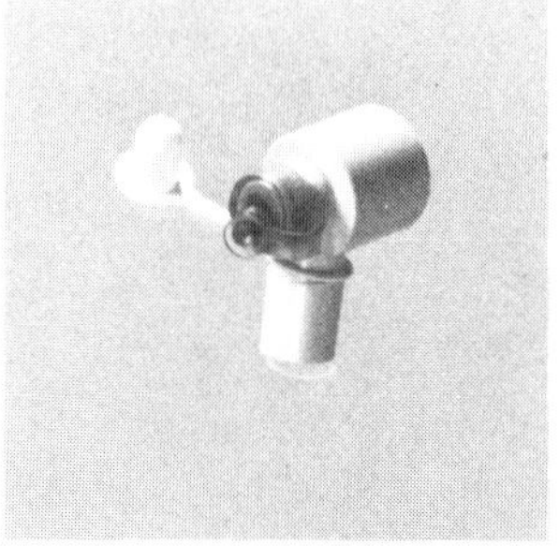

FIG. 1-5. Adapter for an endotracheal tube through which a bronchofiberscope can be inserted while ventilation is maintained.

For rigid bronchoscopy, children and some adults will require a general anesthetic. Intravenous thiopental sodium together with a muscle relaxant is a satisfactory anesthetic combination for these patients. During the bronchoscopic examination, the patient is ventilated with oxygen through the side arm of the ventilating bronchoscope. Flexible bronchoscopy less commonly requires a general anesthetic, but occasionally, a surgeon may order bronchoscopy of a patient who is still anesthetized and intubated after an operation or of a patient requiring mechanical ventilation. This may be done through an adapter (Fig. 1-5). The flexible bronchoscope is inserted through the plastic cap that then maintains a relatively closed system, permitting ventilation to continue.

Technique

Insertion of the Rigid Bronchoscope

Unless the procedure is emergent, any loose teeth should be removed prior to the examination. The patient is positioned supine with the neck fully extended. Sometimes, particularly for a patient with a short, fat neck, an assistant must support the patient's occiput with his hands and move the head as the operator requires. The bronchoscope is introduced into either side of the mouth, usually the patient's right side if the operator is right handed. With the handle anterior, the scope is advanced until the tip of the epiglottis is seen. The end of the bronchoscope is used to elevate the epiglottis and the base of the tongue until the glottis is well visualized. The most common mistake of beginning endoscopists is to advance the scope too far before the vocal cords are recognized and orientation of the bronchoscope with the glottis is determined. When the vocal cords are clearly in view, the handle of the scope is turned to the side and the end of the bronchoscope is advanced between the cords.

Insertion of the Fiberoptic Bronchoscope

The bronchofiberscope can be inserted transnasally, transorally, through a number 8 or larger endotracheal tube, through a rigid bronchoscope, or through a tracheostomy. Although the transnasal approach is currently the most popular, it has the disadvantage that each reinsertion is as difficult as the first. Passing the scope through an endotracheal tube remedies this objection, but insertion of the endotracheal tube may be more traumatic to the patient than insertion of the bronchofiberscope alone. The transoral approach is rarely used because the patient could bite the instrument and damage the fiberglass bundles. Use of a flexible bronchoscope passed through a rigid bronchoscope takes away the major advantages of both scopes and has little to recommend it.

To insert the bronchofiberscope transnasally, lubricate the instrument with 2% lidocaine jelly and insert the scope through the nose into the pharynx, visualizing first the epiglottis, then the vocal cords. With the glottis in view, slowly advance the instrument until the scope passes between the vocal cords into the trachea. It may be necessary to inject 1 or 2 ml of 2% lidocaine solution through the injection port if anesthesia of the trachea or bronchi is incomplete.

Bronchoscopic Examination

The technique of the examination is the same for both types of bronchoscope. Because of the magnification of the bronchofiberscope, disorientation is more likely during its use. If this happens, the operator should withdraw the scope until a recognizable landmark is seen, then again advance the instrument.

During insertion of the scope the vocal cords should be examined for position, mobility, and the presence of any abnormal lesions. As the bronchoscope descends in the trachea, inspect the mucosa and note any abnormal mobility of the tracheal wall, narrowing of the lumen, or evidence of an extraluminal mass. Examine the carina for thickening, fixation, or deviation. Usually, the bronchial tree of the abnormal lung is inspected first in case the examination must be terminated early. No biopsies should be taken until both bronchi have been examined because bleeding could obscure the field.

The mucosa of each lobar, segmental, and if possible subsegmental bronchus should be examined for abnormalities; this is usually not difficult, except for the apical segmental bronchus of the right upper lobe and the apical-posterior bronchus of the left upper lobe. The orifice of the right upper lobe bronchus is found on the lateral side of the right main bronchus just below the level of the carina. The middle lobe bronchus comes off the anterior medial portion of the main bronchus 1.7–2 cm below the orifice of the upper lobe, and the orifice of the bronchus to the superior segment of the lower lobe is found directly posterior at the same level as the middle lobe bronchus. The bronchi of the four basilar segments of the lower lobe extend obliquely downward and are easily examined to the subsegmental level.

The left main bronchus is longer than the right main bronchus and makes a greater angle with the trachea. It bifurcates into the upper lobe bronchus extending laterally and the lower lobe bronchus medially and downward. The upper lobe has two divisions; the upper and the lower (lingula). Both segments of the lingula plus the anterior and apical-posterior segments of the upper division bronchus should be inspected. The examination of the bronchi of the left lower lobe is similar to that of the right except that three basal segmental bronchi will usually be found, rather than four as in the right lung.

Bronchoscopic Biopsy

With either a rigid or a fiberoptic bronchoscope, a biopsy can be performed with biopsy forceps or with a small endobronchial brush. Histologic sections may be made from forceps biopsies, but a brush biopsy usually requires cytologic techniques. A biopsy forceps cannot be passed through the bronchofiberscope if the flexible tip is bent; the forceps must be introduced with the tip straight. When the jaws are visible at the end of the scope, the tip may be flexed. The scope, with the biopsy forceps protruding, can be manipulated into a lobar or segmental bronchus. Even the largest biopsy forceps that will pass through a 2–2.6 mm channel of a fiberoptic bronchoscope yields a specimen of small size, so several biopsies of each lesion or area should be obtained.

This will usually provide tissue sufficient for a histologic diagnosis, occasionally, if a tumor is quite necrotic, a larger cup forceps passed through a rigid bronchoscope is necessary to obtain sufficient tissue.

Small cell undifferentiated carcinoma characteristically infiltrates under the bronchial mucosa for a considerable distance from the primary site. Frequently, the only bronchoscopic finding will be bronchial narrowing and mucosal injection. Transmucosal biopsy of such stenotic areas should always be done even though an intraluminal mass is not visible. Although excessive risk of hemorrhage from biopsy of a bronchial carcinoid has been described, I have not found this to be a danger, particularly with the small biopsy forceps of a fiberoptic bronchoscope. If the purpose of the bronchoscopy is to diagnose and stage a carcinoma of the lung prior to its resection, a biopsy of the site of the proposed bronchial transection is useful. Usually this entails biopsies of the lobar bronchial orifice and of the main carina. Such biopsies should not be full thickness because of the risk of hemorrhage from an adjacent vessel.

Even though visualization of the tracheobronchial tree is much improved with the bronchofiberscope, much disease of the lung occurs outside the area that can be examined and biopsied under direct vision. In such conditions, two techniques, bronchial brushing and transbronchial biopsy, may permit a tissue diagnosis. Both techniques utilize instruments passed through the bronchofiberscope into the correct bronchus and guided into the peripheral lesion under biplane fluoroscopy (Fig. 1-6). The brush is introduced and withdrawn within a catheter, which serves as a protective sheath to prevent contamination of the bronchoscopic channel. With this system, the bronchofiberscope need not be removed after each specimen is obtained.

Transbronchial biopsy may also be made by passing a closed forceps distally until it is within the area to be biopsied, as seen on biplane fluoroscopy.

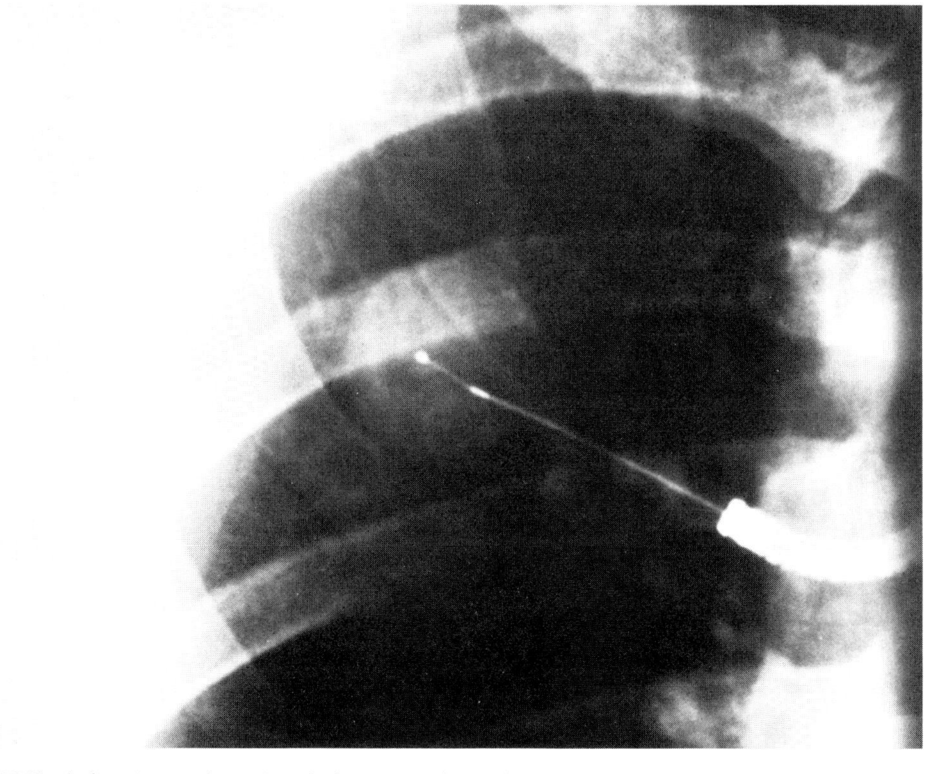

FIG. 1-6. A cytology brush inserted through a bronchofiberscope and positioned in a right upper lobe mass.

The instrument is withdrawn slightly, opened, then advanced until resistance is encountered. If the forceps is still within the correct area, it is closed and withdrawn slowly while the bronchofiberscope is kept in its original position. If the tissue sample is too large to pass through the channel, the jaws of the biopsy forceps are pulled back to the tip of the bronchoscope and the scope with the forceps is removed.

As with any test, the decision-making potential of these procedures depends greatly on their accuracy, in this case on the false negative rate and the rate of biopsy failure. In diagnosing malignancy in 97 patients, Radke and colleagues (18) have reported an overall accuracy of 56% using fiberoptic bronchoscopy with brushing and biopsies guided by biplane fluoroscopy. Of the 55 patients correctly diagnosed, both brushing and biopsy were correct in 27, biopsy alone was positive in 23, and brushing alone was positive in 5. The diagnostic accuracy was 28% if the greatest diameter of the lesion was less than 2 cm and 64% if the greatest diameter was equal to or greater than 2 cm. In a similar study, Ellis (6) had an 81% positive diagnosis on biopsy and a 57% positive diagnosis on brushing of localized carcinomas greater than 4 cm in diameter. With malignancies less than 4 cm in diameter, 58% of the biopsies were positive. The smallest tumor from which he obtained a positive biopsy was 1.5 cm. In 29 patients with diffuse lung disease, he obtained a positive biopsy in 79%.

The most common complication of the bronchoscopy itself, that is, not due to the anesthetic, is bleeding following biopsy. When the risk of hemorrhage is greater than usual, either because of the nature of the lesion to be biopsied or because of a clotting abnormality, the bronchofiberscope should be introduced initially through an endotracheal tube. Most minor bleeding from sites biopsied under direct vision may be controlled by lavage with a dilute solution of epinephrine or by direct application of a pledget soaked in epinephrine. If the bleeding is brisk, the patient must be intubated immediately with an endotracheal tube. If bleeding occurs following a transbronchial biopsy, the bronchofiberscope should be wedged into the lobar or segmental bronchus from which the bleeding comes until a clot forms within the bronchus.

Most massive bleeding results from procedures performed through a rigid bronchoscope. When this occurs, it is imperative that a double-lumen endobronchial tube be inserted to localize the blood to one lung while preparation is made for a thoracotomy. If such a tube is not immediately available, position the patient with the bleeding lung down and insert the bronchoscope into the bronchus of the nonbleeding lung so it may be kept free of blood by suctioning.

Transthoracic Needle Biopsy of the Lung

Interest in needle biopsy techniques for intrapulmonary lesions has been renewed. In patients with a high operative risk, in patients with probable metastatic cancer, or in patients who have a pulmonary infection with an unknown organism, this procedure acquires decision-making potential. Reports of its accuracy have varied from 80% to 96%. Sagel and colleagues (19) found an overall diagnostic accuracy in malignant lung lesions of 87% with one aspiration procedure and 96% with two procedures. Berquist et al. (4) reported an overall accuracy of 82%. However, their ability to obtain adequate tissue for diagnosis was significantly reduced in lesions less than 2 cm in diameter.

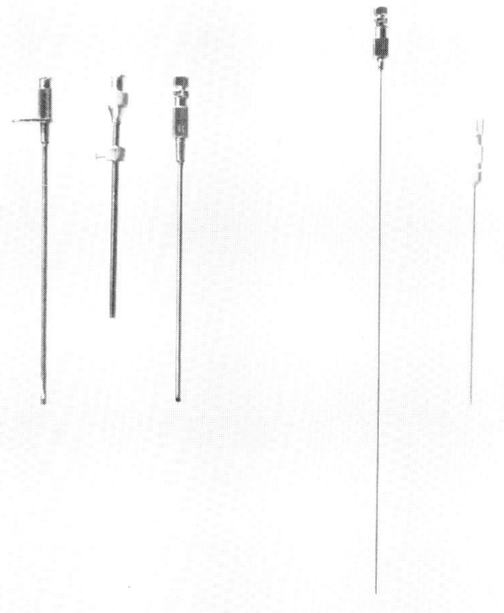

FIG. 1-7. *Right,* an 18-gauge needle. The long needle next to it is a 22-gauge Chiba needle. *Left,* the various parts of a Cope pleural biopsy needle.

The most common complications of this procedure are pneumothorax, which occurs in 14%–55% of patients, and bleeding, which is reported in 3%–10%. Consequently, the contraindications are the presence of a bleeding diathesis and an impaired pulmonary function of a degree that would be life threatening if a unilateral pneumothorax were produced. This is usually an FEV_1 of less than 1 liter.

The patient is placed on a fluoroscopic table in the position that permits the most direct access to the lesion. Using fluoroscopic guidance, a site on the skin overlying the lesion is marked for needle insertion. After the patient's skin has been prepared and the chest wall at the insertion site anesthetized, a small incision is made with a number-11 scalpel blade. Using television-monitored biplane fluoroscopy to check the position, an 18-gauge spinal needle similar to the one on the right in Figure 1-7 is advanced through the chest wall and pleura toward the lesion, but the needle is halted 1–2 cm from the lesion. After the position of the spinal needle has been verified by spot films taken in two projections, a 22-gauge Chiba needle (the long needle next to the spinal needle in Fig. 1-7) is attached to a syringe and advanced through the spinal needle into the lesion. Entry of the needle into the lesion is determined both by the change in resistance to the needle and by biplane fluoroscopy. With continuous suction applied by the syringe, the needle is moved back and forth several times over a distance of 1 cm. The Chiba needle is then withdrawn, and aliquots of the biopsy sample are divided for cytologic and for bacteriologic examination. This procedure is repeated four or five times until the biopsy specimen is adequate.

The risk of a pneumothorax, although still significant, is less with this procedure than with previous needle biopsy techniques, because the pleura is punctured only once by the spinal needle, which remains in place and forms a conduit for the biopsy needle. The absence of reports of chest wall tumor implantation following this procedure suggests that the risk of this complication may also be reduced.

Needle Biopsy of the Parietal Pleura

Although needle biopsy of the parietal pleura, because of its high sampling error, cannot be used to exclude any disease, it is relatively safe and should be considered in any patient with an undiagnosed exudative pleural effusion. The most common indications for the procedure are suspicion of metastatic carcinoma to the pleura or of a granulomatous pleuritis, usually tuberculosis.

To establish the diagnosis in patients with a pleural effusion secondary to metastatic carcinoma involving the pleura, most authors have reported better yields from pleural-fluid cytology than from needle biopsy of the pleura. First et al. (7) found that 43 of 44 patients with confirmatory evidence of carcinoma of the pleura had positive pleural-fluid cytology, while only 16 had a positive pleural needle biopsy. Salyer and co-workers (20) reported a positive needle biopsy on the first attempt in 49% of 95 patients with proven pleural metastasis. After several attempts, a positive biopsy was obtained in 56%, but 72% had a positive diagnosis from pleural-fluid cytology. In 17 of their patients, however, the pleural needle biopsy was positive when the pleural-fluid cytology was not. In 10 collected series, the average yield for diagnosing carcinoma of the pleura from one or more needle biopsies was 54%.

The success rate is better for biopsies performed for tuberculous pleuritis, especially if the tissue is cultured. In 50%–80% of patients with a pleural effusion from tuberculous pleuritis, histologic evidence of tuberculosis can be obtained from a pleural needle biopsy, and tubercle bacilli can be cultured from the biopsy specimen in 55%–76% of patients who have not received antituberculous therapy, whereas the average published figure for positive pleural fluid cultures of tuberculosis is 31.5%. Overall, an average of 72% of patients with tuberculous pleuritis can be diagnosed from a needle biopsy.

Many pleural biopsies are reported to show a "nonspecific pleural reaction." Scerbo et al. (21) have examined the eventual diagnosis in 102 patients with such a biopsy report, a group that formed 68% of their total biopsy experience. Of these patients, 40% were finally shown to have a neoplasm of the pleura, 19% developed tuberculosis, and 16% had a bacterial pneumonia.

In order to avoid damage to the lung, this procedure is usually done only in patients with a pleural effusion. If this practice is followed, complications are rare; the most common are pneumothorax in 1%–4% of biopsies and hemorrhage in less than 1%.

Several needles have been designed for percutaneous biopsy of the parietal pleura. The technique for use of the Cope (5) needle (Fig. 1-7) probably the most popular biopsy needle is as follows. The patient is positioned so the pleural fluid accumulates at the site chosen for the biopsy. Usually this will be just above a rib in the lower portion of the chest with the patient in a sitting position. After the skin is prepared and the chest wall at the insertion site anesthetized, a small nick is made in the skin with a number-11 scalpel blade. The cannula and the inner sharp needle attached to a syringe are inserted until pleural fluid is obtained (Fig. 1-8A). The needle and cannula are then slowly withdrawn just to the point that fluid can no longer be aspirated. The inner needle is removed, and the end of the cannula is occluded with a thumb to prevent aspiration of air into the pleural cavity. Insert the hooked curet attached to a syringe into the cannula (Fig. 1-8B). The hook should always be directed inferiorly to prevent injury to the intercostal blood vessels. Advance the curet until pleural fluid can again be aspirated. The

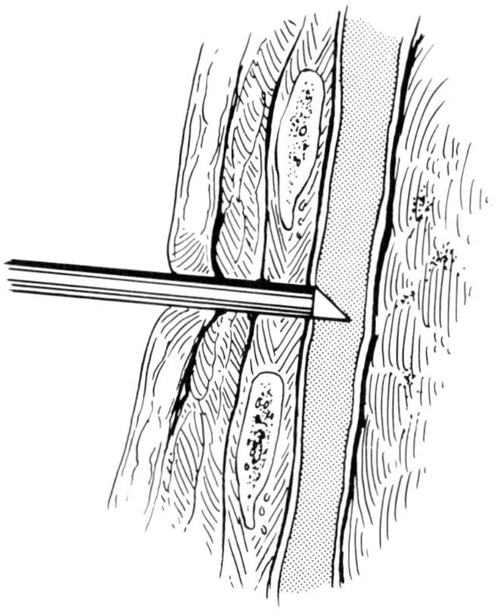

FIG. 1-8A.

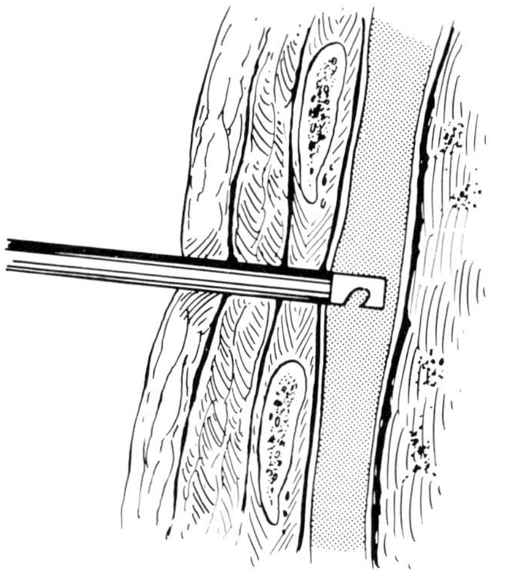

FIG. 1-8B.

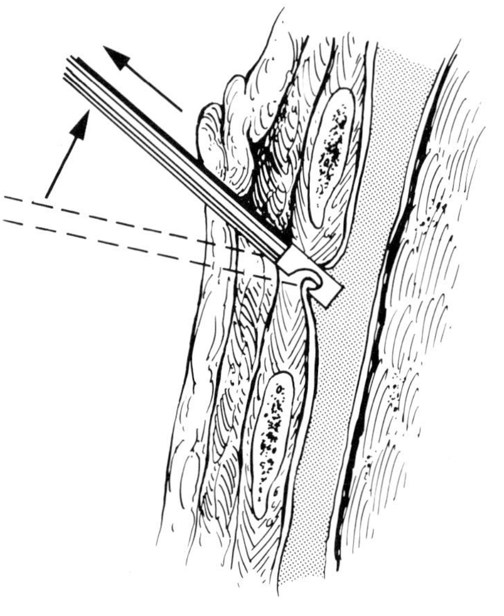

FIG. 1-8C.

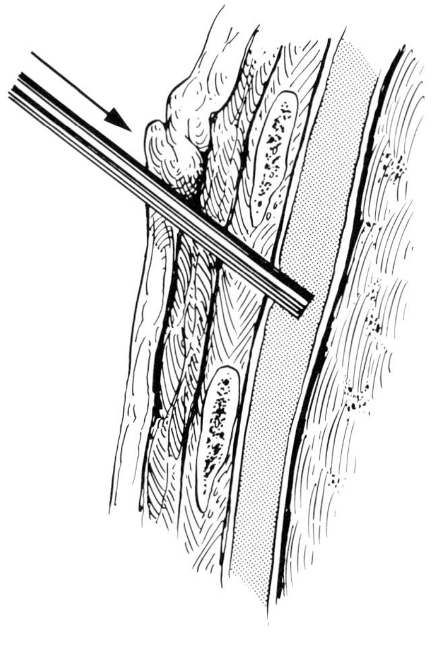

FIG. 1-8D.

outer end of both the cannula and the curet are then elevated (Fig. 1-8C), and the curet is slowly withdrawn until the hook is felt to catch the parietal pleura. Holding the curet in place, slowly advance and rotate the cannula over the end of the curet to cut a piece of the pleura (Fig. 1-8D). The hooked curet with the tissue is withdrawn, but the cannula is left in place until three or four such pieces of tissue have been obtained for histology and culture.

Biopsy of Mediastinal Lymph Nodes

The most common objective of a biopsy of the mediastinal lymph nodes is to evaluate the resectability of a carcinoma of the lung; in addition, the procedure may be used to diagnose sarcoid, lymphoma, or other diseases that involve the lymph nodes in the superior mediastinum. In previous years, scalene lymph node biopsy was widely used to determine the resectability of lung cancer. This procedure is still indicated if a palpable scalene lymph node is found, but it has been largely superseded by pretracheal mediastinoscopy and anterior mediastinotomy, both of which produce a greater yield of positive lymph nodes than does the scalene lymph node biopsy. Ashraf and co-workers (2) reported that 27% of patients with carcinoma of the lung undergoing mediastinoscopy had mediastinal lymph node metastasis. Kirschner (12) found 44.6% to have mediastinal metastasis; this included 36% of patients with adenocarcinoma and 39% of patients with squamous cell carcinoma. Jolly et al. (11) found that in a series of patients with potentially operable cancer of the right lung, 40% were diagnosed by pretracheal mediastinoscopy to have nodal metastasis; of patients with carcinoma of the left lung, left anterior mediastinotomy was positive in 38%.

Nohl-Oser (15) has divided the mediastinal lymph nodes accessible to biopsy by mediastinoscopy, mediastinotomy, or scalene node biopsy into six groups: *Inferior tracheobronchial* lymph nodes are subcarinal. They lie within the pretracheal fascia and can be biopsied during mediastinoscopy without breaking through this fascia. *Right superior tracheobronchial* nodes lie in the angle between the trachea and the right bronchus. They are above the right pulmonary artery and between the azygos vein and the trachea. These nodes are outside the pretracheal fascia, so the fascia must be breached during mediastinoscopy if the nodes are to be biopsied. *Left superior tracheobronchial* lymph nodes lie underneath the arch of the aorta and are associated with the left pulmonary artery and the left recurrent laryngeal nerve. *Anterior tracheal* nodes lie anterior to the lowest part of the trachea below the innominate artery. *Paratracheal* nodes are found anterior and lateral to both the right and left side of the trachea, but they are more numerous on the right side than on the left. On the right they are inferior to the innominate artery and posterior to the inferior vena cava. *Inferior deep cervical* nodes are outside the chest. The medial nodes of this group overlie the scalenus anterior muscle and are removed with the scalene fat pad. Mediastinoscopy permits access to the paratracheal nodes, the right superior tracheobronchial nodes, and the inferior tracheobronchial nodes. A left anterior mediastinotomy must be used to biopsy the left superior tracheobronchial nodes.

The effect of finding carcinoma in the mediastinal lymph nodes on the decision to operate varies greatly among surgeons. Some consider any type of mediastinal spread as a contraindication to resection. At the other extreme, some surgeons do not perform mediastinal lymph node biopsies, because they believe no amount of nodal cancer spread contraindicates resection if the lung and the primary tumor itself can be removed. This difference of opinion

TABLE 1-1 Percent of Patients with Metastasis to Mediastinal Lymph Nodes Surviving Five Years After Resection for Bronchogenic Carcinoma

	Lymph Nodes Obtained By:	
Author	Thoracotomy	Mediastinoscopy
Higgins & Beebe (10)	10.4	
Bergh & Schersten (3)	7	
Paulson & Urschel (16)	7	
Kirsch et al. (13)	15	
Abbey Smith (1)	28.5	
Naruke et al. (14)	18.8	
Gibbons (9)		0
Viikari et al. (22)		0
Pearson et al. (17)		9.5

is due to a lack of detailed survival data about patients with varying degrees of mediastinal lymph node disease. There are reports of long-term survival of patients who had carcinoma in resected mediastinal lymph nodes, but this situation may not be comparable to that of carcinoma in mediastinal lymph nodes found by mediastinoscopy. The data in Table 1-1 represents a comparative summary of available reports, including series with and without postoperative irradiation and drug therapy. It is difficult to apply these data to decision-making for an individual patient because few authors analyze survival statistics by the location or degree of involvement of the positive nodes.

Mediastinoscopy

In addition to the usual contraindications for a general anesthetic, the contraindications to mediastinoscopy are few, but important. Mediastinoscopy can be performed only once because tracheal adhesions develop. Similarly it is unwise to perform mediastinoscopy in a patient who has previously had a sternotomy. If mediastinoscopy is performed on a patient with a large superior mediastinal tumor, the tumor swelling that may result can cause enough tracheal obstruction to require an immediate median sternotomy for relief. Although mediastinoscopy in a patient with obstruction of the superior vena cava may be more bloody than usual, it can be done without undue risk.

Mediastinoscopy is performed using a general anesthetic. With the patient supine and the neck slightly extended by a small roll under the shoulders, make a 3–4 cm transverse incision through the skin and platysma, one finger's breadth above the sternum in the suprasternal notch. Deepen the incision by dividing the tissue in the midline down to the anterior wall of the trachea. If a thyroid ima vein is encountered, it should be ligated and divided. Dissect inferiorly along the anterior wall of the trachea with scissors or hemostat for 1–2 cm, then continue the dissection with a finger, palpating the tissue on both sides of the trachea for firm nodes or other masses.

When finger dissection becomes difficult or has extended as far as possible, insert the mediastinoscope with the handle up. The Carlens mediastinoscope (Fig. 1-9) has a light carrier and a slot on the side of the tube to facilitate the insertion of instruments such as the suction cannula or the biopsy forceps shown in Figure 1-10. Continue the dissection along the anterior wall of the trachea using the suction cannula as a dissector. This dissection will be in the position indicated by the cross section of the mediastinoscope anterior to the trachea in Figure 1-11. One will sometimes encounter heavier fibers of connective tissue between the innominate artery and the trachea. Usually

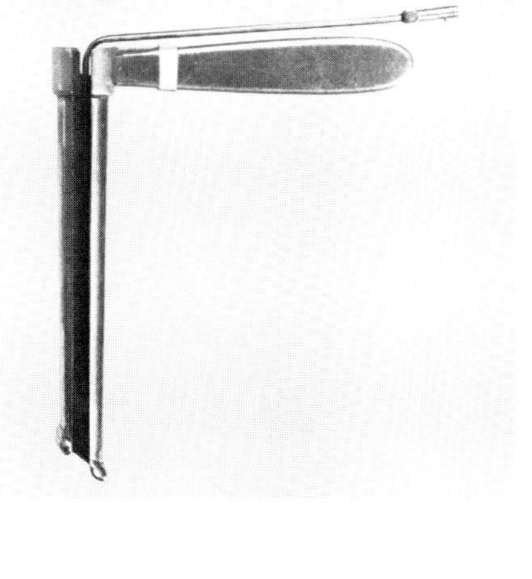

FIG. 1-9. A Carlens mediastinoscope.

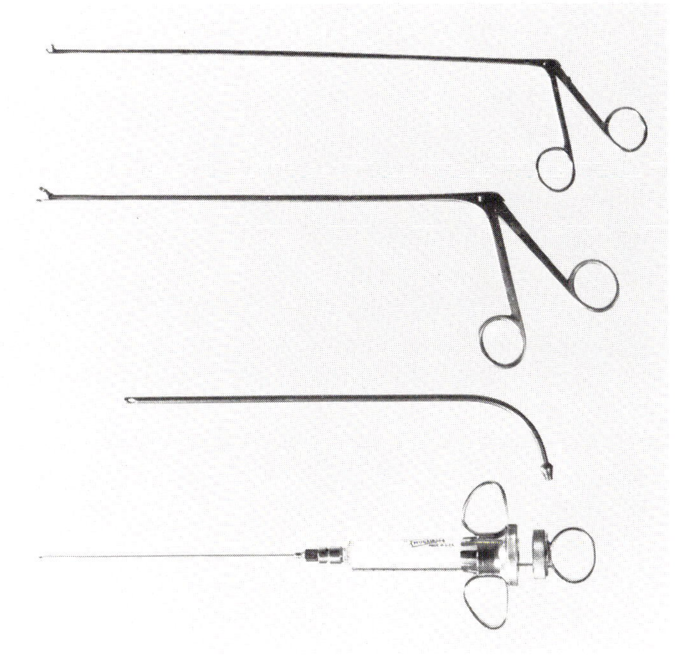

FIG. 1-10. Suction cannula, biopsy forceps, and syringe and needle used to aspirate a structure before biopsy during mediastinoscopy.

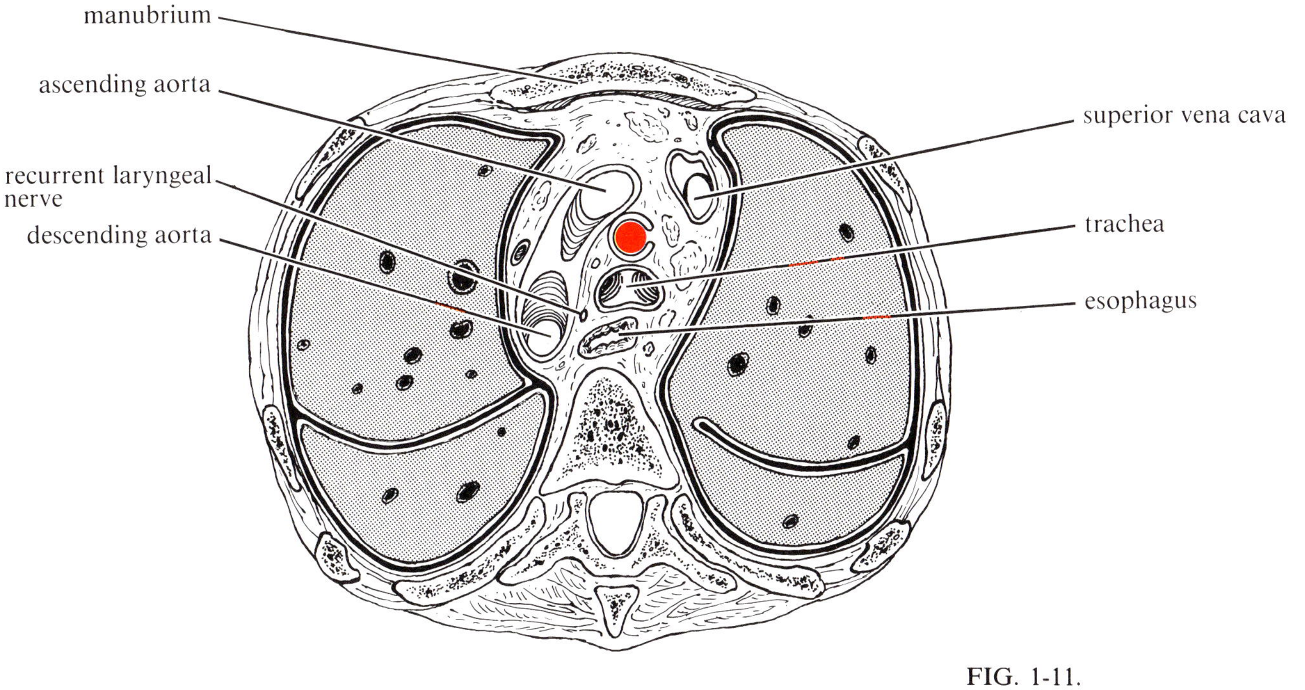

FIG. 1-11.

these can be separated or broken with the suction cannula, but occasionally it will become necessary to place small hemostatic clips and divide the connective tissue.

Below the innominate artery, break through the pretracheal fascia on both sides of the trachea with the suction cannula and identify and biopsy several of the paratracheal lymph nodes that lie anterior-lateral to the trachea. Because lymph nodes and small veins have a similar appearance when partially isolated, any structure, before biopsy, should be aspirated with a syringe and a long needle similar to that in Figure 1-10. Do not extend this dissection behind the trachea at any point, because this may perforate the esophagus.

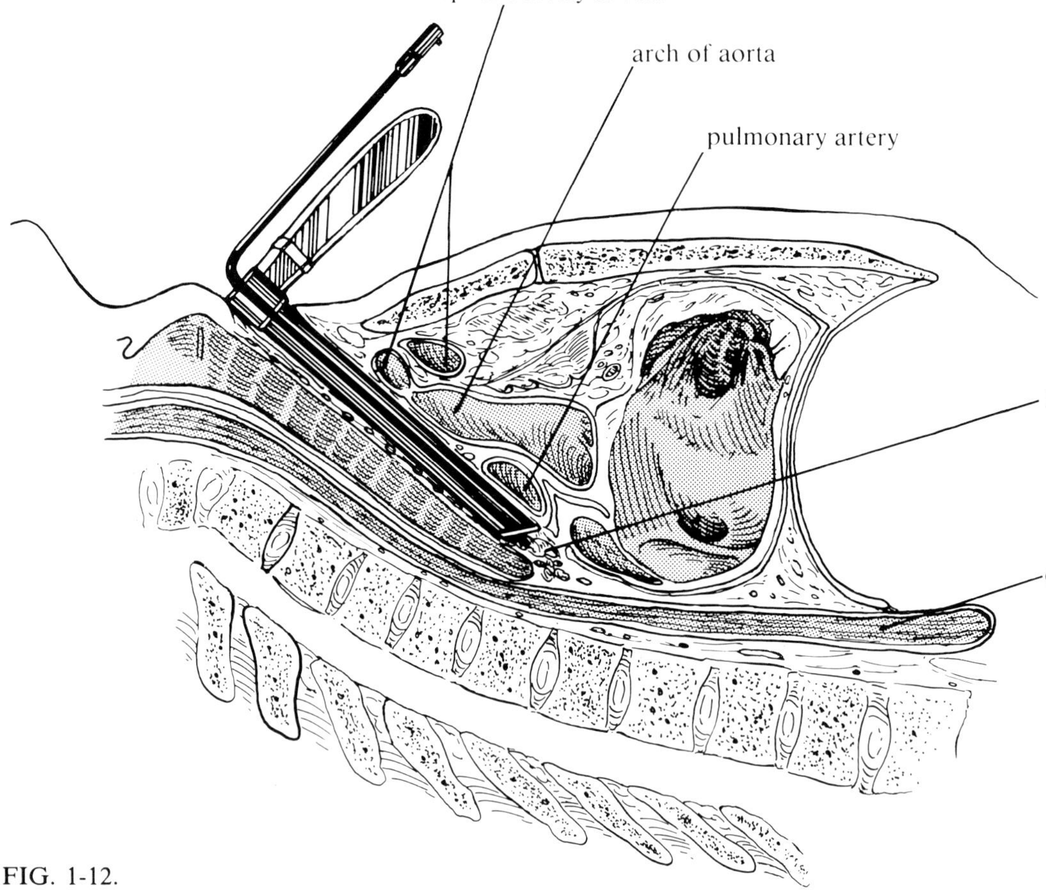

FIG. 1-12.

Dissect out the anterior surface of the carina and the first 1–2 cm of the right main bronchus. Identify and biopsy a right superior tracheobronchial lymph node located just superior to the right main bronchus between the azygos vein and the trachea; then identify and biopsy an inferior tracheobronchial node below the carina. When the mediastinoscope is in position to biopsy the subcarinal nodes, it will be situated as shown in Figure 1-12. It is unnecessary to dissect along the main bronchi to biopsy lymph nodes that can be removed during the resection. Such a dissection provides no decision-making information and causes fibrosis that obliterates the usual planes of dissection.

If bleeding occurs, it often results from tearing a small vein and will usually stop if the mediastinoscope is withdrawn for 2–3 min. If it does not stop, a hemostatic clip should be applied to the bleeding site if it can be visualized. If it cannot be visualized, or if a major vascular structure is lacerated, an immediate thoracotomy is required.

Anterior Mediastinotomy

The patient should be in a supine position and under a general anesthetic. Make a 3-cm vertical incision over the left second interspace just lateral to the edge of the sternum (Fig. 1-13). Part the fibers of the pectoralis major muscle to expose the intercostal muscle. By blunt dissection with a hemostat, separate the fibers of the intercostal muscle from the sternum and the costal cartilages to gain access to the mediastinum (Fig. 1-14). During this dissection, the internal mammary vessels must be either retracted laterally or ligated. If the interspace is too narrow to admit the mediastinoscope, the space should

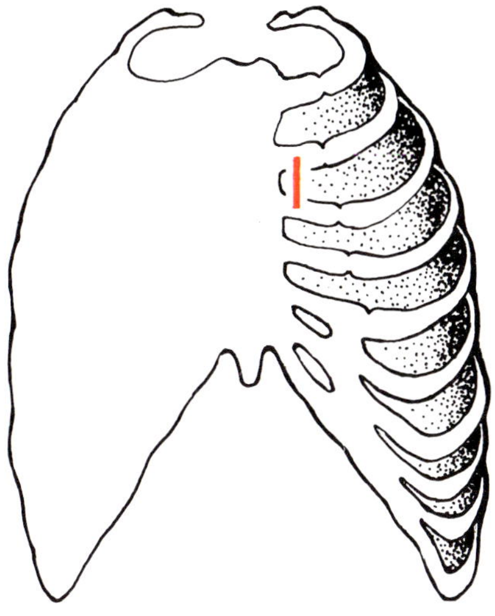

FIG. 1-13.

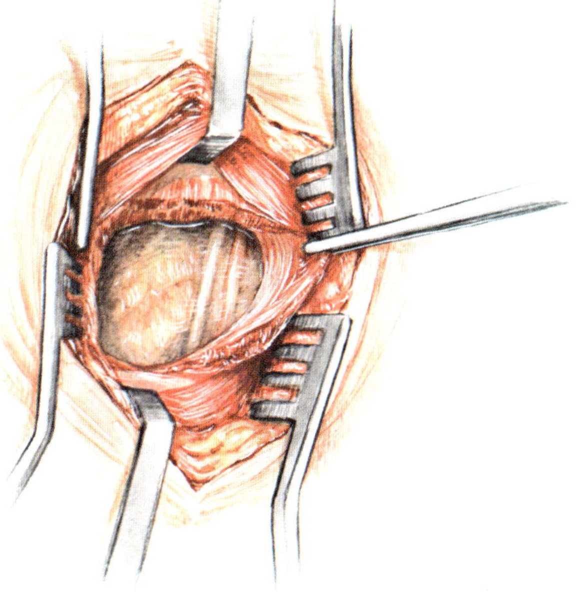

FIG. 1-14.

be enlarged by cutting away a portion of the adjacent costal cartilages with a scalpel. In some patients a reflection of the pleura may be encountered extending medially past the edge of the sternum. Mobilize such a reflection with blunt dissection and retract it laterally. The dissection toward the aortic window through the loose areolar tissue medial to the mediastinal pleura is most easily performed with the finger. This also permits palpation of this region of the mediastinum to identify lymph nodes or other masses. If the pleura remains intact, the phrenic nerve is not encountered during this dissection, but is pushed laterally with the mediastinal pleura. The first structures encountered at the lung hilum will be the left main pulmonary artery and just above it, the ascending aorta. These two structures are usually easily differentiated because the tension is less in the wall of the pulmonary artery than in the aorta.

Insert the mediastinoscope through the interspace opening and advance it to the pulmonary artery. Figure 1-15 shows the mediastinoscope in an intrapleural position, also an acceptable approach. The region between the aorta and the pulmonary artery should be examined, bearing in mind that the vagus nerve, with the recurrent laryngeal nerve, lies superior and posterior to the first portion of the pulmonary artery. A ring of lymph nodes, the left superior tracheobronchial nodes, will be encountered surrounding the first portion of the left main pulmonary artery. These nodes can be dissected out with the suction cannula and biopsied after aspirating each with a syringe and long needle as described for mediastinoscopy. If necessary, the left pleural cavity may be entered and the anterior portion of the left upper lobe and its hilum examined.

If the pleural cavity is not entered, the wound is closed without drains. If the left pleural cavity is entered, a catheter is inserted and the air aspirated as the wound is closed. The catheter can then be removed unless an air leak has been produced.

Scalene Lymph Node Biopsy

This procedure can be performed with either general or local anesthesia. A 4–5 cm transverse incision is made overlying the anterior portion of the sternocleidomastoid muscle about one finger's breadth above the clavicle (Fig. 1-16). Incise the underlying platysma, expose the sternocleidomastoid muscle, retract it laterally, and divide the anterior edge of this muscle for 2–3 cm. Identify the internal jugular vein beneath the anterior edge of the sternocleidomastoid. Identify the omohyoid and reflect this muscle superiorly. Beginning at the level of the omohyoid, dissect down to the scalenus anterior muscle;

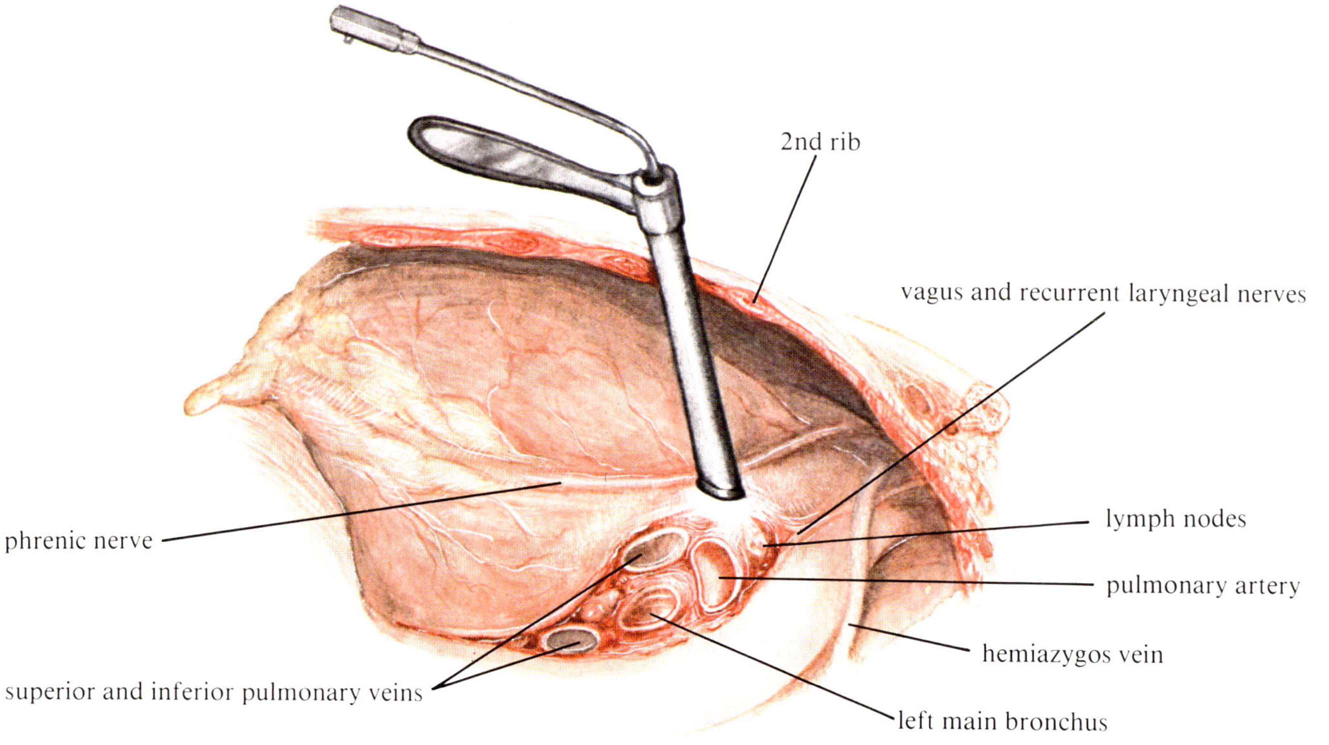

FIG. 1-15.

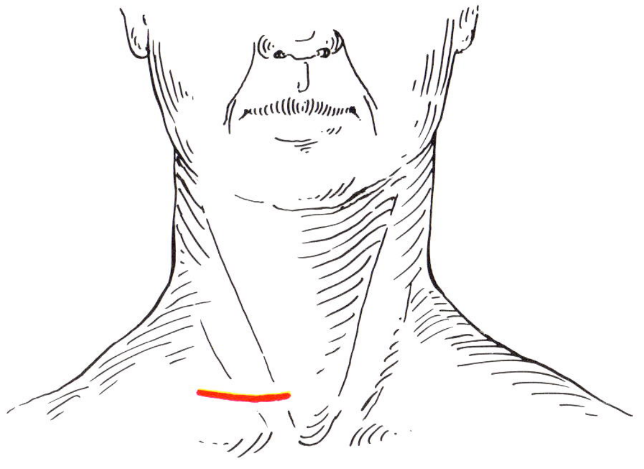

FIG. 1-16.

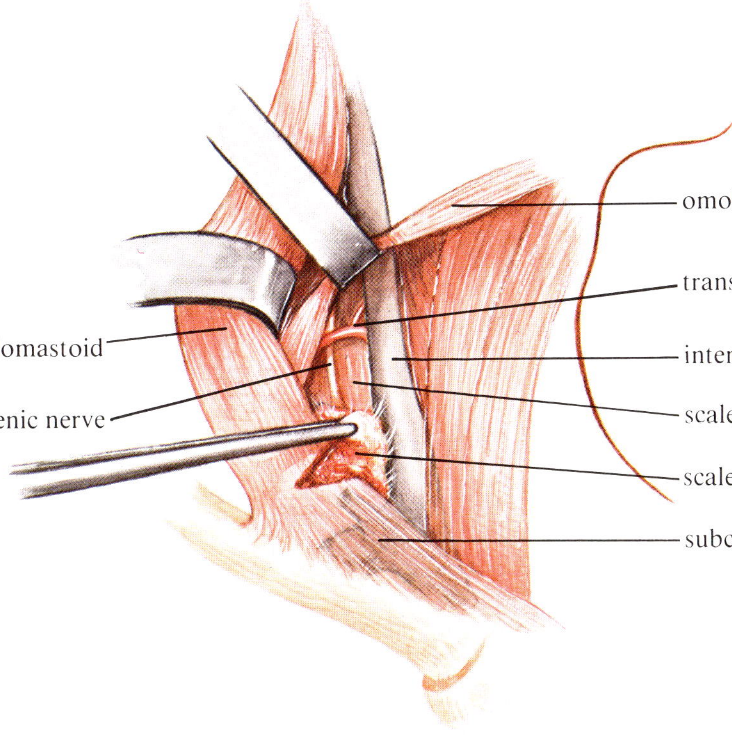

FIG. 1-17.

identify and spare the phrenic nerve, which lies on the superficial surface of this muscle. The scalene fat pad with its contained lymph nodes is then dissected free and removed. The limits of this dissection (Fig. 1-17) are: deep, the phrenic nerve and the scalenus anterior muscle; anterior, the internal jugular vein; superior and lateral, the omohyoid muscle; inferior, the subclavian vein. The transverse cervical artery, which may require ligation and division, is usually encountered just superficial to the scalenus anterior muscle, running transversely across the upper part of this dissection. On the left, the thoracic duct should be identified as it joins the subclavian vein at its junction with the internal jugular vein. If an unrecognized laceration is made in this duct, a troublesome lymph fistula will result. After removal of the scalene fat pad, the sternocleidomastoid muscle and the platysma are closed with absorbable sutures.

References

1. Abbey Smith R: The importance of mediastinal lymph node invasion by pulmonary carcinoma in selection of patients for resection. Ann Thorac Surg 25:5–11, 1978.
2. Ashraf MH, Milsom PL, Walesby RK: Selection by mediastinoscopy and long-term survival in bronchial carcinoma. Ann Thorac Surg 30:208–214, 1980.
3. Bergh NP, Schersten T: Bronchogenic carcinoma: a follow-up study of a surgically treated series with special reference to the prognostic significance of lymph node metastasis. Acta Chir Scand (Suppl) 347, 1965.
4. Berquist TH, Bailey PB, Cortese DA, Miller WE: Transthoracic needle biopsy. Accuracy and complications in relation to location and type of lesion. Mayo Clin Proc 55:475–481, 1980.
5. Cope C: New pleural biopsy needle. JAMA 167:1107–1108, 1958.
6. Ellis JH: Transbronchial lung biopsy via the fiberoptic bronchoscope. Chest 68:524–532, 1975.
7. First B, Kahan AV, Koss LG: Comparison of the diagnostic values of biopsies of the pleura and cytological evaluation of pleural fluids. Am J Clin Pathol 72:48–51, 1979.
8. Fishmann NH, Bronstein MH: Is mediastinoscopy necessary in the evaluation of lung cancer? Ann Thorac Surg 20:678–686, 1975.
9. Gibbons JRP: The value of mediastinoscopy in assessing operability in carcinoma of the lung. Br J Dis Chest 66:162–166, 1972.
10. Higgins GA, Beebe GW: Bronchogenic carcinoma. Arch Surg 94:539–549, 1967.
11. Jolly PC, Li W, Anderson RP: Anterior and cervical mediastinoscopy for determining operability and predicting resectability in lung cancer. J Thorac Cardiovasc Surg 79:366–371, 1980.
12. Kirschner PA: Discussion of article by Ashraf, M.H. et al. Ann Thorac Surg 30:208–214, 1980.
13. Kirsh MM, Kahn DR, Gago O, Lampe I, Fayos JV, Prior M, Moores WY, Haight C, Sloan H: Treatment of bronchogenic carcinoma with mediastinal metastasis. Ann Thorac Surg 12:11–21, 1971.
14. Naruke T, Suemasu K, Ishikawa S: Lymph node mapping and curability at various levels of metastasis in resected lung cancer. J Thorac Cardiovasc Surg 76:832–839, 1978.
15. Nohl-Oser HC: Lymphatics of the lung. *In* Shields TC (ed): General Thoracic Surgery. Philadelphia, Lea and Febiger, 1972.
16. Paulson DL, Urschel HC Jr: Selectivity in the surgical treatment of bronchogenic carcinoma. J Thorac Cardiovasc Surg 62:554–562, 1971.
17. Pearson FG, Nelems JM, Henderson RD, Delarue NC: The role of mediastinoscopy in the selection of treatment for bronchial carcinoma with involvement of superior mediastinal lymph nodes. J Thorac Cardiovasc Surg 64:382–390, 1972.
18. Radke JR, Conway WA, Eyler WR, Kvale PA: Diagnostic accuracy in peripheral lung lesions. Factors predicting success with flexible fiberoptic bronchoscopy. Chest 76:176–179, 1979.
19. Sagel SS, Ferguson TB, Forrest JV, Roper CL, Weldon CS, Clark RE: Percutaneous transthoracic aspiration needle biopsy. Ann Thorac Surg 26:399–405, 1978.
20. Salyer WR, Eggleston JC, Erozan YS: Efficacy of pleural needle biopsy and pleural fluid cytopathology in the diagnosis of malignant neoplasm involving the pleura. Chest 67:536–539, 1975.
21. Scerbo J, Keltz H, Stone DJ: A prospective study of closed pleural biopsies. JAMA 218:377–380, 1971.
22. Viikari SJ, Inberg MV, Puhakka H: The role of mediastinoscopy in the treatment of lung cancer. Bull Soc Int Chir 2:119, 1974.

Preoperative Evaluation and Preparation for Pulmonary Resection

2

Preoperative Evaluation

The decision to recommend any operative procedure to a patient must include weighing the risk from the proposed operation against the risk of the known disease without surgical intervention. In no situation is this more relevant than in treatment for carcinoma of the lung. In addition to an assessment of nutritional status, renal function, liver function, clotting parameters, and other tests commonly performed before any major operation, the evaluation of a patient for pulmonary resection must emphasize the appraisal of pulmonary function, muscle strength, and cardiac function. The problem confronting the surgeon is not to determine whether such a patient has normal pulmonary and cardiac function, nor is it even to determine which patients are considered at increased risk from surgery; rather, it is to screen out those in whom the risk from a given resection is prohibitive.

Estimating the ability of a patient to tolerate a given pulmonary resection is subjective at best. A normal or a grossly abnormal value for preoperative pulmonary function testing is predictive for a group of patients, but neither values between these extremes nor values applied to an individual patient have the necessary accuracy of prediction. The critical values are those found *after* a given resection, but preoperatively these can only be surmised. For this reason, no lower limits for the preoperative values of spirometric tests may be set without knowledge of the stage of the patient's disease. Obviously, a patient with a vital capacity only one-half the usual minimum value will tolerate a pneumonectomy if the lung to be removed is already totally atelectatic. Because the magnitude of error in excluding a patient with carcinoma of the lung from a curative resection that will be tolerated exceeds that of including a patient who will not survive that resection, the direction in which the preoperative evaluation must be weighted is obvious. However, this prejudice should not impede a continued effort to identify those patients who will die from the pulmonary resection necessary for the removal of all obvious cancer. The resection should always be designed to provide the best chance of controlling the disease process, while preserving adequate pulmonary function.

TABLE 2-1 Relative Dry Weights of Lung Lobes as a Percent of Total Lung Weight for Adult Humans

	Right Lung	Left Lung
Upper lobe	19.4	22.4
Middle lobe	8.3	
Lower lobe	25.2	24.7
Total	52.9	47.1

From Schilling (10).

The $FEV_{1.0}$, the maximum volume of air that can be expired in one second, is the most valuable of the spirometric tests. If the postoperative value is less than 0.75 liters, the patient's ability to cough in the postoperative period will be inadequate, and the probability of becoming a pulmonary cripple with respirator dependency is great. The postoperative value for this test may be approximated from 1) the preoperative value, 2) the fraction of the normal lung mass contributed by the lobes to be resected (Table 2-1), and 3) an estimate of the fraction of the diseased lobes that is still being ventilated and perfused, based on chest radiograms and occasionally on ventilation–perfusion scans. Although the vital capacity of the remaining lung may be decreased to 50% or less through the third postoperative day and remain below 60% of the preoperative value to the seventh day, the decrease in the $FEV_{1.0}$ of the remaining lung is not as marked (11).

A low value for pulmonary function studies may be caused solely by pulmonary disease, or it may be due also to a lack of patient training or cooperation. Such spuriously low values may often be detected with an exercise tolerance test. The great value of this test is that little training or understanding is necessary to perform it. If a patient can climb two flights of stairs, totaling 32 steps or so, without stopping and then immediately count to 20 in three or fewer breaths, the patient's pulmonary status is usually adequate to tolerate a pneumonectomy.

For the purpose of predicting survival after a pneumonectomy, measurement of pulmonary arterial pressure before and after ligating the artery to the diseased lung has been the single most accurate test. Rams and his associates (9) found that the mean pulmonary arterial pressure of patients ultimately dying of cardiopulmonary complications after pneumonectomy averaged 25 torr before ligating one pulmonary artery, and rose to 32 torr after ligation the artery. Van Nostrand et al. (13) reviewed the course of 213 patients who had undergone pneumonectomy. They reported a mortality rate of 33% for those patients in whom the mean pulmonary arterial pressure exceeded 32 torr after one pulmonary artery had been ligated, compared to an 8% overall mortality due to cardiopulmonary failure. They also examined the data from the forced expiratory vital capacity, the maximum breathing capacity, and the midexpiratory velocity to determine if any of these preresectional tests would be a better predictor of postoperative death from pulmonary insufficiency than are the $FEV_{1.0}$, the exercise tolerance test, and the mean pulmonary artery pressure. They concluded that none of the former three tests nor a combination of tests would aid in selecting those patients who would be unable to tolerate a pneumonectomy more accurately than do the latter three tests.

The most common cause of diffuse lung disease in adults is chronic obstructive pulmonary disease, which is characterized by prominent abnormalities of the ventilation–perfusion ratio with a consequent decrease in the Pa_{O_2}. When the history or the preresectional spirometric tests disclose a significant degree of respiratory dysfunction, arterial blood oxygen and carbon dioxide tensions should be measured while the patient is breathing room air. If the Pa_{O_2} is above 75–80 torr, the mismatch of ventilation with perfusion is not severe in spite of low values for the spirometric tests. If the Pa_{O_2} is below 60 torr, the risk of a major pulmonary resection is increased unless there is present a significant amount of atelectatic lung that will be removed during the resection. In the absence of this latter situation, if a resection is indicated, consideration should be given to one of a magnitude less than a lobectomy. If the Pa_{CO_2} is above 46 torr, alveolar ventilation is inadequate. When this condition is chronic, the risk from any thoracotomy is high, and the probability of developing respirator dependence is great.

A mismatch of ventilation and perfusion makes gas exchange inefficient and increases the amount of ventilatory work required for a given oxygen uptake. This increased work can be performed by most patients who have adequate nutrition and an average muscle mass, but in some women and debilitated men, the respiratory muscles do not have the strength to sustain this increased effort. The few patients who I have seen die postoperatively from respiratory insufficiency have been in this category and have died from respiratory muscle failure, not inadequate lung tissue. It is often difficult to distinguish these patients prior to surgery. Pulmonary function studies may show only a moderate disability for the patient's size and weight, and there is as yet no available test that measures prolonged respiratory muscle work capacity to fatigue. Peters (8) has emphasized that the ventilatory response to a given stimulus seems to depend primarily on the amount of work required (and probably also on the ability to perform that work). If the work is increased, the ventilatory response to a given fall in Pa_{O_2} or increase in Pa_{CO_2} will be less. Although these patients may tolerate being off a respirator for several hours in the postoperative period, they tire easily, the Pa_{O_2} falls, the Pa_{CO_2} rises, and respiratory arrest often occurs. To obviate such an occurrence, the degree of pulmonary function required for a given resection in debilitated patients should be greater than that in patients with a normal muscle mass.

Pulmonary disease and cardiac disease are joint phenomena in many patients being evaluated for a pulmonary resection. It is necessary frequently to consider the degree of cardiac disability, particularly the chance of a reinfarction, when weighing the risk of such surgery. Tarhan et al. (12) studied the incidence of myocardial infarction following non-cardiac surgery and found that 37% of those patients operated on within three months of a previous myocardial infarction had a reinfarction in the postoperative period. This risk decreased to 16% in patients operated on between three and six months after infarction, then remained at 4%–5% in patients having surgery more than six months after infarction. The mortality rate for reinfarction in the postoperative period was 54%. A similar study was reported by Goldman and co-workers (4). They reported that postoperative cardiac death occurred in 22.7% of those patients operated on within six months following a myocardial infarction, but in only 2.5% of those whose previous infarct was more than six months prior to surgery. Among all preoperative findings, the only ones that correlated with intraoperative or postoperative infarction were: age over 70 years, cardiac dyspnea, orthopnea or edema, a grade II/IV or louder murmur of mitral stenosis, more than five premature ventricular contractions per minute, and a tortuous or calcified aorta. The presence of an S_3 gallop rhythm or jugular venous distension was associated with 18% and 22% risks of postoperative cardiac death. However, those patients with a history of heart failure who were no longer in failure were significantly less likely to develop pulmonary edema than were those patients whose congestive failure was still evident preoperatively.

Based on these and other studies, it seems unwise to perform any pulmonary resection, even for carcinoma of the lung, within three months of a myocardial infarction or a cerebrovascular accident. After three months, although the risk is still increased, a resection may be advisable since the risk of the surgery is probably less than the risk of watching a known carcinoma of the lung for longer than three months. A patient in congestive heart failure should not undergo a pulmonary resection, but if the failure can be successfully treated, the patient may have a resection when he is well compensated.

A situation may arise in which a patient in need of a coronary artery bypass or surgery on the carotid arteries is discovered to have also a carcinoma of the lung. If the carcinoma is resectable, such patients are best treated by performing the coronary artery or carotid artery surgery first and delaying the pulmonary resection for 8–10 weeks. If a patient undergoing a coronary artery bypass has also a small asymptomatic pulmonary nodule, the nodule can be removed by a wedge resection through the median sternotomy at the time of the coronary artery bypass after the heparin effect has been reversed.

Preoperative Preparation

The effort expended in preparing the patient for a pulmonary resection is amply repaid by the consequent decrease in postoperative complications. Among the most important measures is the discontinuation of smoking for at least two weeks prior to surgery. An increase of postoperative complications in cigarette smokers has been amply documented. Chalon et al. (3) have reported postoperative pulmonary complications in 7.9% of nonsmokers, 23% of patients that smoked 10–19 cigarettes per day, 29% who smoked 20–29 cigarettes per day, and 43% who smoked 30 or more cigarettes per day. These complications paralleled the morphologic integrity of the ciliated tracheobronchial epithelial cells seen in smears.

There is disagreement as to whether spirometric tests improve after smoking is stopped, but none as to the improvement in symptomatology. Airway condition may continue to improve for six months after smoking is stopped, but significant improvement is often noticed within a few weeks. Buist and co-workers (1) reported that patients who quit smoking showed within one month a dramatic decrease in pulmonary symptoms such as cough, expectoration, shortness of breath, and wheezing; they postulated that this may be due to a regression of the hypersecretion from the mucous glands in the central airways. My impression is that significant improvement in an abnormal $\text{FEV}_{1.0}$ is also common after smoking is stopped, a view shared by many. McCarthy and colleagues (7) found a significant increase in the $\text{FEV}_{1.0}$, particularly in people in whom the values were abnormal initially; they believed this improvement was due to a decrease in the inflammatory changes in the airway.

Chronic bronchitis is a common associated abnormality in patients who require a pulmonary resection, and such patients are subject to a considerable risk of acute bronchitis and pneumonia. When an acute infection supervenes, there is an increase in cough, hypoxia, and development of a purulent sputum with increased bacterial content. While treatment of such patients with appropriate antibiotics will not eliminate bacteria from the sputum, it will decrease the bacterial content, ameliorate the symptoms, and lessen the risk of postoperative infection. Because the bacteria involved are usually mouth organisms, the most commonly used antibiotic is a penicillin, but determination of specific therapy should include sputum Gram stain and appropriate antibiotic sensitivity studies. Treatment should be continued for 7–10 days; longer periods of antibiotic therapy increase the risk of overgrowth by Gram negative organisms.

A patient's cough in the postoperative period may be ineffective due to pain and sedation. Time spent before surgery teaching the patient how to cough effectively will result in greater cooperation and a more adequate cough with a consequent decrease in the risk of pneumonia.

Antibiotic prophylaxis has been defined as the administration of drugs shortly before, during, or shortly after bacterial contamination. An antibiotic given several hours after contamination constitutes early treatment. Although Hirschmann has written that a decrease in the incidence of postoperative pneumonia has been found in patients given prophylactic antibiotic therapy for colorectal surgery (5), there is no convincing data that confirms the value of prophylactic antibiotic therapy for pulmonary resections. However, many thoracic surgeons, including myself, believe that it is beneficial. Although the risk of a wound infection from a thoracic incision exists, it seems too small to justify the use of antibiotic prophylaxis to decrease it. The danger of postoperative bronchitis, pneumonia, or a peribronchial stump abscess, however, is real. It is my practice to give 1 g cefazolin on call to the operating room and a second 1 g dose 4 hours later. The administration of this drug is then discontinued. Cefazolin, rather than one of the other cephalosporins, is used because it produces a high serum level and has a prolonged serum half-life.

The risk of a serious cardiac arrhythmia developing subsequent to a pneumonectomy in a patient with a preoperative normal sinus rhythm is about 10%. Because arrhythmias such as atrial flutter or atrial fibrillation may be associated with a ventricular tachycardia, congestive heart failure may evolve unless the arrhythmia is quickly controlled. In order to prevent this complication, the prophylactic administration of digitalis is advocated by many thoracic surgeons. Wheat and Burford (14) reported that 29% of their patients who had a pneumonectomy without preoperative digitalization developed a cardiac complication, but only 15% of those who were digitalized developed the complication. Burman (2) also found that the preoperative digitalization of patients undergoing a pneumonectomy reduced the rate of postoperative cardiac arrhythmias from 30% to 12.9%. A dissenting opinion is held by Juler et al. (6), who did not find a decrease in the rate of postoperative arrhythmias in patients digitalized preoperatively. It is my practice to give 75% of a digitalizing dose preoperatively to patients with the potential for a pneumonectomy. Then in the event that an arrhythmia with a tachycardia does develop, the time necessary to slow the heart rate is shortened considerably and the risk of congestive heart failure developing is decreased.

References

1. Buist AS, Sexton GJ, Nagy JM, Ross BB: The effect of smoking cessation and modification on lung function. Am Rev Respir Dis 114:115–122, 1976.
2. Burman SO: Digitalis and thoracic surgery. J Thorac Cardiovasc Surg 50:873–881, 1965.
3. Chalon J, Taygab MA, Ramanathan S: Cytology of the respiratory epithelium as a predictor of respiratory complications after operation. Chest 67:32–35, 1975.
4. Goldman L, Caldera DL, Southwick FS, Nussbaum SR, Murray B, O'Malley TA, Goroll AH, Caplan CH, Nolan J, Burke DS, Krogstad D, Carabello B, Slater EE: Cardiac risk factors and complications in non-cardiac surgery. Medicine 57:357–370, 1978.

5. Hirschmann JV: Rational antibiotic prophylaxis. Hosp Prac 16:105–128, 1981.
6. Juler GL, Stemmer EA, Connolly JE: Complications of prophylactic digitalization in thoracic surgical patients. J Thorac Cardiovasc Surg 58:352–360, 1969.
7. McCarthy DS, Craig DB, Cherniack RM: Effect of modification of the smoking habit on lung function. Am Rev Respir Dis 114:103–113, 1976.
8. Peters RM: Management of surgically treated patients with limited pulmonary reserve. Am J Surg 138:379–383, 1979.
9. Rams JJ, Harrison RW, Fry WA, Moulder PV, Adams WE: Operative pulmonary artery pressure measurements as a guide to postoperative management and prognosis following pneumonectomy. Dis Chest 41:85–90, 1962.
10. Schilling JA: Pulmonary resection and sequelae of thoracic surgery. *In* Fenn WO, Rahn H (eds): Handbook of Physiology: Respiration. Washington, D.C., American Physiological Society, 1965.
11. Smith TC, Cook FD, DeKornfeld TJ, Siebecker KL: Pulmonary function in the immediate postoperative period. J Thorac Surg 39:788–798, 1960.
12. Tarhan S, Moffitt EA, Taylor WF, Giuliani ER: Myocardial infarction after general anesthesia. JAMA 220:1451–1454, 1972.
13. Van Nostrand D, Kjelsberg MO, Humphrey EW: Presectional evaluation of risk from pneumonectomy. Surg Gynecol Obstet 127:306–312, 1968.
14. Wheat MW, Burford TH: Digitalis in surgery: extension of classical indications. J Thorac Cardiovasc Surg 41:162–168, 1961.

Indications for Pulmonary Resection

3

Neoplasia

In the United States, patients with carcinoma of the lung, or with a pulmonary abnormality suspected of being carcinoma of the lung, comprise 50% or more of general thoracic surgery practice. Table 3-1 gives the 1977 World Health Organization classification of lung tumors; although several other schemata have been published, most are variations of this one. In contrast to series collected prior to 1970 in which squamous cell carcinoma was the predominant cell type, current data indicate the most common malignant tumor of the lung in both men and women is adenocarcinoma (11, 51). The term "bronchogenic" carcinoma has been used in the past to refer to malignant tumors of classes 1–5 and the term "bronchial adenoma" to classes 6 and 7. Both terms are inappropriate. The tumors of classes 1–5 may arise from cells not in the bronchi, while tumors not in these classes may arise from a bronchus. An adenoma, on the other hand, implies a benign tumor, but the tumors in classes 6 and 7 are malignant and must be treated as such.

The several histologic types of carcinoma of the lung have a predilection for different parts of the lung. The lung, as seen on a radiogram, may be divided into two zones: the central zone, that part occupied by the main, lobar, segmental, and first-order subsegmental bronchi, all available to inspection with a fiberoptic bronchoscope; and the peripheral zone, the rest of the lung parenchyma. Of squamous cell carcinomas, 65% occur in the central zone. Of the one-third that occur in the peripheral zone, approximately 30% will have cavitated when discovered. Of small cell undifferentiated carcinomas, 85%–90% occur in the central zone. Often, however, they cause only narrowing of the involved bronchus by submucosal infiltration and have no intraluminal mass, thus bronchoscopic biopsy of these tumors may be difficult. Of adenocarcinomas, 75% occur in the peripheral zone. The large cell undifferentiated group is comprised of poorly differentiated squamous cell carcinoma, poorly differentiated adenocarcinoma, and a truly undifferentiated set. They occur more frequently in the peripheral zone.

TABLE 3-1–World Health Organization Histologic Classification of Lung Tumors (52)

I. Epithelial tumors
  A. Benign
    1. Papillomas
      a. Squamous cell papilloma
      b. "Transitional" papilloma
    2. Adenomas
      a. Pleomorphic adenoma ("mixed" tumor)
      b. Monomorphic adenomas
      c. Others
  B. Dysplasia and carcinoma in situ
  C. Malignant
    1. Squamous cell carcinoma (epidermoid carcinoma)
      Variant:
      a. Spindle cell carcinoma
    2. Small cell carcinoma
      a. Oat-cell carcinoma
      b. Intermediate cell type
      c. Combined oat-cell carcinomas
    3. Adenocarcinoma
      a. Acinar adenocarcinoma
      b. Papillary adenocarcinoma
      c. Bronchiolo-alveolar carcinoma
      d. Solid carcinoma with mucus formation
    4. Large cell carcinoma
      Variants:
      a. Giant cell carcinoma
      b. Clear cell carcinoma
    5. Adenosquamous carcinoma
    6. Carcinoid tumor
    7. Bronchial gland carcinomas
      a. Adenoid cystic carcinoma
      b. Mucoepidermoid carcinoma
      c. Others
    8. Others
II. Soft tissue tumors
III. Mesothelial tumors
  A. Benign mesothelioma
  B. Malignant mesothelioma
    1. Epithelial
    2. Fibrous (spindle-cell)
    3. Biphasic
IV. Miscellaneous tumors
  A. Benign
  B. Malignant
    1. Carcinosarcoma
    2. Pulmonary blastoma
    3. Malignant melanoma
    4. Malignant lymphomas
    5. Others
V. Secondary tumors
VI. Unclassified tumors
VII. Tumor-like lesions
  A. Hamartoma
  B. Lymphoproliferative lesions
  C. Tumorlet
  D. Eosinophilic granuloma
  E. "Sclerosing hemangioma"
  F. Inflammatory pseudotumor
  G. Others

Staging of a lung cancer is based on a description of its anatomic extent, utilizing generally accepted categories. Table 3-2 gives the staging method of the American Joint Committee for Cancer Staging and End-Results Reporting. The status of lung cancer in every relevant patient seen by a thoracic surgeon should be staged at least twice, once preoperatively and once postoperatively when the final pathology report is available. Such a procedure is useful both in assessing results and in planning therapy.

Rationale of the Therapeutic Approach for Carcinoma of the Lung

The decision to perform a pulmonary resection is based on answers to three questions:

1. Is there a significant possibility that the patient has a carcinoma of the lung?
2. Is there a significant possibility that the patient might have a protracted survival because of a resection?
3. Can the patient survive the necessary resection?

The information needed to answer question 3 was discussed in Chapter 2. The other two are answered here.

Probability of Carcinoma

One of the common decisions required of a thoracic surgeon is whether or not to recomend surgery to a patient with a solitary pulmonary nodule. Such a decision must be made by weighing the risk of the surgery against the

TABLE 3-2 Staging of Lung Cancer by the American Joint Committee for Cancer Staging and End-Results Reporting (2)

a. Stage

Stage			
Occult carcinoma			
	Tx	N_0	M_0
Stage 1			
	TIS	N_0	M_0
	T_1	N_0	M_0
	T_1	N_1	M_0
	T_2	N_0	M_0
Stage 2			
	T_2	N_1	M_0
Stage 3			
	T_3 any N or M		
	N_2 any T or M		
	M_1 any T or N		

b. TNM classification

TNM classification	Definition
Primary tumor (T)	
T_x	Tumor proven by the presence of malignant cells in bronchopulmonary secretions, but not visualized roentgenographically or bronchoscopically; or any tumor that cannot be assessed
T_0	No evidence of primary tumor
TIS	Carcinoma in situ
T_1	Tumor 3.0 cm or less in greatest diameter, surrounded by lung or visceral pleura, and without evidence of invasion proximal to a lobar bronchus at bronchoscopy
T_2	Tumor more than 3.0 cm in greatest diameter or a tumor of any size that either invades the visceral pleura or has associated atelectasis or obstructive pneumonitis extending to the hilar region. At bronchoscopy, the proximal extent of demonstrable tumor must be within a lobar bronchus or at least 2.0 cm distal to the carina. Any associated atelectasis or obstructive pneumonitis must involve less than an entire lung, and there must be no pleural effusion
T_3	Tumor of any size with direct extension into an adjacent structure, such as the parietal pleura, the chest wall, the diaphragm, or the mediastinum, or a tumor demonstrated bronchoscopically to involve a main bronchus less than 2.0 cm distal to the carina; or any tumor associated with atelectasis or obstructive pneumonitis of an entire lung or pleural effusion
Nodal involvement (N)	
N_0	No demonstrable metastasis to regional lymph nodes
N_1	Metastasis to lymph nodes in the peribronchial or the ipsilateral hilar region, or both, including direct extension.
N_2	Metastasis to lymph nodes in the mediastinum
Distant metastasis (M)	
M_x	Not assessed
M_0	No (known) distant metastasis
M_1	Distant metastasis present

risk of malignancy in the nodule. Data relevant to question one above are given in Tables 3-3 and 3-4, reproduced from Steele's monograph (47). The incidence of malignancy in resected pulmonary nodules of men is listed as a function of size of the nodule and age of the patient. Data of similar detail are not available for women. The Connecticut Tumor Registry of 1978 reported the number of cancers of the lung in men to be 2.25 times that in women, but in persons under age 45, the incidence in men was only 1.14 times that in women. Additionally, a greater fraction of carcinoma of the lung in women presents as a peripheral tumor, so Tables 3-3 and 3-4 may also approximate the risk of cancer for women born after 1934.

TABLE 3-3 Risk in Men of Malignancy of Resected Pulmonary Nodules by Size of the Nodule

	Greatest diameter (cm)					
	1.0 or less	1.5–2.0	2.5–3.0	3.5–4.0	4.5–5.0	5.5–6.0
Primary carcinomas	7%	21%	51%	68%	82%	90%
Metastatic malignancy		4%	3%	6%		5%
Hamartomas	8%	13%	7%	1.3%	7%	
Tuberculosis	21%	17%	17%	14%	7%	
Histoplasmosis	51%	28%	8%	6%	2%	5%
Coccidioidomycosis	13%	17%	14%	4%	2%	

From Steele (47). Courtesy of Charles C Thomas, Publisher, Springfield, Illinois.

The risk of death from an excisional biopsy of a lung nodule in Steele's report was 0.4%. Data that indicate the chance of malignancy in an individual lung nodule to be less than the risk of an excisional biopsy are:

1. Evidence that the nodule was present and *unchanged* two or more years previously
2. Demonstration of diffuse or concentric calcification within the lesion, such as that shown by tomography in Figure 3-1

The presence of one small area of calcium in a nodule is not evidence that it is benign. A carcinoma can grow around a previously calcified granuloma as well as it can grow around any other structure. It is the pattern of calcification that is important. Siegelman et al. (45) have described the use of thin section computerized tomography to calculate a representative density or CT number for pulmonary nodules. They found the highest representative CT number for any malignant lesion to be 147H, while 20 of 33 benign lesions had a representative CT number of 164H or greater. If this finding can be confirmed, the test will significantly increase our ability to accurately exclude some benign nodules as indications for thoracotomy.

The use of a given diagnostic procedure should depend upon the probability of obtaining data with decision-making potential, that is, data that warrant making a decision *not* to operate if cancer is not demonstrated. If the overall probability of cancer in a given nodule is 35% and the risk of death from an excisional biopsy is 0.4%, it makes little sense to employ in a decision-making capacity either a transbronchial brush biopsy with a 30% error rate

TABLE 3-4 Risk in Men of Malignancy of Resected Pulmonary Nodules by Age of the Patients

Ages	Carcinomas	Total patients in age group	Percentage carcinomas in age group
25–29	1	39	(2)
30–34	2	53	(4)
35–39	13	100	(13)
40–44	18	120	(15)
45–49	27	105	(26)
50–59	56	135	(41)
60–69	127	253	(50)
70–79	31	44	(70)
80–83	5	5	(100)

From Steele (47). Courtesy of Charles C Thomas, Publisher, Springfield, Illinois.

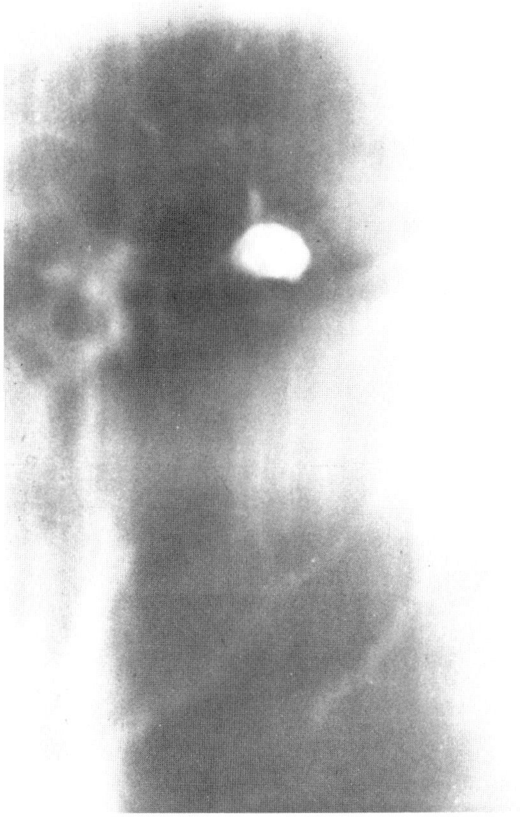

FIG. 3-1. Tomogram of a granuloma showing concentric calcification within a lung nodule.

or a percutaneous needle biopsy with an 8%–15% error rate. However, in a patient whose risk of operative death is 10%–15%, such procedures do acquire decision-making potential and should be employed.

Patients with a solitary pulmonary nodule who are completely asymptomatic, who have no abnormal physical findings, and who have no portentous abnormalities in the routine laboratory examinations of urine, stool, or blood should not have a system search by x-ray, hunting for an undiscovered primary carcinoma below the diaphragm. The cost to benefit ratio is so low that it can not be justified; fewer than 1% of such patients will have an undiscovered primary malignancy. Even in patients who have had a previous nonpulmonary malignancy, a solitary pulmonary nodule is not necessarily a metastasis. In a review of 142 patients who developed a solitary pulmonary nodule and had had a previous squamous cell carcinoma of the head or neck, Cahan (8) found all except five to be new primary carcinomas of the lung; of 72 similar patients who had had a previous carcinoma of the breast, 43 had nodules that were carcinoma of the lung (9).

Carcinoma of the lung may present as an area of pneumonia with no discernible pulmonary mass. Any patient with recurrent pneumonia in the same lobe or with a single area of unresolved pneumonia (defined as a new pulmonary infiltrate that does not completely clear after five weeks of adequate therapy) ought to be suspected of harboring a small carcinoma that partially obstructs a bronchus. Such patients should undergo fiberoptic bronchoscopy.

Carcinoma of the lung is more common in patients who have had tuberculosis or other pathologic conditions that result in lung scarring. Because of this scarring, however, the detection of a carcinoma may be difficult. Indications that such a patient may have developed carcinoma are:

1. Clearing of pulmonary disease in one area of the lung during therapy, while infiltrates or masses are enlarging in another
2. Progressively enlarging nodular densities that arise during treatment
3. Unilateral hilar enlargement
4. X-ray evidence of progression of the disease with a persistently negative sputum

Determining Operability

The answer to question two, "Is there a significant possibility that the patient might have a protracted survival because of a resection?" involves a search for the reasons of inoperability listed in Table 3-5. Half of all patients found to have a carcinoma of the lung will be inoperable because of distant metastasis or metastasis to the mediastinal lymph nodes at the time of diagnosis. These metastases will usually be evident from the history, the physical examination, or the routine laboratory or x-ray examinations. Because of the inaccuracy of liver scans and the low yield of bone and brain scans in asymptomatic patients with non-small cell carcinoma of the lung, the routine use of these tests to screen patients preoperatively cannot be recommended.

All patients suspected of harboring a carcinoma of the lung should have bronchoscopy preoperatively. A biopsy can be obtained from patients with central tumors, thus saving the time required for a frozen section diagnosis during the thoracotomy. In addition, bronchoscopy permits the surgeon to determine the degree of proximal bronchial involvement and thereby to define the least resection possible. The carina between the two main bronchi should be biopsied in any patient with stage 2 or 3 disease. Although it is advisable to resect the trachea and carina when tumors arise in these areas, such resections for carcinomas extending from within the lung across the carina have not produced long-term survival. Such a finding is indicative of inoperability. The bronchial tree of patients with peripheral tumors should be inspected for the presence of simultaneous second primary carcinomas, which occur in 2%–4% of patients.

Pretracheal mediastinoscopy or mediastinotomy is recommended preoperatively for patients with T_2 or T_3 carcinomas. The yield from routine mediastinoscopy in patients with T_1 carcinoma has been too small to justify its use. Only 5%–8% of patients with T_1 carcinomas will have positive mediastinal lymph nodes (44). The findings at mediastinoscopy that indicate inoperability are 1) metastasis to the highest right-sided mediastinal lymph nodes, 2) metastasis to the left mediastinal lymph nodes above the arch of the aorta, 3) metastasis to contralateral mediastinal lymph nodes, and 4) carcinoma that is not confined within the capsule of a lymph node.

A pleural effusion associated with a carcinoma of the lung places the patient in stage 3, and at least one center has reported no survivors five

TABLE 3-5 Reasons for Inoperability in Patients with Lung Cancer

1. Distant metastasis
2. Involvement of the trachea or the contralateral main bronchus with carcinoma
3. Mediastinal lymph node metastasis
4. Superior vena caval obstruction
5. Malignant cells in a pleural effusion
6. Recurrent laryngeal nerve paralysis from carcinoma
7. Histology is oat cell carcinoma

years after a pulmonary resection for carcinoma in patients with a pleural effusion (5). However, I have followed patients who underwent resection of a carcinoma of the lung with a pleural effusion secondary to an obstructive pneumonia and who survived for well over five years following the resection. Some surgeons consider any patient with bloody pleural fluid inoperable, but it is relatively common to lacerate an intercostal vessel during a thoracentesis and thus produce a spuriously bloody fluid. For these reasons I have confined the indication of inoperability to the finding of malignant cells in the pleural fluid. This interpretation should be made by a pathologist experienced in cytology, because the confusion of reactive mesothelial cells with malignant cells in pleural fluid is a frequent error.

Paralysis of the left recurrent laryngeal nerve by a carcinoma is evidence of inoperability. However, since older patients may develop an idiopathic left vocal cord paresis, the surgeon must be certain that the vocal cord paralysis in a patient with a carcinoma of the lung is due to the carcinoma. This can be established by radiographic evidence of a mass in the aortic window or by an examination of the region of the aortic window by a left mediastinotomy.

The consensus at present is that small cell undifferentiated carcinoma diagnosed prior to thoracotomy is evidence of inoperability. The few reported patients surviving long-term after resection of this disease usually had small peripheral tumors and no evidence of lymph node metastasis. However, in the past several years the literature on this tumor has become less clear. It is well known that carcinoids may be misdiagnosed as small cell undifferentiated carcinoma and that sampling errors and biopsy artifacts can result in an erroneous diagnosis. Now a type of carcinoid has been defined, termed atypical carcinoid, that has a prognosis intermediate between typical carcinoids and small cell undifferentiated carcinoma (3). In addition, the claim has been made that some tumors diagnosed by light microscopy as small cell carcinoma turn out to be poorly differentiated squamous cell or adenocarcinoma when examined by electron microscopy (29). Atypical carcinoids and poorly differentiated squamous and adenocarcinoma should be resected, but it is still probably wisest to consider inoperable those patients who are diagnosed to have typical oat cell carcinoma.

In addition to the above indications of inoperability, local spread of the carcinoma, discovered during the thoracotomy, may make the tumor unresectable. Common findings warranting such a decision are: implants of carcinoma on the pleura, invasion of the esophagus or the vertebral bodies, involvement of the pulmonary artery trunk or the pulmonary artery to the opposite lung, invasion of the left atrium that cannot be safely resected, extensive invasion of the superior or inferior vena cava, and an extension of the carcinoma that would require a pneumonectomy for complete removal in a patient that could tolerate only a lobectomy.

Table 3-6 gives the initial treatment categories of 2353 men at the Minneapolis Veterans Administration Medical Center from 1947 through 1975 having carcinoma of the lung. Only 26.9% had a resection with curative intent. The reasons for the inoperability of the other 1385 patients are given in Table 3-7.

Selection of Operation

At thoracotomy, peripheral undiagnosed lung nodules should be removed by wedge resection. However, if a nodule is deep within the substance of the lobe, a more formal segmental resection may be required to remove it. On those rare occasions when a lesion visible on the chest radiograph cannot be found, the segment in which it was seen should be totally removed. Although

TABLE 3-6 Initial Treatment Category for Patients with Carcinoma of the Lung. Minneapolis Veterans Administration Medical Center, 1947–1975

Total patients	2353	(100%)
Operable	954	(40.5%)
Resectable for cure	632	(26.9%)
Resected for palliation	63	(2.7%)

a lobectomy may be performed to take out an undiagnosed abnormality, lesions that would require a pneumonectomy for complete removal should be biopsied before the resection, using a Tru-Cut or similar type biopsy needle. A pneumonectomy without prior histologic diagnosis is unacceptable.

The choice of resection for carcinoma of the lung has become increasingly more conservative. Prior to the 1960s, a pneumonectomy was thought to provide the greatest opportunity for cure of any cancer of the lung. Although there have been no well-controlled randomized studies on the subject, for patients whose carcinomas can be completely removed by a lobectomy, published reports show that the chance for long-term survival is not increased by a pneumonectomy. Additionally, unless death supervenes, any patient undergoing a penumonectomy will develop progressive cardiac and pulmonary disability.

At present a lobectomy should be considered the operation of choice for any carcinoma that can be completely removed by this resection. Carcinomas arising in one lobe but extending across a fissure into the parenchyma of a second lobe can be removed by a combination lobectomy and wedge resection of the involved area in the second lobe, leaving this area in continuity with the primary tumor mass. For those patients with a carcinoma of the upper lobes near or involving the main bronchus, a lobectomy with a sleeve resection of the main bronchus and reanastomosis to the carina of the lower and middle lobes on the right, or the lower lobe on the left, is an attractive alternative to a pneumonectomy and provides an equal opportunity for long-term survival. A pneumonectomy should be reserved for those patients in which all of the tumor will not be removed either by a lobectomy or by a lobectomy plus a resection of the main bronchus. The reason for the latter is usually that either the artery to the lower lobe or the parenchyma of both lobes is involved with the carcinoma.

At times a carcinoma will involve contiguous structures that can be resected en bloc with a portion of the lung. If the chest wall has been invaded,

TABLE 3-7 Cause for Inoperability of Patients with Carcinoma of the Lung. Minneapolis Veterans Administration Medical Center, 1947–1975

Total patients inoperable	1385	(100%)
Evidence of distant metastasis	433	(31.3%)
Nodal metastasis on mediastinoscopy or scalene node biopsy	291	(21%)
Tumor past the carina	78	(5.6%)
Vocal cord paralysis	38	(2.7%)
Superior vena caval obstruction	32	(2.3%)
Inadequate pulmonary function	111	(8.0%)
Inadequate cardiac function	38	(2.7%)
Debility	84	(6.1%)
Other	280	(20%)

the diseased area may be removed. If the pericardium is involved, the involved area may be resected and the pulmonary veins or artery ligated and divided within the pericardium. If necessary, a portion of the left atrium may also be removed, but care must be taken to interfere neither with the drainage from the pulmonary veins of the opposite lung nor with the action of the mitral valve. An extensive mediastinal lymph node dissection also can be done, removing the lymph nodes from beneath the carina and both main bronchi. On the right side, thosc superior mediastinal lymph nodes along the esophagus, between the trachea and superior vena cava, and anterior to the vena cava can be removed below the level of the subclavian artery, but on the left side, the dissection is usually limited by the arch of the aorta.

In 1955, Brock and Whytehead (6) suggested the routine use of a "radical pneumonectomy" that consisted of the intrapericardial division of the pulmonary vessels, the excision of a perihilar area of pericardium, and an extensive mediastinal lymph node dissection. Although the published series of this procedure are small, routine use seems to be associated with no significant increase in survival, but rather with an increase in complication rate (22).

Many patients with carcinoma of the lung have chronic obstructive pulmonary disease of a degree so advanced that even a lobectomy would leave them a respiratory cripple. If these patients have a peripheral T_1 carcinoma, it should be removed by a generous wedge resection, or for a more proximal tumor, by a formal segmental resection. Jensik et al. (24) have reported data for survival following this procedure that differ little from those for survival after a lobectomy.

Prognosis of Carcinoma of the Lung

The noun "cure" has been greatly misused in the medical literature. The logical and most understood definition of this word is *the return of a group of patients to a normal survival experience for the age, race, and sex.* However, in the medical literature whether or not a treatment is a cure has been determined by counting the number of patients alive at some period (three, five, or ten years) following the treatment. The following data, from Humphrey et al. (21), show a different method for analyzing survival.

In Figure 3-2, the survival curve of 1123 men who had a pulmonary resection with curative intent for squamous cell carcinoma of the lung at one of 29 Veterans Administration Medical Centers is shown for 14 years following surgery. The survival curve (Fig. 3-2) is biphasic, but by using exponential analysis, the curve has been separated into two population groups. The high-risk group is comprised of patients dying at a rapid rate, 54.1% per year, and represents 56% of all patients. Patients in the low-risk group died at a slower rate, 9.7% per year, and comprise 44% of all patients in the study. If one were to equate the low-risk group with cure, then the rate of death should be equal to that of the expected annual mortality, 4.2% for men of the same age and race, according to United States vital statistics (shown by the heavy solid line in Fig. 3-2). But this is not the case. At 14 years after resection, this low-risk group had an excess death rate of 5.7% per year or 2.15 times the expected rate. In the period 8–14 years after resection the greatest cause of death in the low-risk group was carcinoma of the lung. The death rate from lung cancer in this group is 9.87 times the standard rate.

The survival curve for 246 men who underwent resection for adenocarcinoma of the lung is plotted in Figure 3-3. The high-risk population, comprising 53% of the total, died at the rate of 57.5% per year. The low-risk population, 47% of the total, died at 12.1% per year, which rate is slightly greater than

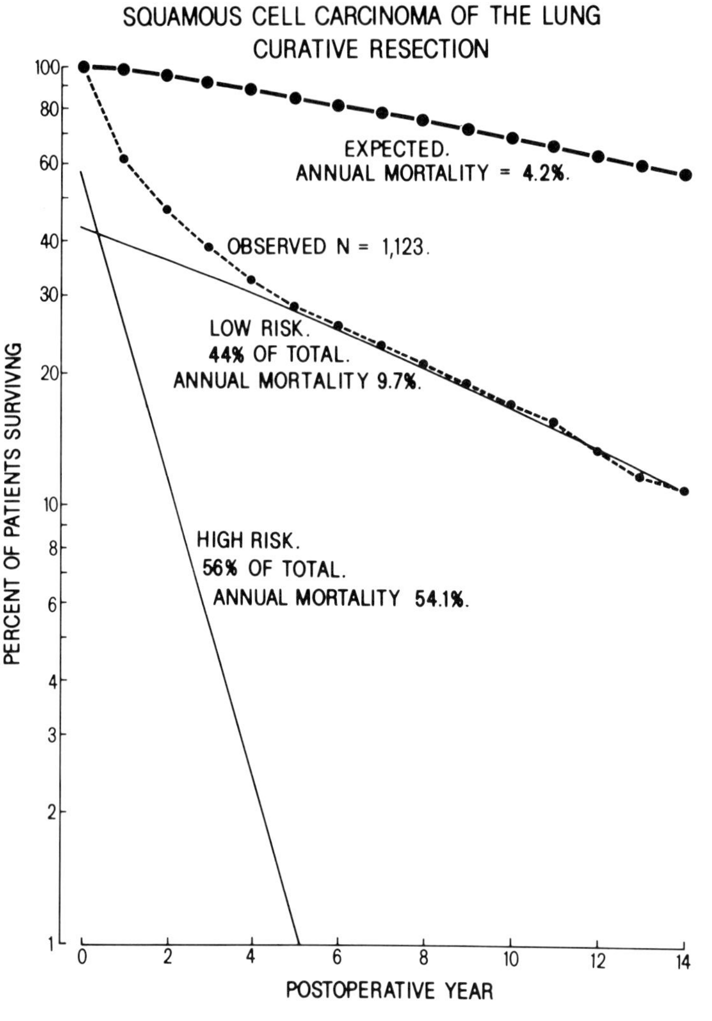

FIG. 3-2. The light dashed line represents the average observed survival of 1123 men undergoing curative resection for squamous cell carcinoma of the lung. The heavy dashed line represents the average expected survival assuming exposure to death rates for men in the United States. The light solid lines are the extrapolated and subtraction curves. By permission of Surgery, Gynecology & Obstetrics.

that for the group with squamous cell carcinoma and considerably greater than the expected mortality of 4% per year. In this low-risk group of men, deaths from carcinoma of the lung beyond the eighth postoperative year were 9.44 times the expected.

The data from a 12-year follow-up study of patients with small asymptomatic cancers from the solitary pulonary nodule study of Steele (47) are plotted in Figure 3-4. The slopes of the survival curves for this group of patients are remarkably similar to those for the over-all survival of men undergoing curative resection of squamous cell carcinoma or adenocarcinoma of the lung. Only the relative size of the two risk groups is different. In this population of patients with small cancers, the high-risk group, comprising 36% of the total, died at the rate of 60.1% percent per year. The low-risk group, comprising 64% of the total, died at the rate of 10.3% per year. The expected annual mortality for this low-risk group is 3.7% per year.

These data indicate that no group of patients with squamous cell carcinoma or adenocarcinoma of the lung, even when as small as that in the solitary pulmonary nodule study, may be labeled "cured." These data should not be interpreted as suggesting that a resection does not influence the course of many patients with carcinoma of the lung. If the mortalities of the high-risk groups are assumed to be somewhat comparable to those of untreated patients, it is evident that converting patients from a group dying at the rate of 50%–60% per year to one dying at 10% a year is worthwhile, but it should not be confused with cure.

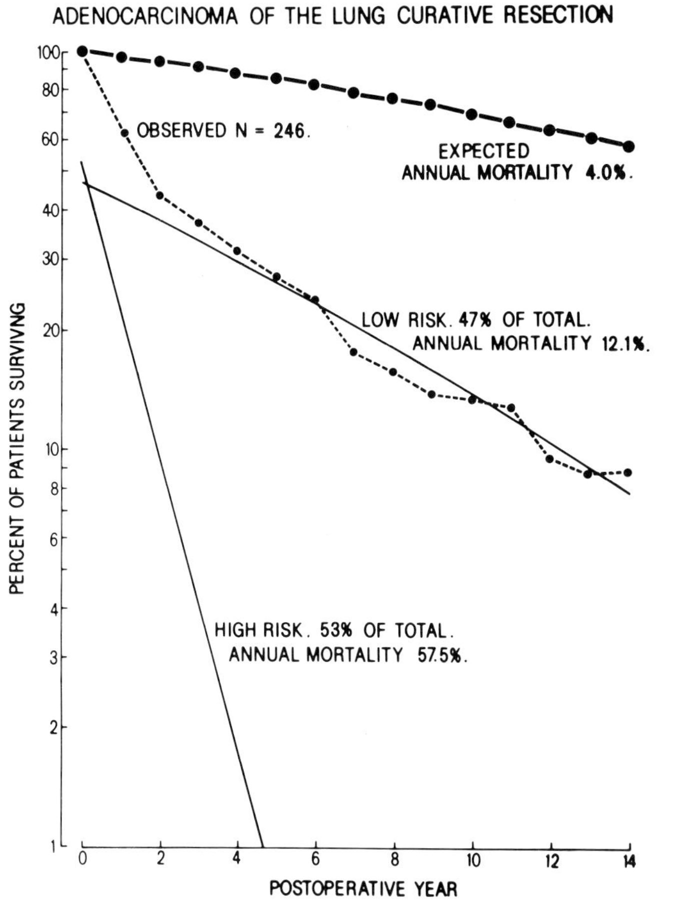

FIG. 3-3. The light dashed line represents the average observed survival for 246 men undergoing curative resection for adenocarcinoma of the lung. The heavy dashed line represents the average expected survival rate assuming exposure to death rates for men in the United States. The light solid lines are the extrapolated and subtraction curves. By permission of Surgery, Gynecology & Obstetrics.

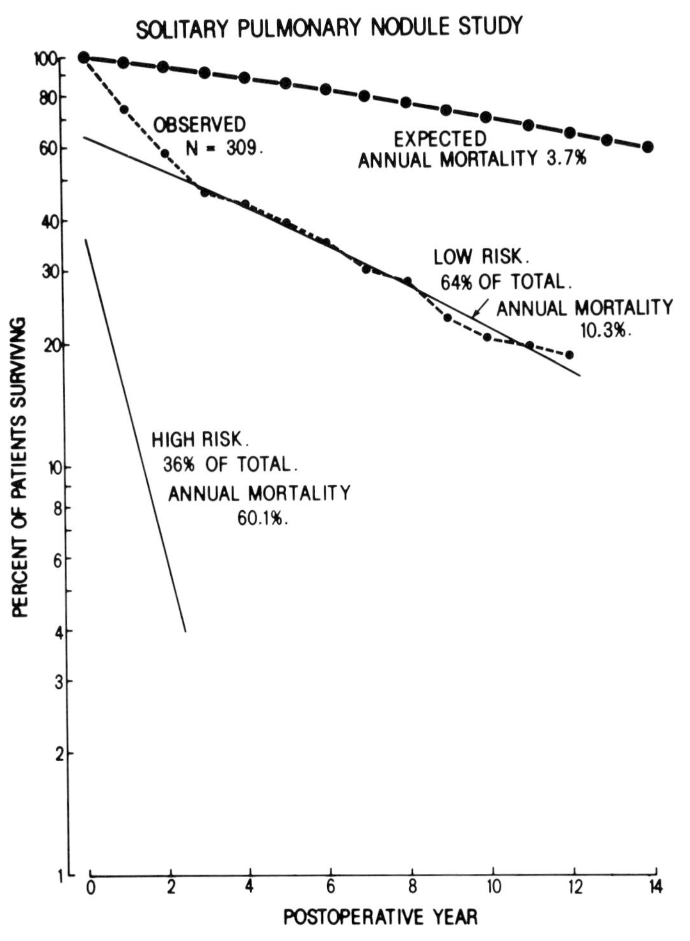

FIG. 3-4. The light dashed line represents the average observed survival of 309 men undergoing a resection of primary cancer of the lung that presented as an asymptomatic pulmonary nodule. The heavy dashed line represents the average expected survival assuming exposure to death rates for men in the United States. The light solid lines are the extrapolated and subtraction curves. By permission of Surgery, Gynecology & Obstetrics.

Adjuvant Therapy for Carcinoma of the Lung

The poor prognosis for long-term survival of patients with carcinoma of the lung has prompted many trials of adjuvant therapy for surgery, given either before or after the resection. Three categories of adjuvant therapy have been used, preoperative or postoperative radiation, chemotherapy, and immunostimulation.

Preoperative radiation therapy as an adjuvant was suggested in 1955 by Bromley and Szur (7) and in 1960 by Bloedorn and Cowley (4). To test this proposal, the Veterans Administration Surgical Oncology group conducted a randomized study (43), comparing the use in 86 men of 4000–6000 rads of radiation given to the primary tumor and the mediastinum over a 4–6 week period, followed by resection one month later, to the use in 90 men of a resection alone, performed as soon as possible after the diagnosis. All of these patients had had a preoperative histologic diagnosis of carcinoma of the lung. Although there was no significant difference in the 30-day postoperative mortality rate between the two groups, there was a significant difference in the late survival. At 36 months after resection, 29% of the patients having only surgery were alive, but only 19% of the patients receiving preoperative radiation followed by surgery were alive. At 54 months, the survival rates were 21% for the surgery only group and 12.5% for the preoperative radiation plus surgery group. The median survival of the surgery only patients was 495 days, while that for the patients receiving preoperative radiation was 240 days.

These data suggest strongly that the routine use of preoperative radiation therapy for carcinoma of the lung is ill advised. At present, the only indication for its use seems to be in the therapy of superior sulcus tumors. Paulson advises the use of 3000 rads to the tumor given in ten fractions, followed by a resection within 3–6 weeks (40). With this regimen he reports a 35% 5-year survival. Even this procedure, however, has not been subjected to a randomized study.

The use of postoperative radiation therapy for patients with carcinoma of the lung remains controversial. Paterson and Russell (39) reported no significant difference in the survival of those patients given 4500 rads to the mediastinum postoperatively and those treated by resection alone. However, both Kirsh et al. (28) and Green et al. (18) have reported in nonrandomized selected series an increased 5-year survival rate in patients given postoperative radiation therapy. Prior to general acceptance, this procedure requires a prospective randomized study to determine its value.

The list of anticancer drugs given to patients in attempts to find a successful adjuvant after a resection for carcinoma of the lung is long indeed. Over a 24-year period, the Veterans Administration Surgical Oncology group has entered more than 3800 patients with cancer of the lung into six different treatment protocols designed to detect possible benefit from nitrogen mustard, cyclophosphamide, cyclophosphamide alternated with methotrexate, and CCNU plus hydroxyurea, all given as adjuvants to surgery. None of these drugs or combination of drugs has been effective in decreasing the long-term mortality rate, nor are there other reports of significant differences between a treated and a control group from any randomized study conducted on non-small cell carcinoma of the lung.

McKneally et al. (32) have reported that the intrapleural administration of 10^7 units of BCG (bacille Calmette Gúerin) in the early postoperative period appeared to prolong survival and reduce the rate of tumor recurrence in patients with stage 1 lung cancer when compared to control patients. Attempts by Lowe et al. (30) and others to repeat these results have so far been unsuccessful.

TABLE 3-8 Cumulative Survival at Five Years for Resection of Pulmonary Metastases

Primary site	Mountain et al. (35)	Muzzall & Humphrey (36)	Wilkins et al. (49)
Head and Neck	(34) 30%		
Breast	(21) 14%		(9) 52.7%
Colon–rectum	(28) 28%	(5) 40%	(35) 25.4%
Urinary tract	(16) 50%	(5) 20%	(28) 44.2%
Male genital	(11) 37%		(14) 41.9%
Uterus and uterine cervix	(31) 19%	(1) 100%	(9) 39.5%
Sarcoma		(5) 60%	(21) 21.3%
Other	(18) 31%		
Melanoma		(4) 0%	(9) 0%

The obvious conclusion from all of these trials is that at present, there is no therapy that when given in addition to a surgical resection will increase the chance of a long-term survival for a patient with a non-small cell carcinoma of the lung.

Pulmonary Metastasis From Nonpulmonary Malignancy

For a patient who has had a previous malignancy and later develops a growing solitary pulmonary nodule, two important questions must be answered. First, is the nodule a metastasis from the previous malignancy or a new carcinoma of the lung? Second, if the nodule is a metastasis, is there a significant chance that resection of the nodule will prolong the patient's life? Data bearing on the first question have been presented earlier in this chapter. The data for survival 5 years after resection of solitary pulmonary metastases are summarized for three series in Table 3-8. The overall 5-year survival for these highly selected patients has been about 30%. Even the presence of several pulmonary metastases should not be construed to be beyond surgical therapy. The survival of patients having more than one metastasis removed has been reported to be similar to that of patients with solitary metastases.

The selection of patients for resection of pulmonary metastases is based on the following criteria:

1. The disease at the primary site must be controlled.
2. No metastases outside of the lungs are demonstrable.
3. All apparent disease in the chest must be completely resectable.
4. The risk of the resection must not be excessive.

Several authors have contended that if the length of the disease-free interval between the primary resection and the appearance of the pulmonary metastasis is greater than 12–36 months, the prognosis is improved. Morton and colleagues have reported the length of the doubling time of the metastasis to be an important variable in prognosis (25,34). In these series, patients with a tumor doubling time greater than 40 days had a 63% 5-year survival after resection of pulmonary metastases, whereas no patient with a tumor doubling time less than 40 days survived beyond 30 months.

The resection of pulmonary metastases should conserve as much lung tissue as possible, while still removing all apparent tumor. Usually such metastases can be adequately treated by a wedge resection, although occasionally a lobectomy will be required for a centrally located lesion. This conservative type of operation permits additional resections to be performed for metastases that may appear in the future. Patients with simultaneous bilateral metastases are best explored through a median sternotomy. This incision gives adequate exposure and is associated with less morbidity than are two posterior lateral thoracotomies.

Bacterial Infections

Primary Lung Abscess

Pyogenic lung abscess can result from disease processes such as septic emboli, cavitating pneumonias, tracheoesophageal fistulae, or infected pulmonary cysts, but at present, they are most commonly due in adults to aspiration in a person with a depressed cough reflex and with poor dental hygiene. This etiology results in a characteristic localization and spectrum of pathogens. The abscess is usually localized to the superior segment of the lower lobes or to regions termed the axillary subsegments that are parts of the anterior and posterior segments of the upper lobes. The pathogens characteristically include anaerobic bacteria together with nonspecific oral and upper respiratory tract bacteria. In infants and young children, the most common pathogen is a staphylococcus.

Occasionally it may be difficult to distinguish between a primary lung abscess and a cavitating carcinoma or between a subpleural lung abscess and an empyema cavity. A cavitating carcinoma of the lung usually has an irregular cavity, while that of a pyogenic abscess is usually smooth. The false negative rate of either a transbronchial biopsy or a percutaneous needle biopsy is relatively higher for cavitating carcinomas than for noncavitating carcinomas, so a negative biopsy cannot be used to rule out carcinoma. If the diagnosis remains in doubt, that is an indication for resection. Computerized tomography has been helpful in differentiating between a subpleural lung abscess and an empyema. The distinction between these two becomes important if drainage of the latter by a tube thoracostomy is proposed. Drainage of a lung abscess across a free pleural cavity may result in an empyema.

Most abscess cavities will heal with adequate nonoperative management, which includes appropriate and prolonged antibiotic therapy together with adequate drainage. Antibiotic therapy should be continued until the cavity is closed or at least until it is thin walled and less than 2 cm in diameter. Typically, a lung abscess will drain adequately through a communicating bronchus; however, if toxicity persists or if the cavity does not decrease in size with appropriate antibiotic therapy, drainage by other means must be instituted. Connors et al. (10) have reported the successful use of a #8 coronary angiocatheter with a teflon guide, introduced into the appropriate bronchus through rigid bronchoscope, to aspirate the contents of such a cavity. Alternatively the abscess may be drained by tube thoracostomy if the areas of parietal and visceral pleura through which the thoracostomy will be done are adherent to one another. If the pleura is not adherent, the wound is packed with iodoform gauze after a 2–3 cm length of rib has been removed. Three or four days later the wound is reexplored and a tube thoracostomy performed. Such drainage will often result in a dramatic decrease in toxicity and improvement in the patient's course. All patients with a lung abscess should undergo bronchoscopy; it can establish the presence either of an associated carcinoma or of an intrabronchial foreign body.

The complications of a lung abscess are massive hemoptysis; rupture into the pleural space, producing an empyema; dissemination, producing a brain abscess; or metastatic infection in the opposite lung. Although the latter complication may be treated by thoracostomy drainage, the development of massive hemoptysis, the suspicion of carcinoma, or the failure of an abscess to close on adequate nonoperative therapy are indications for a resection. Some abscess cavities require several months to close. An empirical rule is that a resection should be considered if during any 3–4 week period, a cavity shows absolutely no decrease in size with adequate antibiotic therapy. With current endoscopic techniques and antibiotic therapy, resection is rarely indicated. In a recent series reported by Estera et al. (15), only 10% of patients underwent a resection. Other authors have reported 0–15% resection rates.

To prevent aspiration of infectious material into the contralateral lung, patients with a lung abscess have been operated on in the prone or supine position, but now, the use of a double lumen endobronchial tube permits the utilization of a standard posterior–lateral incision. Care must be taken to place accurately the tube before the patient is turned into the lateral position, or the abscess may empty into the dependent lung. The least resection that will permit a bronchial closure through healthy tissue should be performed. Usually this can be done with a segmental resection or a lobectomy.

Bronchiectasis

Bronchiectasis is a disease characterized by infection of the bronchial wall and peribronchial pneumonia severe enough to cause destruction and dilatation of the bronchi. It most commonly occurs in the basilar segments of the lower lobes, and onset is usually during childhood. Early changes, such as the bronchial dilatation that occurs in children following an episode of pneumonia, are reversible. In the latter states, however, the bronchi are replaced by fibrous tubes, there is hypertrophy of the bronchial arteries, and left to right intrapulmonary shunting may become significant.

The importance of bronchiectasis as a cause of disability has decreased significantly over the past 30 years. The classic description of a patient with this condition—malnourished, febrile and cyanotic with clubbing of the digits—is no longer relevant, nor does patient classification by the bronchographic appearance into such categories as cylindrical or saccula bronchiectasis contribute to our management of the disease. At present, most patients with bronchiectasis are asymptomatic until a secondary infection occurs in the bronchi; then they become febrile, develop a cough, and produce large volumes of foul-smelling sputum. Such episodes may occur frequently during the winter months, and at such times hemoptysis is common.

Although hemoptysis has been reported in 45%–65% of patients with bronchiectasis, it is rarely life threatening. Patients with bronchiectasis are now most usefully classified etiologically into two categories: 1) those patients with systemic abnormalities that either have affected or have the potential for affecting the entire lung (examples are cystic fibrosis, α_1-antitrypsin deficiency, dysglobulinemia, neutrophil abnormalities, pansinusitis, Kartagener's syndrome, and the Williams–Campbell syndrome); and 2) those patients whose bronchiectasis has been caused by a localized abnormality such as an antecedent specific pulmonary infection, obstruction of a bronchus either by a foreign body or by external compression from lymph nodes, or from aspiration due to a remedial cause.

Most patients with bronchiectasis can be managed nonoperatively. The only two indications for surgery are failure of medical therapy and massive hemoptysis, the latter occurring rarely. The group that benefits most frequently from a resection is comprised of young patients who have frequent episodes of pneumonia in spite of adequate medical therapy. These patients should be considered for a resection if they satisfy the following criteria:

1. The bronchiectasis is localized to one lung and can be removed by, at most, a lobectomy.
2. The area of bronchiectasis is significant, that is, more than one segment is involved.
3. The patient does not have a systemic disease that would be expected to produce bronchiectasis in the remaining lung after the surgical resection.

Prior to surgery, patients should undergo bronchoscopy to determine whether a foreign body or an intrabronchial tumor is present. Bronchograms of both lungs should be done to determine the extent of the disease and to map out the portion to be resected. Determination of the magnitude of resection must be based on the bronchograms, because frequently the external surface of the involved lung appears perfectly normal. Bronchograms should not be performed during an acute infection, and due to the risk of pneumonitis following a bronchogram, bilateral examinations should not be performed simultaneously, but should be staged with an interval of two weeks. Radiograms of the nasal sinuses should be obtained before deciding whether or not to operate.

Other Bacterial Infections

Actinomycosis

Actinomycosis is an infection of endogenous orgin caused by the bacterium *Actinomyces israeli.* Its principal interest to the thoracic surgeon is its ability to mimic carcinoma. In the lung it causes a chronic inflammation with dense fibrosis and may extend through the chest wall, destroying ribs and producing chronically draining sinus tracts. Surgery is infrequently required for an empyema or for chest wall disease, the treatment of choice is high-dose penicillin therapy continued for one to three months.

Bacterial Pneumonias

Antibiotic therapy is the primary treatment for bacterial pneumonias, but occasionally certain organisms, such as a *Klebsiella,* that are characterized by the production of numerous small cavities, will not respond well to antibiotic therapy and will spread to the opposite lung by transbronchial aspiration. If evidence of such spread develops, the involved lobe may require resection to prevent further destruction of the opposite lung.

Severe bacterial pneumonia may destroy a major portion of the parenchyma of the involved lobe. Such lobes will organize and heal by fibrosis and contraction to leave a small airless remnant. These destroyed lobes do not require removal unless they become the site of chronic or recurrent infection, or hemorrhage, but the bronchi must be thoroughly examined to rule out the presence of an intrabronchial tumor.

Tuberculosis

Improvement in the management of tuberculosis during the past 30 years is one of the most dramatic achievements of modern medicine. This has been due primarily to the development of an effective chemotherapeutic regimen. Over this 30-year period the annual attack rate has decreased from approximately 50 per 100,000 to the present rate of 13 per 100,000. There is, however, still a reservoir of tuberculosis in the United States that is estimated to be 7% of the population. The disease is particularly prevalent among the elderly, among individuals in institutions, among recent imigrants from South East Asia, and among the malnourished.

TABLE 3-9 Mycobacteria Causing Human Pulmonary Disease

1. Mammalian tuberculous mycobacteria
   a. *M. tuberculosis*
   b. *M. bovis*
2. Nontuberculous (atypical) myocobacteria
   a. *M. kansasii*
   b. *M. avium–M. intracellulare* complex (Battey)
   c. *M. scrofulaceum*
   d. *M. xenopi*
   e. *M. simiae*
   f. *M. szulgai*
   g. *M. fortuitum* } *M. fortuitum* complex
   h. *M. chelonei* }

A listing of the mycobacteria that cause human pulmonary disease is given in Table 3-9. The vast majority of human tuberculosis is caused by the bacillus *Mycobacterium tuberculosis;* however, pulmonary disease caused by the nontuberculous mycobacteria is being encountered with increasing frequency. Indeed, with the decrease in the attack rate and with the marked susceptibility to drug therapy of *M. tuberculosis,* and because the nontuberculous mycobacteria as a group are less sensitive to drug therapy, the cases referred to a thoracic surgeon at present are most commonly caused by nontuberculous organisms.

M. tuberculosis is not found free in nature, it is contagious from person to person, and it can infect apparently normal lung tissue. Nontuberculous mycobacteria are usually not transmitted from person to person, but are acquired from the environment; disease caused by these organisms usually occurs in individuals with some type of preexisting chronic lung disease. Wolinsky (50) believes that preexisting lung lesions are almost always present in *M. fortuitum, M. chelonei,* and *M. scrofulaceum disease,* in most cases of *M. avium-intracellulare* disease, and in one-half of the cases of *M. kansasii* disease. Pulmonary disease caused by *M. fortuitum–M. chelonei* is frequently associated with chronic aspiration in patients with esophageal disease, particularly achalasia.

Most tuberculous infections are contracted by inhalation of the bacillus, so they are manifested originally and subsequently in the lungs. It is estimated that 5% of persons newly infected will develop tuberculosis within one year of exposure, and an additional 5% will develop the disease sometime later. Pulmonary tuberculosis is usually classified into two major categories: primary and postprimary. As pointed out by many authors, primary tuberculosis is no longer confined to children.

The earliest evidence of disease in adults is usually a small area of inflammation in the apical or posterior segments of the upper lobes, less commonly in the superior segment of the lower lobes. The characteristic lesion is a granuloma, which consists of a caseous center surrounded by tuberculous granulation tissue. In time, the caseous center undergoes fibrous encapsulation and may calcify. If the disease progresses, cavitation and increased tissue destruction occur. The primary lesion in children is generally subpleural, and in contrast to adults, it is associated with enlarged hilar and mediastinal lymph nodes, the well-known Ghon complex.

Tuberculosis may present in many clinical forms, advanced fibrocaseous disease (the most common form), tuberculous pneumonia, tuberculous endobronchitis, acute hematogenous (miliary) tuberculosis, extrapulmonary tuberculosis, and mixed tuberculous and bacterial empyema from the rupture of a caseous focus of disease into the pleural cavity. If widespread pleural involvement producing a tuberculous pleural effusion occurs, it is soon after the primary infection, at a time when radiologic evidence of pulmonary parenchymal involvement is usually absent. For this reason, tuberculosis must be suspected in all unexplained exudative pleural effusions. Life-threatening hemorrhage occurs occasionally in patients with extensive cavitary disease and seems to happen soon after the onset of therapy.

Because life-threatening complications may occur following a pulmonary resection, it is as important for a surgeon to refrain from operating on an untreated patient with active tuberculosis as it is to operate on a patient with a carcinoma that mimics tuberculosis. The diagnosis of tuberculosis is made by the radiographic appearance, by the tuberculin skin test reactivity, and by culturing the organism or finding it on a smear or section of sputum or other material taken from the patient. For sound decision-making, the risk of error, both false-positive and false-negative, must be known for each diagnostic procedure.

The clinical and radiographic presentation of tuberculosis is not always characteristic. It has been reported (31) that 44% of tuberculosis patients admitted to a large urban teaching hospital were misdiagnosed. Stead and Dutt (46) found that recently the radiographic appearance of new tuberculous infections among residents and employees of a nursing home was quite atypical in that the principal involvement was often in the middle and lower lung fields, but Hadlock et al. (19) reported radiographic findings atypical of either primary or postprimary tuberculosis in only 8% of his patients. It is generally agreed that the radiographic findings of tuberculosis and those of carcinoma of the lung are remarkably similar. McQuarrie et al. (33) found that in those patients who were diagnosed to have tuberculosis but in fact had a lung carcinoma, this similarity caused an average delay of 8 months from the development of pulmonary changes due to the carcinoma until its diagnosis.

A positive skin test does not necessarily mean a patient has tuberculosis, but does a negative skin text exclude tuberculosis? The tuberculin skin test performed with intermediate strength PPD, 5TU per 0.1 ml, was designed to detect 99.6% of patients with active tuberculosis; however, recent reports do not show this degree of accuracy. Hyde (23) reported that only 81% of 100 patients with proven active pulmonary tuberculosis developed 10 mm or more reaction to PPD-5TU and 10% developed no reaction at all. Khan et al. (27) found that only 78% of patients with newly diagnosed pulmonary tuberculosis had a positive reaction to PPD-5TU. It is known that patients with far-advanced, severe tuberculosis may lose cutaneous sensitivity to tuberculin, but patients with Hodgkins disease or other lymphomas, patients undergoing steroid therapy, and some patients for unknown causes may also be unreactive. Weak reactions to tuberculin may be due to one of the nontuberculous mycobacteria. These findings indicate that a negative skin test cannot be relied upon to exlude tuberculosis.

It is difficult to determine the error entailed in assuming that a patient with a radiographic chest lesion resembling tuberculosis, but with negative smears and cultures for tuberculosis, does not have tuberculosis. It has been stated (1) that in known cases of pulmonary tuberculosis, one sputum culture gives a 75% chance of a positive result, and that only 5% or 6% of all cases cannot be diagnosed by sputum or gastric smears and cultures. Wells et al. (48) reported 75% of their patients with cavitary tuberculosis had sputum positive on culture, and of these, one-third had sputum positive on smear for acid-fast organisms. Khan and co-workers (27) found that of those patients with sputum positive on culture for tuberculosis, 24% had multiple negative sputum smears for acid-fast bacteria. They also reported that certain lesions were associated with a greater difficulty in obtaining positive cultures for tuberculosis. Of six patients with tuberculosis of the lower lung fields, only two yielded sputum positive on smear or culture, and of eight patients with discrete tuberculomas, sputum smears and cultures were negative in all. Fiberoptic bronchoscopy and biopsy in these latter eight patients permitted a diagnosis of tuberculosis in only two. The possibility of environmental contamination compounds this problem in patients with a possible infection due to one of the nontuberculous mycobacteria. A single, nonrepeatable positive sputum culture of one of these organisms is of little significance.

Therapy

The treatment of pulmonary disease caused by *M. tuberculosis* is almost totally medical. The present 9-month regimen of isoniazid and rifampin for drug-sensitive cases results in a treatment failure rate of only 1% and a late relapse rate of 1% (46). Since a high incidence of isoniazid-resistent disease is found in Southeast Asia, streptomycin and pyrazinamide instead of isoniazid are usually used with rifampin in patients who contract their disease in that area.

The indications for surgery in pulmonary disease caused by *M. tuberculosis* are few. They are suspicion of malignancy, bronchopleural fistula with empyema, and rarely, persistent or life-threatening hemoptysis. The only situation in which immediate surgery, without preoperative drug therapy, is indicated is that of massive hemorrhage shortly after diagnosis. Any patient who develops hemoptysis of more than 600–700 ml and either continues to bleed or stops and then rebleeds should have an immediate resection of the lobe harboring the bleeding site. The reported mortality of delaying surgery in such patients is high.

In all other situations, the patient should receive at least three weeks of therapy with two *effective* drugs prior to any pulmonary resection for tuberculosis. If the patient has developed a resistent organism while being treated with the primary drugs, it is our practice to give three new secondary drugs for three weeks before the resection. A surgeon should be especially wary of resecting or doing an incisional biopsy of a cavitary lesion that could be either carcinoma or tuberculosis without prior chemotherapy. Such lesions, if tuberculosis, may contain up to 10^9 bacteria, and persistent bronchopleural fistula with an empyema commonly develop in the postoperative period.

The response to drug treatment is not as successful if the pulmonary disease is due to nontuberculous mycobacteria. *M. kansasii* usually responds well to appropriate drug therapy, but surgery still plays a significant role in the treatment of disease caused by the other mycobacteria, particularly *M. avium-intracellulare.* For this disease, resection, after a period of adequate drug treatment, is indicated for localized residuals with continuing positive sputum. The preoperative preparation described previously should be used.

A pulmonary resection for tuberculosis does not differ from resections for other conditions, with the following exceptions. The pleural cavity is often obliterated by dense, very vascular adhesions. Dividing these adhesions may cause extensive blood loss unless the bleeding points are controlled by cautery or ligature. If the intrapleural dissection becomes too difficult, the lobe may be dissected free in the plane of the endothoracic fascia. All disease usually cannot and need not be removed. Only those areas containing cavities or large caseous foci should be resected. For the indications given above, this usually requires a lobectomy.

Fungal Disease

Coccidioidomycosis

Coccidioidomycosis is caused by the dimorphic fungus *Coccidioides immitis,* which is prevalent in the southwestern United States, in Mexico, and Central and South America, but now also occurs in isolated cases around the world. The organism exists as a saprophyte in the soil and releases the infectious form, the arthrospore, into the air. The arthrospores are inhaled into the lungs where they develop into the parasitic form, doubly refractile spherules containing multiple endospores. Although the arthrospores are very infective, the endospores are not, therefore coccidioidomycosis is not directly transmissible from person to person, but can be transmitted by dressings from draining skin lesions or plaster casts on which the mycelial phase of the fungus has developed. The skin test is helpful only in ruling out coccidioidomycosis; the disease is diagnosed by culturing *Coccidioides immitis* or by demonstrating the endosporulating spherules in body fluids or tissue sections.

Following inhalation of the arthrospores, 40% of the patients who convert their skin test will develop symptomatic pulmonary coccidioidomycosis (13). The symptoms range from influenza-like to those of a suppurative pneumonia and are often associated with erythema nodosum, erythema multiforme, and articular symptoms. Pulmonary infiltrates on a roentgenographic examination are frequent; approximately 20% of patients develop hilar adenopathy and approximately 20% will have some evidence of a pleural effusion. Usually the symptoms persist for two to three weeks, but if the roentgenographic abnormalities are present for more than eight weeks, the patient is considered to have persistent coccidioidomycosis (13).

While a principal cause of death and disability from this disease is the extrapulmonary dissemination, thoracic surgeons are most frequently concerned with treatment of the persistent forms of pulmonary coccidioidomycosis. These may be solid nodules, thick-walled cavities, or the classical thin-walled cavities. With time, 50% of the cavities will close, but the larger the cavity, the less likely it is to close. These cavities may rupture into the pleural cavity, producing a bronchopleural fistula and a pyopneumothorax; they may become secondarily infected, particularly with *Aspergillus,* they may disseminate, and they may produce hemoptysis. While hemoptysis is common, it is rarely serious.

The most common reason for a pulmonary resection of this disease is to establish the diagnosis of a solitary pulmonary nodule that could be malignant, but aside from this, little agreement exists about the indications for resection. Other commonly accepted indications are 1) significant pulmonary hemorrhage, 2) a cavity that rapidly enlarges during therapy, 3) a secondarily infected cavity, and 4) a cavity that has ruptured through the pleura. Some authors have suggested that a persistent subpleural cavity or a persistent cavity larger than 4–5 cm in diameter also should be resected.

Prior to 1960, a high incidence of bronchopleural fistulae was reported following segmental resections for coccidioidomycosis. This complication was thought to result from satellites of disease that cross segmental or lobar planes. Consequently, a lobectomy was suggested as the minimal operation. Findlay and Melick (16) have also advocated the administration of 400–600 mg amphotericin-B preoperatively and 300–500 mg postoperatively. With this regimen they were able to decrease the postoperative complication rate from 15% to below 5%. Nelson (37), however, disputes the necessity for perioperative amphotericin-B. The evidence presented to support either of these two opinions is not strong. However, if care is taken not to cut across palpable disease, it is possible using current surgical techniques to perform a wedge or segmental resection for localized disease with an acceptable low morbidity rate. Empyemas caused by coccidioidomycosis should be treated by a decortication.

Histoplasmosis

Histoplasma capsulatum, the organism responsible for the disease histoplasmosis, is a dimorphic fungus that exists in a mycelial form in soil and as a yeast in humans. It occurs in the temperate zone throughout the world, but is most common in the central United States. The fungus, which is found in high concentration in soil contaminated by bird or bat excreta, releases the infecting agent, an airborne spore. This spore is inhaled into the lungs where local growth of the yeast phase occurs.

Most patients infected by *H. capsulatum* remain asymptomatic and develop no significant clinical abnormalities. The sites of infection in the lung and the regional lymph nodes develop areas of caseous necrosis, which later calcify. These calcifications of histoplasmosis are similar to but more extensive than those of tuberculosis. Large calcified mediastinal lymph nodes are very characteristic of histoplasmosis. Although histoplasmosis can occur in an acute form and occurs rarely in a disseminated form, chronic pulmonary histoplasmosis is usually the form that concerns the surgeon. Goodwin and associates (17) believe that chronic histoplasmosis is an opportunistic infection always superimposed on pulmonary centrilobular or bullous emphysema. Because affected patients are usually disabled from chronic obstructive pulmonary disease, because amphotericin-B and the newer drug ketoconazole are effective treatment, and because surgical therapy is no better than amphotericin alone in reducing the number of relapses and deaths (17), the role of surgery in this disease has become that of correcting the anatomic abnormalities resulting from histoplasmosis rather than that of treating the *H. capsulatum* infection itself. The common indications for surgery are 1) the diagnosis of a solitary pulmonary nodule, 2) a secondarily infected cavity, 3) bronchial bleeding or obstruction secondary to calcified hilar lymph nodes, and 4) mediastinal granulomata and fibrosing mediastinitis.

A calcified lymph node may erode the wall of a bronchus and cause repeated hemoptysis. Such an erosion will appear by bronchoscopy to be a mucosal ulcer, occasionally with a piece of calcium protruding through it. These pieces of calcium should not be removed by bronchoscopy because sometimes the lymph node has also eroded an adjacent artery. The removal of such a lymph node during thoracotomy may also be hazardous, particularly above the left upper lobe bronchus, because it can be intimately adherent to the wall of the pulmonary artery. If a fistula from the bronchus is not encountered and if the bronchus is not stenotic, an acceptable procedure is to morselate and remove the calcified interior of the lymph node and leave the capsule undisturbed. If a fistula exists, either a lobectomy or a bronchoplasty, depending upon the location of the lesion, should be done. Occasionally these calcified nodes or portions of them will be completely extruded into the lumen of the bronchus and coughed up as a broncholith. No therapy is required for this unless hemorrhage or stenosis of a major bronchus occurs.

Enlarged lymph nodes may compress or angulate a bronchus and cause distal atelectasis. The middle lobe bronchus is particularly vulnerable to such obstruction, and isolated atelectasis of this lobe without intrinsic pathology has been termed the middle lobe syndrome. Usually patients with this condition are asymptomatic and surgery is not indicated. However, if recurrent infection develops, resection of the atelectatic lobe is indicated.

A large mediastinal granuloma may result in fibrosing mediastinitis, constrictive pericarditis, or an esophageal fistula to the mass of lymph nodes or to the trachea or bronchi. Fibrosing mediastinitis may cause obstruction of the superior vena cava or the trachea. In time, a patient can usually compensate for superior vena caval obstruction by the development of collateral venous channels, but esophageal, tracheal, or pericardial abnormalities secondary to this type of mediastinal disease will usually require surgical correction.

Blastomycosis

The disease blastomycosis is caused by the dimorphic fungus *Blastomyces dermatitidis,* which exists in nature, probably in soil, as a mycelium. The mycelial form releases spores that may become airborne and are the infective particles of *B. dermatitidis.* Within the mammalian body, it is converted to a yeast form, which is relatively easily identified in tissue sections by its characteristic single thick-necked buds. Because of the lack of a reliable skin test, the endemic area of blastomycosis has been less accurately identified than has those of the other major mycotic infections, but in North America it seems to be somewhat similar to the endemic area of histoplasmosis. It may also be found in the northern part of South America and in Africa (42).

Although the presenting symptoms may vary, the portal of entry for this organism in humans is nearly always the lung. The patient may develop an acute, self-limited penumonia or may remain asymptomatic and later note the insidious onset of chronic pulmonary blastomycosis that clinically and radiographically resembles bronchogenic carcinoma or cavitating tuberculosis. The disease may disseminate to other organs. Most common is a cutaneous form in which the patient presents with cutaneous ulcers that begin as nodules or furuncle-like lesions. These ulcers have a serpiginous border with a raised and crusted surface, but little surrounding erythema. The prognosis of this form is usually good.

The treatment of blastomycosis is primarily medical. In spite of its toxicity, the drug most commonly used at present is amphotericin-B, although ketoconazole, considerably less toxic than amphotericin, will probably become the treatment of choice in the future. On occasion, a thoracotomy must be done for diagnosis, but aside from this, no clear-cut indication for a pulmonary resection in the treatment of blastomycosis exists now. An empyema caused by *B. dermatitidis* should be treated by a decortication in addition to adequate drug therapy, since most such empyemas do not respond well to drainage alone.

Aspergillosis

Fungi of the genus *Aspergillus* are ubiquitous. They are frequent contaminants in the bacteriology laboratory and can be cultured from the sputum of patients with a wide range of pulmonary diseases who show no evidence of aspergillosis. Consequently the isolation of the fungus from the sputum is not accepted as conclusive evidence of aspergillosis. The serum precipitin test for *A. fumigatus* has been shown to be both specific and sensitive for demonstrating antibodies and will confirm the recent growth of the fungus in the body. Eastridge reported the serum precipitins to be positive in 92%–100% of patients with an aspergilloma (14). However, tissue invasion by the fungus must be demonstrated to confirm the diagnosis. Most clinical infections are caused by *A. fumigatus,* but rarely *A. flavus, A. niger,* or *A. nidulous* may also cause human infections.

Four types of aspergillosis are recognized: 1) bronchial with allergic manifestations, 2) intracavitary or saprophytic, 3) invasive or pneumonic, and 4) disseminated. The invasive and disseminated forms are usually seen only in patients who are immunosuppressed either from drug therapy or from a malignancy. A pulmonary resection is appropriate only for the intracavitary form or the pneumonic form in an immunosuppressed patient. The intracavitary form is characterized by a mycetoma or fungus ball, a tangled mass of mycelia that forms either within the lumen or is closely applied to the wall of a preexisting cavity. On a chest roentgenogram, the mycetoma appears as a uniform density partially surrounded by a crescent of air, which changes with a change in the position of the patient. The inner wall of the cavity is composed of vascular granulation tissue and fungi. Any persistent pulmonary cavity can become colonized with *Aspergillus,* but the most frequent association is with tuberculous cavities. The British Tuberculosis Association has reported that aspergillomas occur in 15% of open negative cavities greater than 2.5 cm in diameter (41).

Patients with aspergilloma are prone to develop pulmonary hemorrhage of severe degree. Eastridge and colleagues (14) reported that of 55 patients with pulmonary aspergillosis that they reviewed, 62% developed signficant hemoptysis. Of those patients with hemoptysis, 44% could not undergo surgery because of pulmonary insufficiency and 28% of them died of massive hemoptysis. Karas et al. (26) found that 64% of their 34 patients with an aspergilloma developed hemoptysis and 35% of these had massive hemoptysis. Three of their patients died of massive hemoptysis. Because systemic antifungal therapy has little effect on an aspergilloma, any patient with this disease who develops significant hemoptysis should be considered for resection of the cavity. Most patients with intracavitary aspergillosis are in an advanced stage of some chronic pulmonary disease and have a degree of pulmonary insufficiency. The resection, therefore, should be as conservative as possible. While a lobectomy will be occasionally necessary to remove the cavity, if the cavity can be completely removed by a wedge resection, there is no evidence that the result of a lobectomy would be superior. There is also no evidence that adjuvant antifungal drug therapy following a resection is necessary in nonimmunosuppressed individuals, but aspergillosis occurring in immunosuppressed patients must be treated aggressively by both early resection and drug therapy. In my experience, a cavernostomy has not been a successful temporizing measure. Bleeding from the walls of the cavity usually continues in spite of drainage and the removal of the aspergilloma.

Because of cachexia and significant pulmonary insufficiency, many of these patients will be unable to withstand any type of pulmonary resection. Eastridge (14) has reported the successful treatment of a few such patients by the instillation of sodium iodide and amphotericin-B directly into the cavity through a semipermanent Odman catheter inserted into the trachea through the cricothyroid membrane and advanced into the cavity under fluoroscopy. Others, however, have found this to be only a temporary measure; the cavity has usually become recolonized with time.

Fungal Pneumonia in Immunosuppressed Patients

The increased utilization of immunosuppressive drug regimen for the treatment of leukemia and for organ transplantation has resulted in a rising incidence of life-threatening pulmonary infections by organisms not commonly pathogenic for humans. In addition to the pneumonic form of aspergillosis previously discussed, phycomycosis, genera Mucor and Rhizopus, and the fungus *Al-*

lescheria boydii, the cause of madura foot, have both caused fatal infections. These organisms are difficult to culture so the diagnosis is often not suspected. Phycomycosis is somewhat sensitive to amphotericin B; *A. boydii,* however, is not, but may be sensitive to miconazole or ketoconazole.

Successful therapy of a necrotizing pneumonia or pulmonary abscess caused by one of these organisms in a patient with leukemia depends upon the induction of a remission. The best reported results have followed a resection of the involved lobe after the bone marrow has returned to normal, plus the administration of appropriate drug therapy.

Congenital Disorders

Pulmonary Sequestration

Pulmonary sequestration is an uncommon developmental abnormality consisting of a region of nonfunctioning lung tissue composed of multiple cysts and with an anomalous systemic arterial supply. Two forms of pulmonary sequestration have been identified: intralobar sequestration in which the abnormal tissue occurs within the substance of an otherwise normal lung lobe, and extralobar sequestration in which the abnormal tissue is separated from the rest of the lung and invested with its own pleural covering. Both forms occur four to six times more commonly on the left than on the right side. Intralobar sequestration occurs most commonly in the posterior basal region of the left lower lobe and extralobar sequestration in the posterior mediastinum near the left costophrenic sulcus.

The arterial supply to an area of sequestration arises from the descending aorta or one of its branches. Multiple arteries occur in 15%–20% of patients. In 80%–to 90% of patients, the origin of the artery is supradiaphragmatic, but in 10%–20% it arises below the diaphragm. Because these arteries are often relatively large, if one arising below the diaphragm is inadvertently cut and it retracts out of sight, the blood loss can be catastrophic. The venous drainage from extralobar sequestration is usually to a systemic vein, commonly the azygos or hemiazygos, while the venous drainage from intralobar sequestration is usually to the inferior pulmonary vein. Because of the left to left shunt involving a large artery in this latter situation, congestive heart failure can occur in the neonatal period (38).

Intralobar sequestration is four to five times more common than extralobar sequestration and is also more likely to be symptomatic. Bronchial communication, uncommon in extralobar sequestration, occurs frequently with intralobar sequestration; as a result recurrent localized pulmonary infections in the latter condition are common. Extralobar sequestration is often discovered as an incidental finding during the repair of a diaphragmatic hernia, which occurs in 30%–50% of patients with this type of sequestration.

Aortography and selective arteriography to demonstrate an anomalous systemic artery can provide a definitive diagnosis and are advocated as routine by some authors, but neither these examinations nor others, such as bronchoscopy, bronchograms, or lung scans, have decision-making potential in a patient symptomatic from the condition. In such patients, either newborn or adult, the proper treatment for intralobar sequestration is lobectomy, and for extralobar sequestration it is excision of the lesion. In the 15% of asymptomatic adults with a sequestration of the lung, the suspicion of a malignancy is usually raised. If the presence of an abnormal systemic artery to the lesion can be demonstrated, the probability of malignancy is decreased to less than the risk of a thoracotomy. Although data on the risk of symptoms developing are not available, observation of such patients may well be justified. If such a lesion is encountered during a thoracotomy performed for another reason, however, it should be excised.

Cystic Adenomatoid Malformation

Cystic adenomatoid malformation of the lung is a congenital cystic disease that commonly affects only one lobe. It usually consists of an enlarged, nonfunctioning lobe filled with smooth-walled cysts of varying sizes that contain air or a mucoid fluid and with solid areas composed of gland-like spaces lined by cuboidal or columnar epithelium. The diseased area may communicate with the tracheobronchial tree through malformed air passages lacking cartilage. The relationship of this condition to pulmonary sequestration and other lung bud anomalies has been discussed by Haller et al. (20).

If this condition is symptomatic in infancy, respiratory distress is usually secondary to compression of normal lung tissue by the overexpanded diseased lobe. In older children or adults, the disease usually presents as a chronic pulmonary infection or is discovered on a routine chest radiogram or during a thoracotomy performed for some other condition. In infants this condition may necessitate an emergency operation to relieve the respiratory distress. No matter what the manner of presentation, the diseased tissue should be removed by a lobectomy. Procedures of lesser magnitude have not been successful.

Lung Cysts

Congenital pulmonary cysts may be single or multiple, but because multiple cysts are commonly due to mucoviscidosis (cystic fibrosis) or to the remnants of a staphylococcal pneumonia and do not require surgical therapy, this discussion is confined to solitary cysts. Cysts differ from bulla in that the former have an epithelial lining and the latter do not.

In infants, the usual symptom of this condition is respiratory distress caused from compression of the normal lung by a rapidly expanding cyst. These tension cysts may also enlarge slowly and may not cause symptoms until later in childhood. Some cysts do not enlarge significantly and present in later years as an abscess, a hematoma, an air-containing structure that may be misdiagnosed as a bulla, or if fluid filled, as a mass of unknown etiology. If the cyst is infected, chronicity may be the only feature distinguishing the cyst from an aspiration lung abscess.

The treatment of these cysts requires total excision. An attempt to treat one by unroofing it will lead to a recurrence as soon as the cyst walls become sealed against the parietal pleura. It is thus important that cysts be distinguished from bullae. The excision will usually require a lobectomy either because the cyst is large, the surrounding inflammation is extensive, or because the cyst is not truly solitary, but is associated with adjacent cysts of smaller size.

Lobar Emphysema

Congenital lobar emphysema is an abnormality of unknown etiology characterized by a massive overdistension of one lobe. Rarely, more than one lobe may be involved. The infant is usually normal at birth, but over the ensuing four to five days, the lobe becomes hyperinflated and a mediastinal shift to the contralateral side occurs along with compression of the normal lung; the child develops increasing symptoms of respiratory distress.

The most frequent site for lobar emphysema is the left upper lobe, with the right middle lobe next in frequency. The diagnosis is usually made from the symptoms and the chest radiogram, which shows a marked radiolucency of the involved area with a shift of the mediastinum toward the opposite side. Care must be taken not to mistake the compressed normal lung for primary atelectasis and the radiolucent area for compensatory overexpansion. Because congenital heart lesions occur frequently in these patients, a careful cardiovascular evaluation should be done prior to surgery if possible.

The treatment of choice for this condition is a lobectomy, performed as soon as possible after the diagnosis has been made. Because the lobe is grossly normal, except for distension, the dissection is not complicated. A thoracotomy is often life saving. As soon as the thorax is opened and the chest decompressed, the patient's ventilation will improve. After the lobe has been removed, most children will have no further respiratory symptoms.

Arteriovenous Malformation

Pulmonary arteriovenous malformations are rare congenital lesions composed of abnormal vascular channels with arteriovenous communications causing right to left shunts. They may be associated with the Rendu–Osler–Weber syndrome or may occur as isolated events in the lung. They are multiple in one-third of patients and single in two-thirds.

Most patients with pulmonary arteriovenous malformations are asymptomatic and the lesion is found incidentally on a chest radiogram taken for some other reason. Patients with the Rendu–Osler–Weber syndrome may have symptoms related to that condition, but the most common symptom of a pulmonary arteriovenous malformation itself is dyspnea.

The chest radiogram is the most important diagnostic aid. The lesion will appear as an isolated coin lesion if single, and as several rounded lesions, usually in the lower lobe, if multiple. Often an enlarged afferent vessel connecting the lesion with the hilus can be seen. A pulmonary angiogram is of great value in confirming the diagnosis if the lesion is suspected of being a carcinoma.

The most common operation for this malformation has been a wedge resection or a lobectomy. Dines et al. (12) have given the following indications for pulmonary resection in this condition: 1) patients with symptoms and large shunts, 2) patients with enlarging lesions, 3) patients with multiple lesions if the lesions are sufficiently localized that the volume of the shunt can be reduced by a conservative resection, and 4) patients who have a fistula with a systemic blood supply.

References

1. Allen AR, Harmon RWJ, Klacson LJ, Stewart KM Jr: Accuracy of the confirmatory diagnosis of tuberculosis. Am J Med 22:904–914, 1957.
2. American Joint Committee for Cancer Staging and End-Results Reporting: System for Staging of Lung Cancer, 1979.
3. Arrigoni MG, Woolner LB, Bernatz PE: Atypical carcinoid tumors of the lung. J Thorac Cardiovasc Surg 64:413–421, 1972.
4. Bloedorn FG, Cowley RA: Irradiation and surgery in treatment of bronchogenic carcinoma. Surg Gynecol Obstet 111:141–146, 1960.
5. Brinkman GL: The significance of pleural effusion complicating otherwise operable bronchogenic carcinoma. Dis Chest 36:152–154, 1959.
6. Brock R, Whytehead LL: Radical pneumonectomy for bronchial carcinoma. Br J Surg 43:8, 1955.
7. Bromley LL, Szur L: Combined radiotherapy and resection for carcinoma of the bronchus: experiences with 66 patients. Lancet 2:937–941, 1955.
8. Cahan WG: Multiple primary cancers, one of which is lung. Surg Clin North Am 49:323–335, 1965.

9. Cahan WG, Castro EB: Significance of a solitary lung shadow in patients with breast cancer. Ann Surg 181:137–143, 1975.
10. Connors JP, Roper CL, Ferguson TB: Transbronchial catheterization of pulmonary abscess. Ann Thorac Surg 19:254–260, 1975.
11. Cox JD, Yesner RA: Adenocarcinoma of the lung: recent results from the Veterans Administration lung group. Am Rev Respir Dis 120:1025–1029, 1979.
12. Dines DE, Arms RA, Bernatz PE, Gomes MR: Pulmonary arteriovenous fistulas. Mayo Clin Proc 49:460–465, 1974.
13. Drutz DJ, Catanzaro A: Coccidioidomycosis. Am Rev Respir Dis 117:559–585, 727–771, 1978.
14. Eastridge CE, Young JM, Cole F, Gourley R, Pate JW: Pulmonary aspergillosis. Ann Thorac Surg 13:397–403, 1972.
15. Estera AS, Platt MR, Mills LI, Shaw RS: Primary lung abscess. J Thorac Cardiovasc Surg 79:275–282, 1980.
16. Findlay FM, Melick DW: Treatment of cavitary coccidioidomycosis. *In* Ajello L (ed): Coccidioidomycosis, University of Arizona Press.
17. Goodwin RA Jr, Des Prez RM: Histoplasmosis. Am Rev Respir Dis 117:929–956, 1978.
18. Green N, Kurohara SS, George FW, Crews QE Jr: Postresection irradiation for primary lung cancer. Radiology 116:405–407, 1975.
19. Hadlock FP, Park SK, Awe RJ, Rivera M: Unusual radiographic findings in adult pulmonary tuberculosis. AJR 134:1015–1018, 1980.
20. Haller JA, Golladay ES, Pickard LR, Tepas JJ, Shorter NA, Shermeta DW: Surgical management of lung bud anomalies. Lobar emphysema, bronchogenic cyst, cystic adenomatoid malformation and intralobar pulmonary sequestration. Ann Thorac Surg 28:33–43, 1978.
21. Humphrey EW, Keehn RJ, Higgins GA Jr, Shields TW: The long term survival of patients with visceral carcinoma. Surg Gynecol Obstet 149:385–394, 1979.
22. Humphrey EW, Rao K, VanNostrand D: Current therapy of carcinoma of the lung. *In* Ariel JM (ed): Progress in Clinical Cancer. New York, Grune and Stratton, 1966.
23. Hyde L: Clinical significance of the tuberculin test. Am Rev Respir Dis 105:453–454, 1972.
24. Jensik RJ, Faber LP, Kittle CF: Segmental resection for bronchogenic carcinoma. Ann Thorac Surg 28:475–483, 1979.
25. Joseph WL, Morton DL, Adkins PC: Prognostic significance of tumor doubling time in evaluating operability in pulmonary metastatic disease. J Thorac Cardiovasc Surg 61:23, 1971.
26. Karas A, Hankins JR, Attar S, Miller JE, McLaughin JE: Pulmonary aspergillosis: an analysis of forty-one cases. Ann Thorac Surg 22:1–7, 1976.
27. Khan MA, Kovnat DM, Bachus B, Whitcomb ME, Brody JS, Snider GL: Clinical and roentgenographic spectrum of pulmonary tuberculosis in the adult. Am J Med 62:31–38, 1977.
28. Kirsh MM, Rotman H, Argenta L, Bove E, Cimmino V, Toshian J, Ferguson P, Sloan H: Carcinoma of the lung: results of treatment over ten years. Ann Thorac Surg 21:371–377, 1976.
29. Li W, Hammer SP, Jolly PC, Hill LD, Anderson RP: Unpredictable course of small cell undifferentiated lung carcinoma. J Thorac Cardiovasc Surg 81:34–43, 1981.
30. Lowe J, Shore DF, Iles PB, Langman MJS, Baldwin RW: Intrapleural BCG in operable lung cancer. Lancet 1:11–14, 1980.
31. MacGregor RR: A year's experience with tuberculosis in a private urban teaching hospital in the postsanatorium era. Am J Med 58:221, 1975.
32. McKneally MF, Mauer C, Lininger L, Kausel HW, McIlduff JB, Older TM, Foster ED, Alley RD: Four year follow-up on the Albany experience with intrapleural BCG in lung cancer. J Thorac Cardiovasc Surg 81:485–492, 1981.
33. McQuarrie DG, Nicoloff DM, Van Nostrand D, Rao K, Humphrey EW: Tuberculosis and carcinoma of the lung. Dis Chest 54:29–34, 1968.

34. Morton DL, Joseph WL, Ketcham AS, Geelhoed GW, Adkins PC: Surgical resection and adjunctive immunotherapy for selected patients with multiple pulmonary metastasis. *In:* Najarian JS, Delaney JP (eds): Advances In Cancer Surgery. New York, Stratton Intercontinental Medical Book Corp., 1976.
35. Mountain CF, Khalil KG, Hermes KE, Frazier OH: The contribution of surgery to the management of carcinomatous pulmonary metastasis. Cancer 41:833–840, 1978.
36. Muzzall HA, Humphrey EW: Pulmonary resection for metastatic cancer. Minn Med 47:1234–1237, 1964.
37. Nelson AR: The surgical treatment of pulmonary coccidioidomycosis. Curr Prob Surg, October 1974.
38. O'Mara CS, Baker RR, Jeyasingham K: Pulmonary sequestration. Surg Gynecol Obstet 147:609–616, 1978.
39. Paterson R, Russell MH: Clinical trials in malignant disease. Part IV—lung cancer. Value of postoperative radiotherapy. Clin Radiol 13:141–144, 1962.
40. Paulson DL: Carcinomas in the superior pulmonary sulcus. J Thorac Cardiovasc Surg 70:1095–1104, 1975.
41. The Research Committee of the British Tuberculosis Association. Aspergillus in persistent lung cavities after tuberculosis. Tubercle 49:1, 1968.
42. Sarosi GA, Davies SF: Blastomycosis. Am Rev Respir Dis 120:911–938, 1979.
43. Shields TW, Higgins GA, Lawton R, Heilbrunn A, Keehn RJ: Preoperative x-ray therapy as an adjuvant in the treatment of bronchogenic carcinoma. J Thorac Cardiovasc Surg 59:49–61, 1970.
44. Shields TW, Humphrey EW, Matthews M, Eastridge CE, Keehn RJ: Pathological stage grouping of patients with resected carcinoma of the lung. J Thorac Cardiovasc Surg 80:400–405, 1980.
45. Siegelman SS, Zerhouni EA, Leo FP, Khouri NF, Stitik FP: CT of the solitary pulmonary nodule. AJR 135:1–13, 1980.
46. Stead WW, Dutt AK: What's new in tuberculosis? Am J Med 71:1–4, 1981.
47. Steele JD: The solitary pulmonary nodule. Springfield, Charles C Thomas, 1964.
48. Wells RF, Stead WW, Tsai SH: Determining the activity of pulmonary tuberculosis. Minn Med 40:538–541, 1957.
49. Wilkins EW, Head JM, Burke JF: Pulmonary resection for metastatic neoplasms in the lung. Am J Surg 135:480–483, 1978.
50. Wolinsky E: Nontuberculous mycobacteria and associated diseases. Am Rev Respir Dis 119:107–159, 1979.
51. Vincent RG, Pickren JW, Lane WW: The changing histopathology of lung cancer. A review of 1682 cases. Cancer 39:1647–1655, 1977.
52. Yesner R (Chairman), Sobin L et al: Histological typing of lung tumors, revised. Geneva, World Health Organization, 1977.

Resectional Procedures

4

Thoracic Incisions

The rigidity of the thoracic wall and the relatively fixed position of the thoracic viscera make the patient's position on the operating table and the location and type of incision more critical for operative procedures in the chest than for those in the abdomen. The thoracic incision should be chosen to give the best exposure of that region in which the greatest technical difficulty is expected, in spite of the location of the disease. For operations on the lung this will usually be the hilus. The anterior portion of a lateral thoracic skin incision should be placed below the breast in women to avoid disfigurement, even when one of the higher ribs or interspaces is to be used for entry into the chest.

This section describes the major general-purpose thoracic incisions. Those incisions used only for specific procedures, such as drainage of the pleural cavity or thoracoplasty, will be found in the sections describing those procedures.

Posterior Lateral Thoracotomy

A posterior lateral thoracotomy is the most commonly used incision for operations on the lung, the esophagus, and the posterior mediastinum. Although it is not the incision of choice for operations on the anterior mediastinum, if the exact location of an anterior lesion near the center of the thorax is unknown, this incision is also a good choice. It is easier to perform most operations on the anterior mediastinum, including a thymectomy, through this approach than it is to perform a lobectomy or pneumonectomy through a median sternotomy.

Operations on the lung are usually done through the bed of the fifth rib or through the fifth interspace; however, if a prior three-rib thoracoplasty has been performed to reduce the residual pleural space, lung operations can be done through the bed of the fourth rib. Surgery on the diaphragm or on the esophageal hiatus is usually done through a seventh rib or seventh inter-

Portions of this chapter have been modified from Edward W. Humphrey, Right upper lobectomy, *Surgical Techniques Illustrated* Vol. 3 No. 2, 1978, pp. 61–70, and Edward W. Humphrey, Left lower lobectomy, *Surgical Techniques Illustrated* Vol. 4 No. 2, 1980.

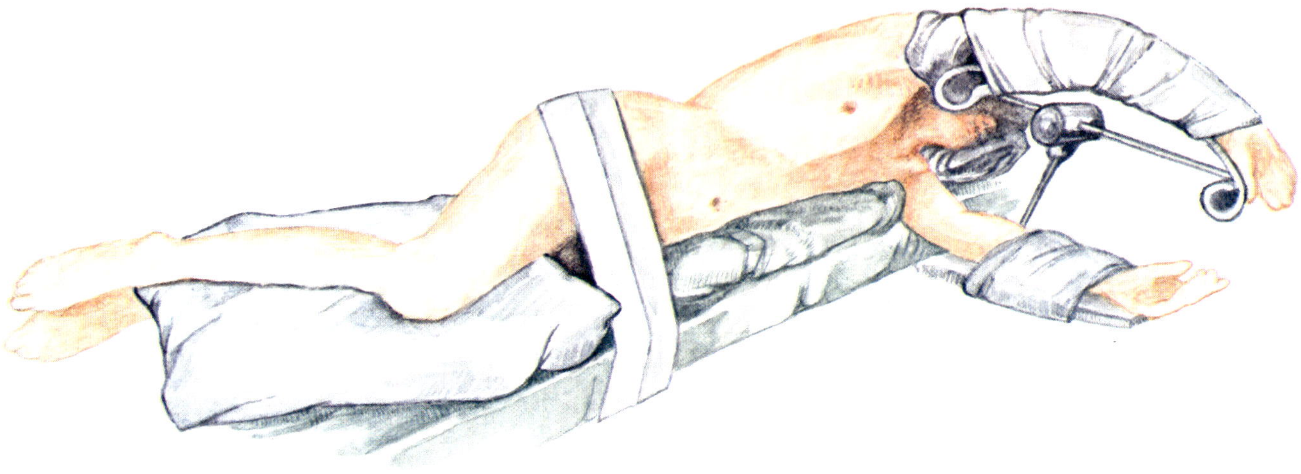

FIG. 4-1.

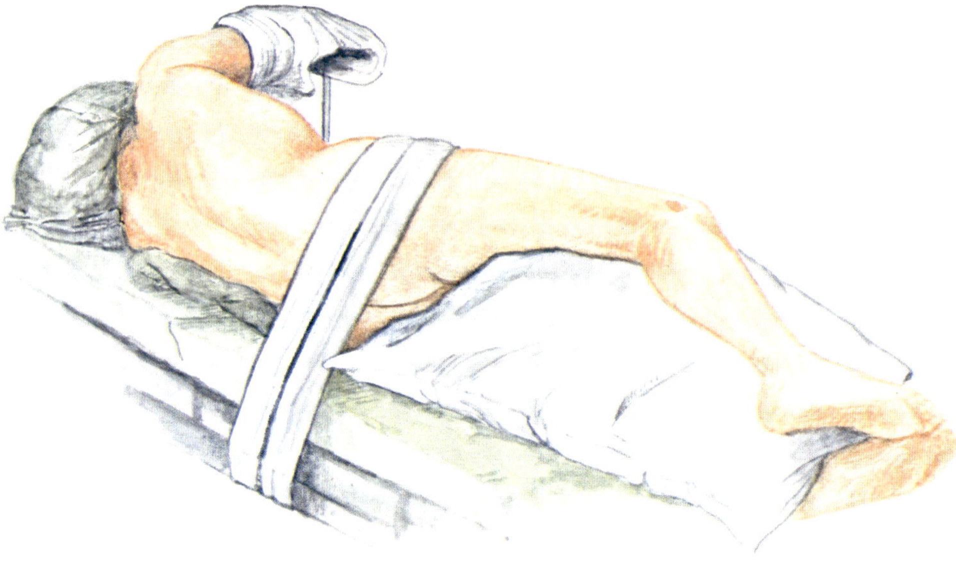

FIG. 4-2.

space incision, while operations on the thoracic esophagus are most easily done through the sixth rib or sixth interspace. The chosen rib is identified either by counting anteriorly at the sternal end of the ribs, beginning with the second, which normally articulates with the sternal angle, or after the shoulder girdle muscles have been divided, by counting down from the first rib, which can be palpated by inserting a hand under the scapula.

The patient is positioned in the straight lateral decubitus (Fig. 4-1), and small sand bags are placed against the front and back of the chest. The lower leg is slightly flexed at the hip and the knee, and a pillow is put between the legs to avoid development of pressure necrosis. Figure 4-2 is a posterior view of the patient fixed in position by a wide strap of adhesive tape passed over the hips and fastened to each side of the operating table. The arms are usually placed on supports perpendicular to the table and level with each shoulder, but in operations that involve exposure of the first three ribs, it is often helpful to internally rotate the upper arm and with the elbow bent, secure the hand and forearm either at the patient's hip or near the head. This makes retraction of the scapula relatively easy because the weight of the arm will pull the scapula forward. Such a position is illustrated in Figure 6-6. If a support for the upper arm is used, the arm and shoulder are fixed to the support with a wide strip of adhesive tape or an elastic bandage. This

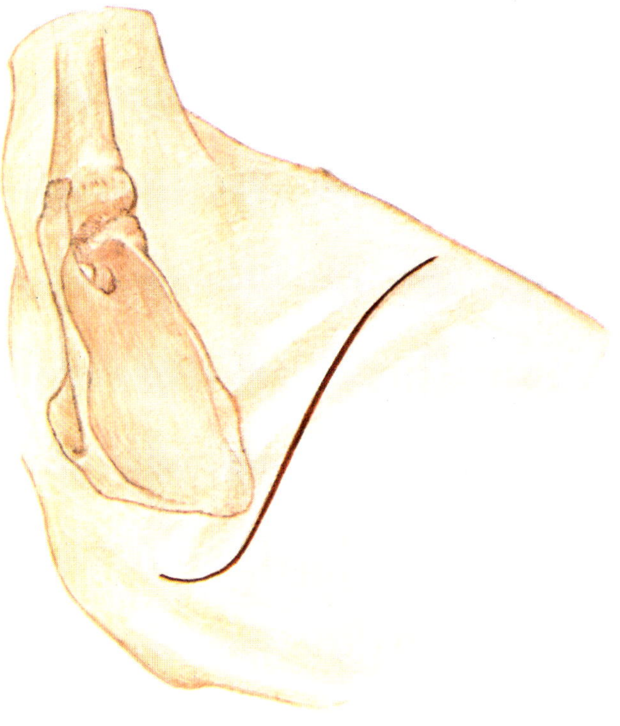

FIG. 4-3.

fixation of both pelvis and arms permits the table to be tilted in either direction without the patient's rolling off.

Prior to incising the skin, it is helpful to make on the skin several scratches across the course of the proposed incision to aid in the accurate reapproximation of the skin during closure. The skin incision begins just lateral to the nipple line immediately over the rib or interspace through which the chest will be entered. Figure 4-3 illustrates the incision used to enter the chest through the fifth rib. It extends posteriorly two or three finger breaths below the inferior angle of the scapula, then superiorly for 5–10 cm midway between the spinous processes of the vertebra and the vertebral border of the scapula.

Figure 4-4 shows the musculature of the lateral chest. The three muscles that must be divided if the chest is entered through any interspace or rib above the seventh are the latissimus dorsi, a portion of the serratus anterior, and a portion of the trapezius. The latissimus dorsi is the most superficial muscle underlying the central portion of this incision. It inserts along the bicipital grove of the humerus and is inervated by the thoracodorsal nerve, which enters the muscle over the inferior part of the axilla (see Fig. 6-28). After the fascia anterior and posterior to this muscle has been incised and the plane of cleavage between the muscle and the chest wall developed, two fingers of one hand are passed beneath the muscle and outward pressure is exerted to arrest any bleeding that may occur as the muscle is divided. It may be cut with either a knife or the cutting cautery, but the larger vessels should be ligated or coagulated individually as they are encountered. The third or inferior division of the serratus anterior muscle, which originates from ribs four to nine and inserts on the inferior angle of the scapula, must be partially divided. This is best accomplished by splitting the muscle fibers anteriorly over the rib or interspace through which the chest will be entered, then cutting the fibers arising from lower ribs at a point near the scapula to prevent injury to the long thoracic nerve. Finally, the fibers of the trapezius that underlie the incision and insert on the medial end of the spine of the scapula are divided. If the rhomboid muscles are extensively mobilized, it is usually not necessary to divide them unless the upper four ribs must be exposed.

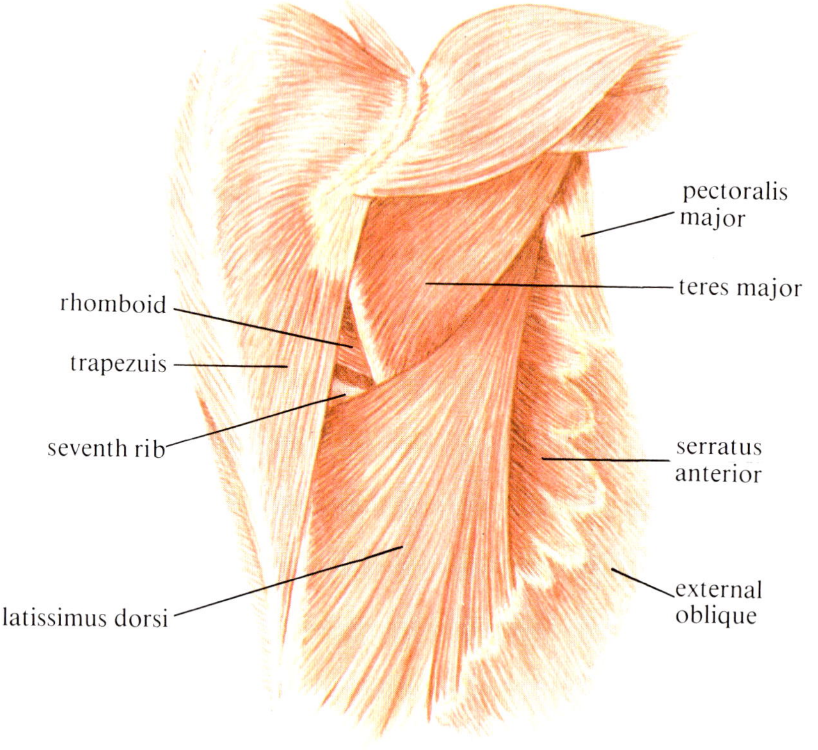

FIG. 4-4.

The chest may be entered through either the periosteal bed of a resected or an unresected rib or through an intercostal space. Although these methods differ little in the exposure obtained, it is my impression that incisions without a rib resection are more frequently complicated by fracture of the ribs adjacent to the incision. If a rib is to be resected, the periosteum is divided with cautery along the middle of the rib from one end of the incision to the other

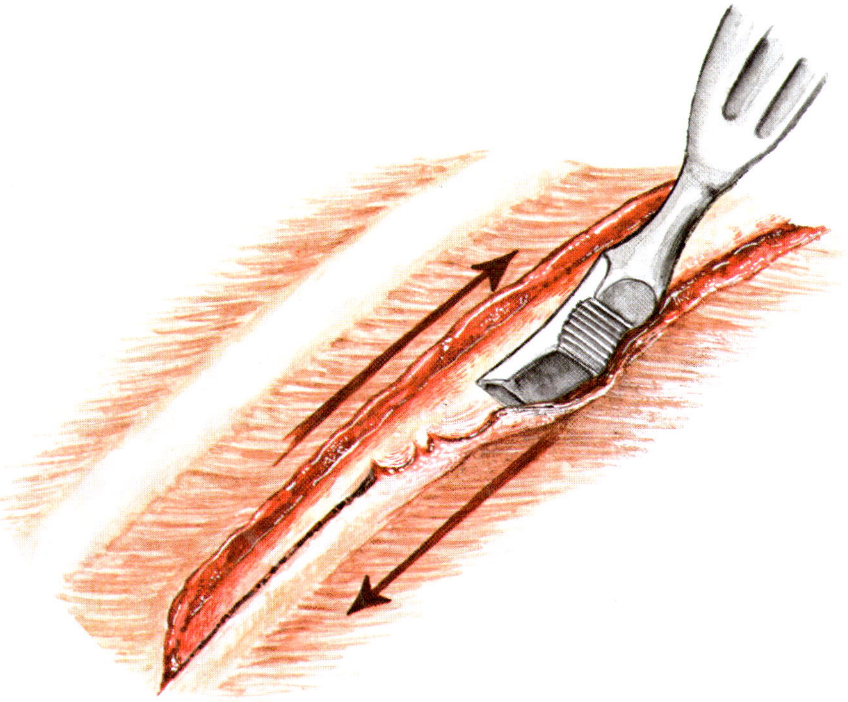

FIG. 4-5.

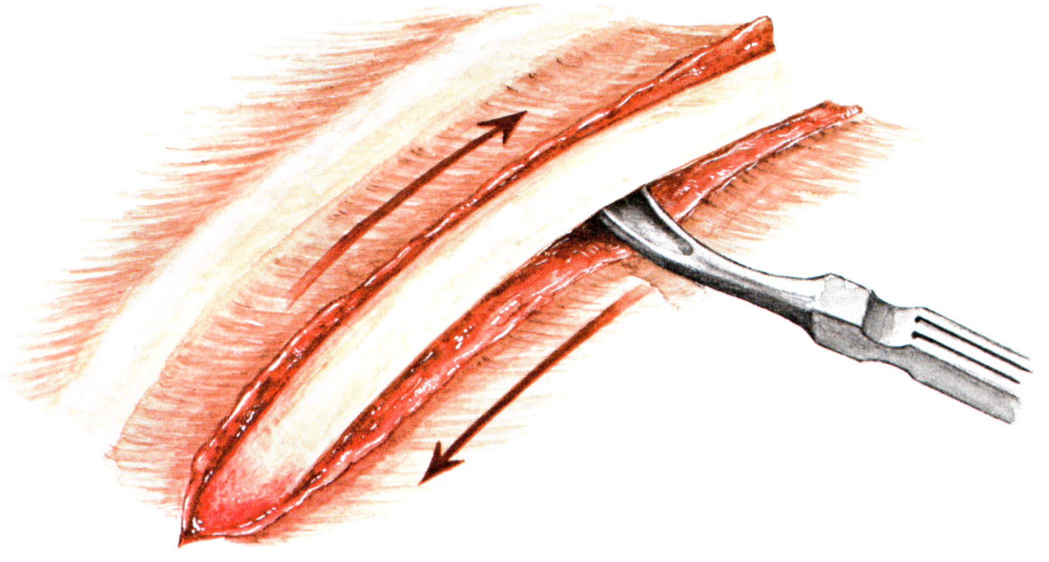

FIG. 4-6.

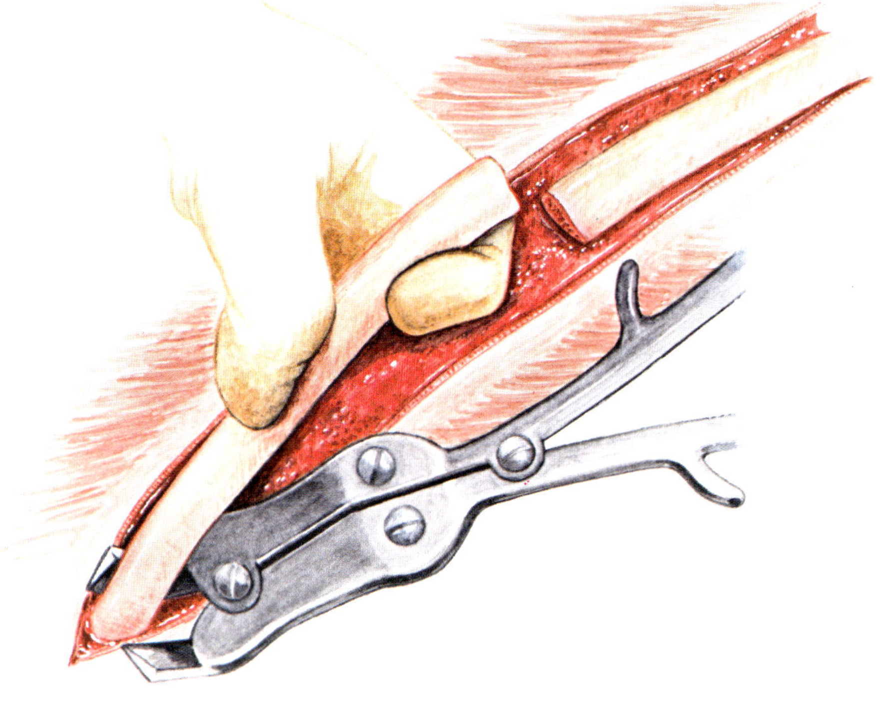

FIG. 4-7.

and separated from the outer surface of the rib with the Alexander periosteal elevator, an end-cutting instrument (Fig. 4-5). This instrument is also used to separate the periosteum and intercostal muscle fibers from both rib margins, working from posterior to anterior on the superior margin and from anterior to posterior on the inferior margin. Figure 4-6 illustrates the use of a Hedblom periosteal elevator, a side-cutting instrument, to separate the periosteum from the inner surface of the rib. Figure 4-7 shows the division of the rib with the Horsley double action rib shears. The length removed should be slightly longer than the muscle incision so that the cut ends of the rib will be covered by muscle. This both facilitates closure and prevents the surgeon's gloves from being torn by the rib ends. With the rib removed, an incision is made

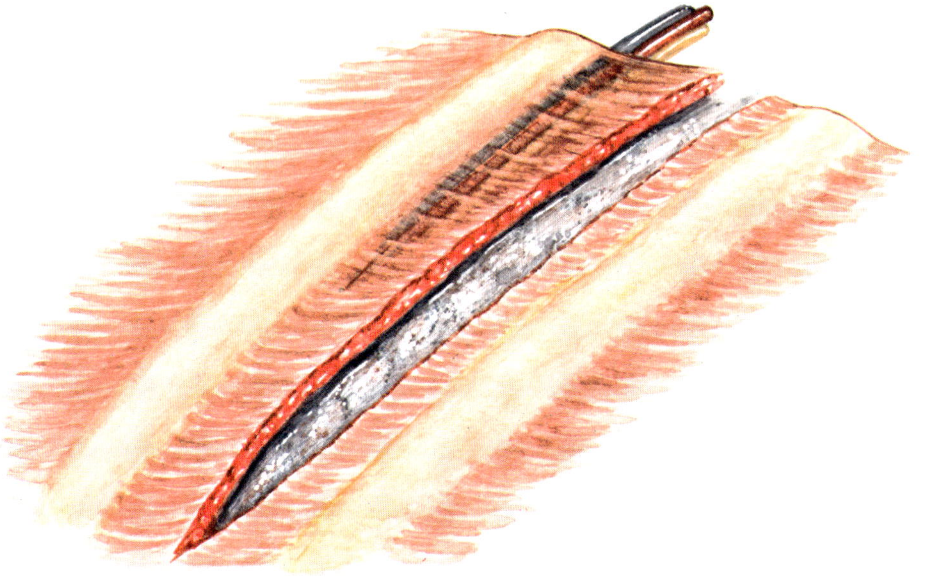

FIG. 4-8.

with a scalpel through the periosteum to expose the parietal pleura. If the chest is to be entered without resecting a rib, the intercostal muscles in the center of the interspace are incised to expose the pleura over the length of the incision (Fig. 4-8).

Provided the pleural cavity under the incision is relatively free of adhesions, the lung surface will be seen to move and the pleura can be safely incised at one point, then divided the full length of the incision with scissors or scalpel (Fig. 4-9). The risk of lacerating the lung during entry is decreased if the anesthesiologist decreases the ventilatory pressure while the pleura is being opened. If the pleural cavity under the incision is obliterated by adhesions, they must be divided as the pleural incision is extended. The syndrome

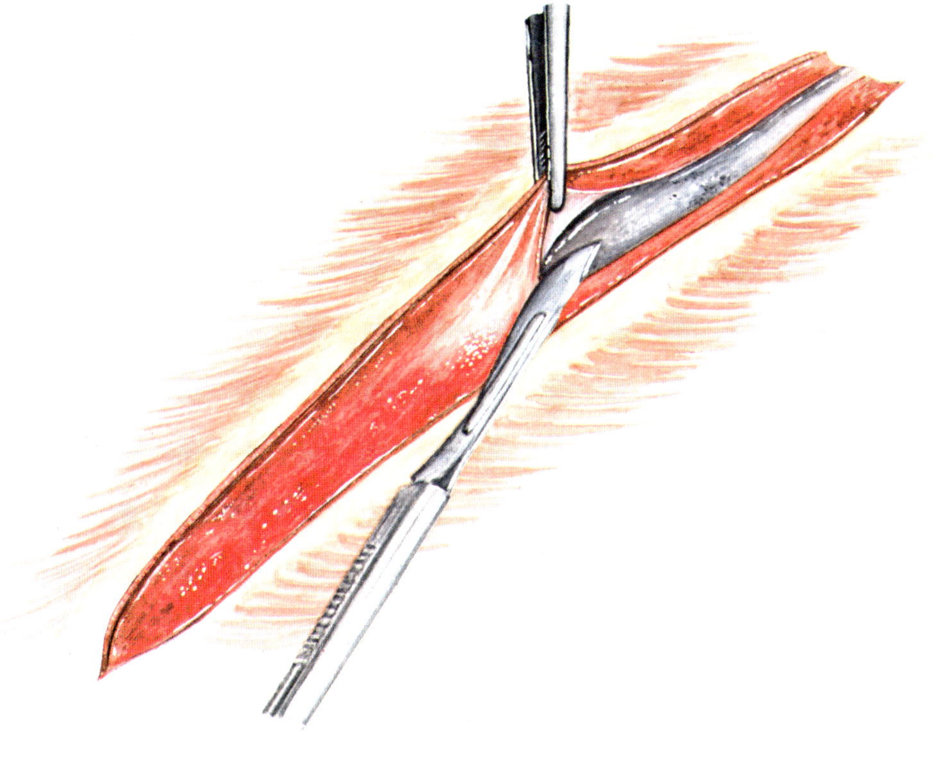

FIG. 4-9.

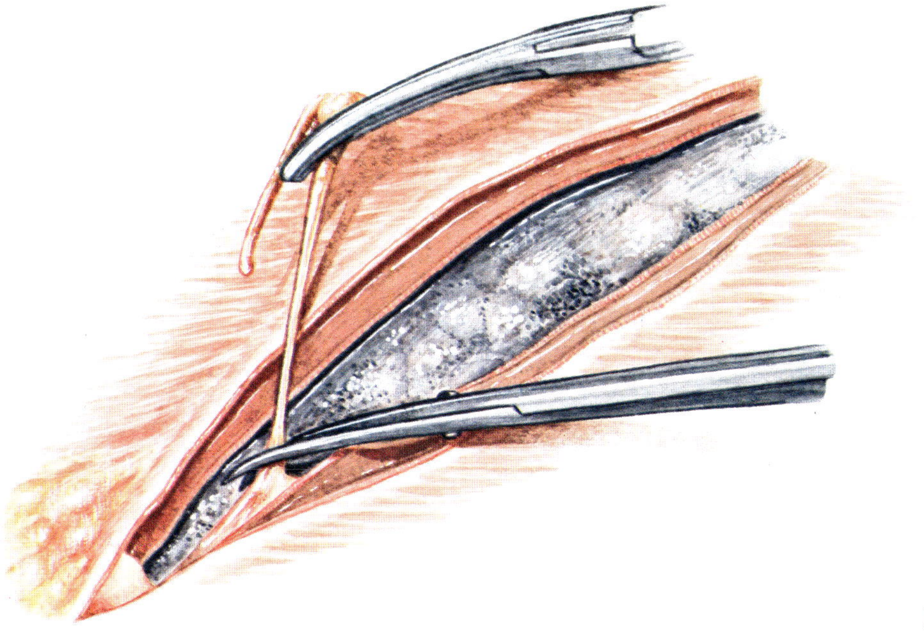

FIG. 4-10.

of chronic post-thoracotomy pain may be caused by traction on the posterior root of the spinal cord via the intercostal nerve when a rib spreader is used. Figure 4-10 illustrates a method that prevents this traction by dividing or removing the intercostal nerve, under the rib resected or the interspace entered, at the posterior limit of the incision prior to the insertion of the rib spreader. Figures 4-11, 4-12, 4-13, and 4-14 are illustrations of some of the commonly used thoracic surgical instruments that are referred to in this book. The rib spreader most commonly used during a posterior–lateral thoracotomy is the Finochietto because its superior blade is long enough also to retract the scapula; prior to its introduction, moist gauze pads should be placed over the wound edges.

Before the thoracotomy incision is closed, the intercostal nerve above and below the nerve that was divided should be blocked with a local anesthetic,

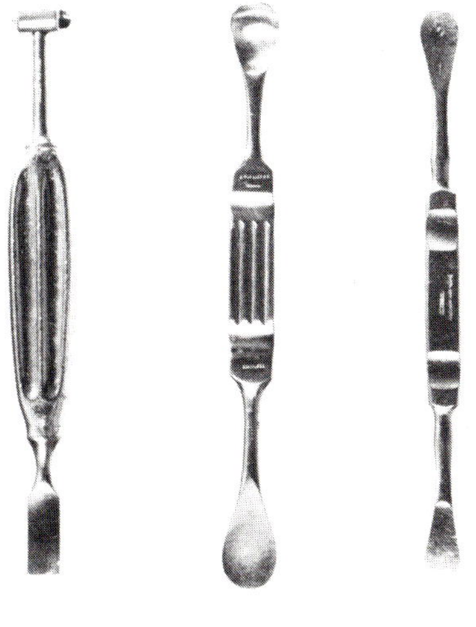

FIG. 4-11. Periosteal elevators. *Left to right:* Alexander, large Hedblom, and small Hedblom.

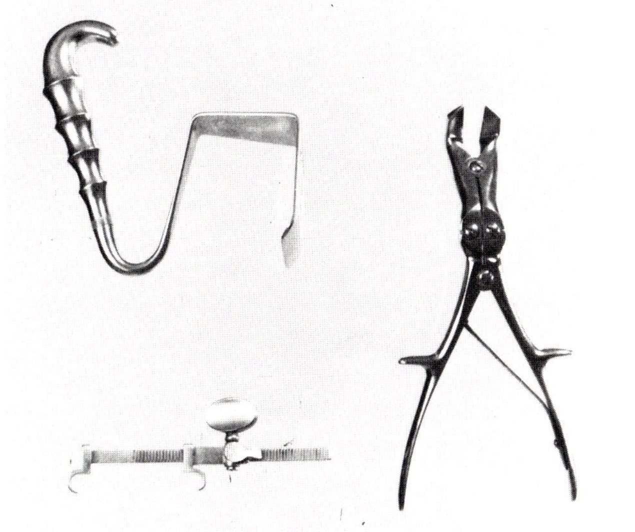

FIG. 4-12. *Upper left,* Davidson scapula retractor. *Lower left,* Bailey rib contractor. *Right,* Horsley rib shears.

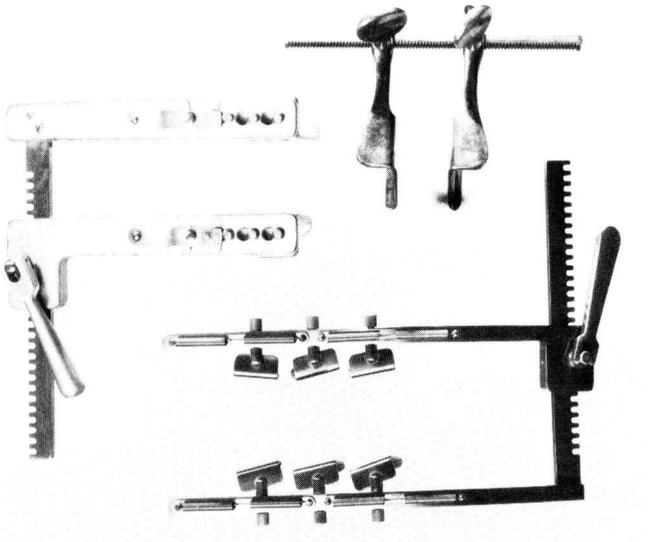

FIG. 4-13. *Left,* Burford–Finochietto rib spreader. *Upper right,* Tuffier rib spreader. *Lower right,* Favaloro–Morse sternal retractor.

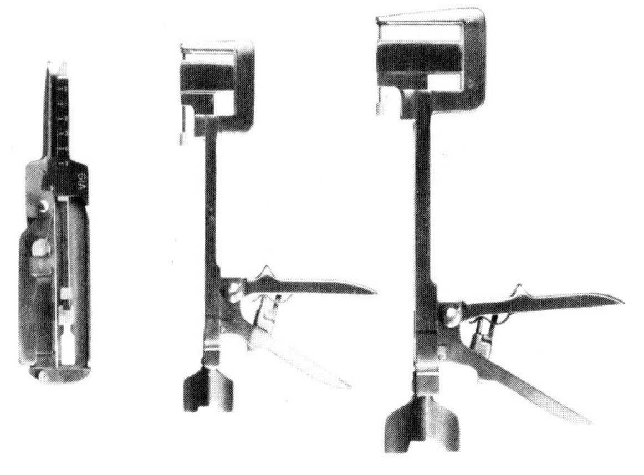

FIG. 4-14. Staplers. *Left to right:* GIA, TA-30, and TA-55.

and intercostal suction catheters should be placed. If these catheters are located too close to the diaphragm, there is a risk of forming adhesions that could limit diaphragmatic excursion, while if they are placed too close to the incision, there is a risk of a wound infection developing from the tube track. The best procedure is that illustrated in Figure 4-15. The cut edge of the latissimus dorsi below the incision should be grasped with two Allis tissue forceps by the assistant and stretched into its usual position so the catheters will not deform the muscle or the skin. Then make a skin opening over the fourth interspace below the incision, and tunnel the tubes over the adjacent rib to enter the pleural cavity through the third interspace below the incision. These catheters should be fixed in position by 2–0 nonabsorbable cutaneous sutures.

To close either an interspace incision or one through the bed of a resected rib, first place four or five pericostal sutures of #1 chromic gut around the two adjacent ribs; then loosely lace together the intercostal muscles, and periosteum if a rib was resected, with a running suture of the same material. The pleura is not closed separately, but is caught in the intercostal muscle suture. Two Bailey rib approximators are used to bring together the two ribs adjacent to the incision (Fig. 4-16) so that the intercostal muscle suture can be pulled tight and the pericostal sutures tied. The muscles of the shoulder girdle are each reapproximated in two layers, the deep fascia of the muscle with interrupted 2–0 or 3–0 nonabsorbable sutures and the superficial fascia with a running 2–0 absorbable suture. Great care must be taken that this reapproximation is done in the correct anatomic position, both to assure good shoulder function and to avoid cosmetic deformity.

Anterior Thoracotomy

Anterior thoracotomy is now used principally for operations on the anterior and apical portions of the upper lobes less than a lobectomy and on the upper mediastinum for some relatively minor procedures. In the past, it was utilized for certain cardiac procedures, but these are now performed mostly through other approaches. Compared to the standard posterior lateral incision, its advantages are that the opening and closing of the incision is quicker and it does not result in as much interference with a patient's respiratory

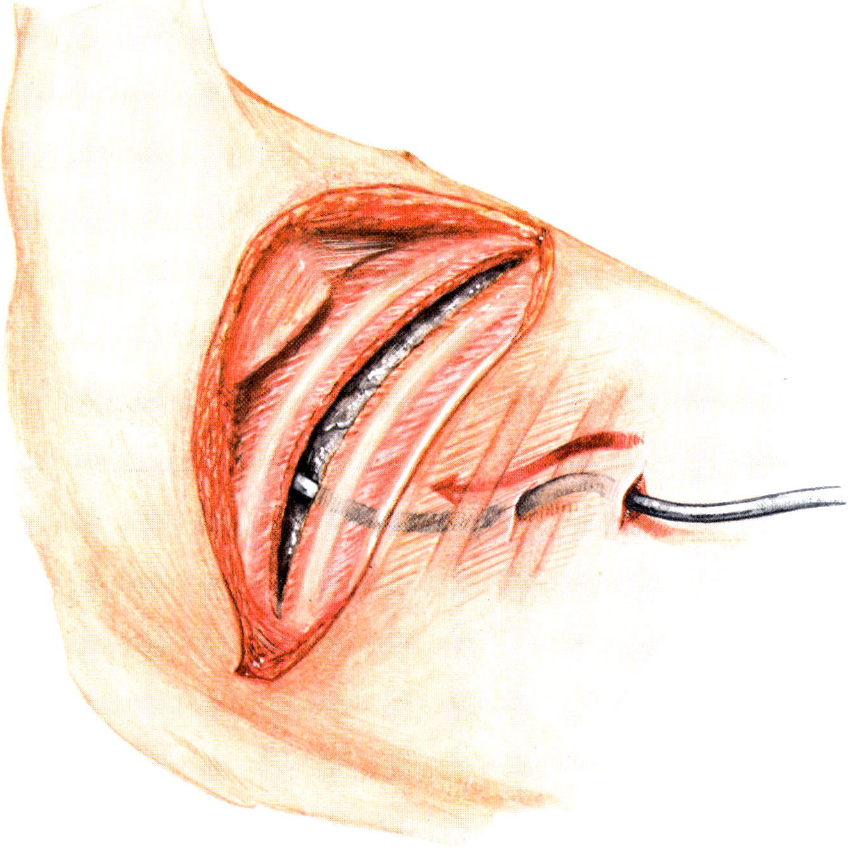

FIG. 4-15.

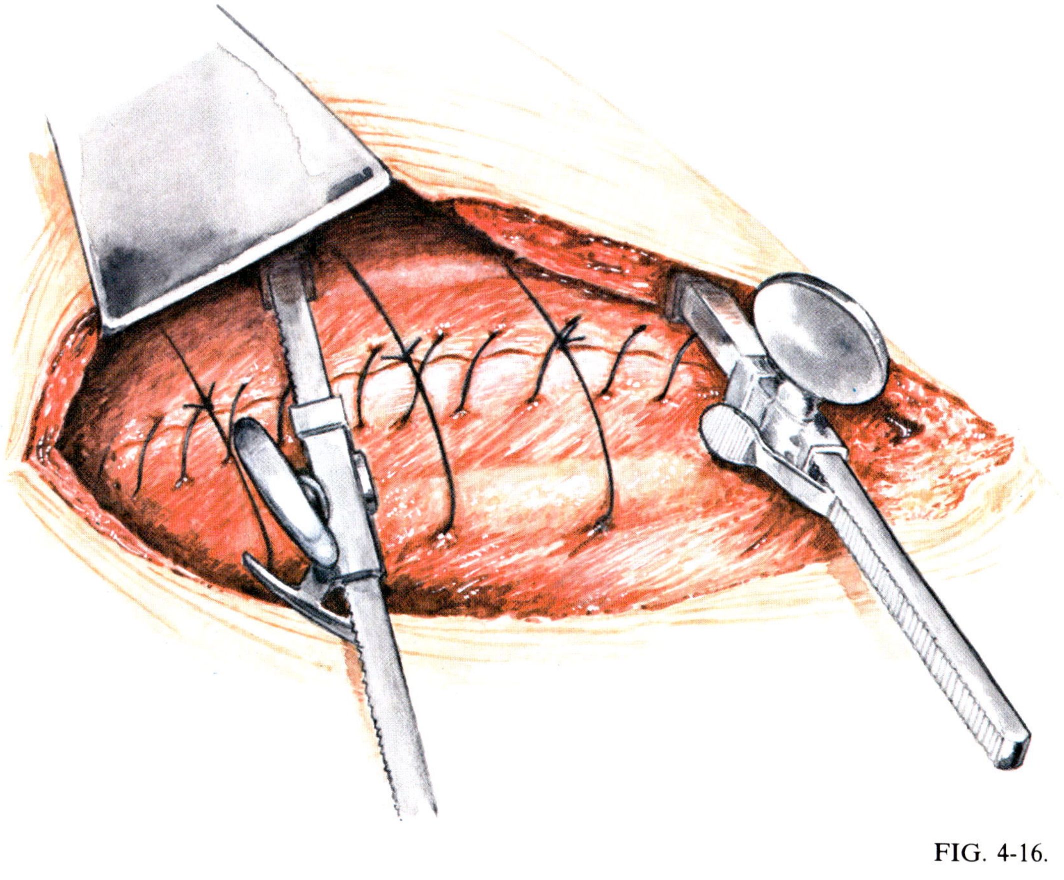

FIG. 4-16.

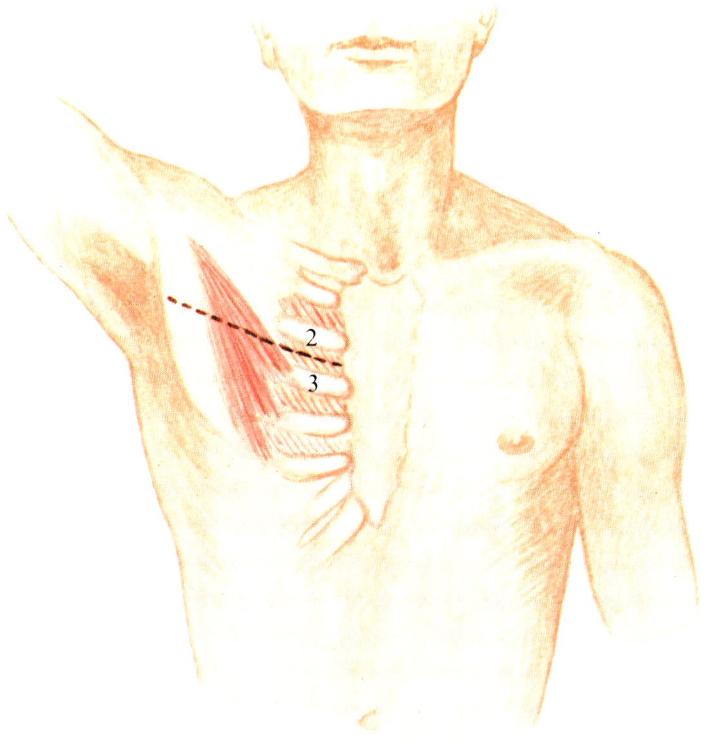

FIG. 4-17.

function. Because the patient is supine, drainage of material from the diseased lung to the dependent lung is decreased, but with double lumen endobronchial tubes, such drainage can now be prevented during a lateral decubitus position so it no longer remains a reason for using an anterior thoracotomy.

The patient's arm may be internally rotated with the elbow bent and the hand secured under the hip or it may be extended above the straight lateral position on an arm support, but without excessive stretch on the brachial plexus. The skin incision is made over the interspace selected and extended from the sternum to the anterior axillary line. Figure 4-17 depicts the usual incision for operations on the upper lobe.The pleural cavity is entered through the second or third interspace. At this level the fibers of the pectoralis major run relatively parallel to the ribs and can be separated rather than cut to expose the interspace, but usually some fibers of the pectoralis minor must be divided at the lateral end of the incision (the dotted line in Fig. 4-18).

As the intercostal muscles are being incised to expose the pleura, the internal mammary artery should not be divided inadvertently. This artery runs about 1 cm lateral to the sternum between the transversus thoracis muscles, the pleura, and the internal intercostal muscle. If divided without prior control, and if immediate entry into the pleural cavity is not possible due to adhesions between the lung and the parietal pleura under the incision, there may be considerable blood loss before the artery can be controlled.

After the pleural cavity has been entered and the lung permitted to fall away from the chest wall, the edges of the incision should be covered with moist gauze pads and a rib spreader inserted. Since the scapula does not need to be retracted and the overall depth of the incision is less, than in a posterior-lateral thoracotomy, a smaller rib spreader, such as a Tuffier, serves well. When greater exposure is required, it may be obtained by dividing the costal cartilage of an adjacent rib and the intervening soft tissue. If this

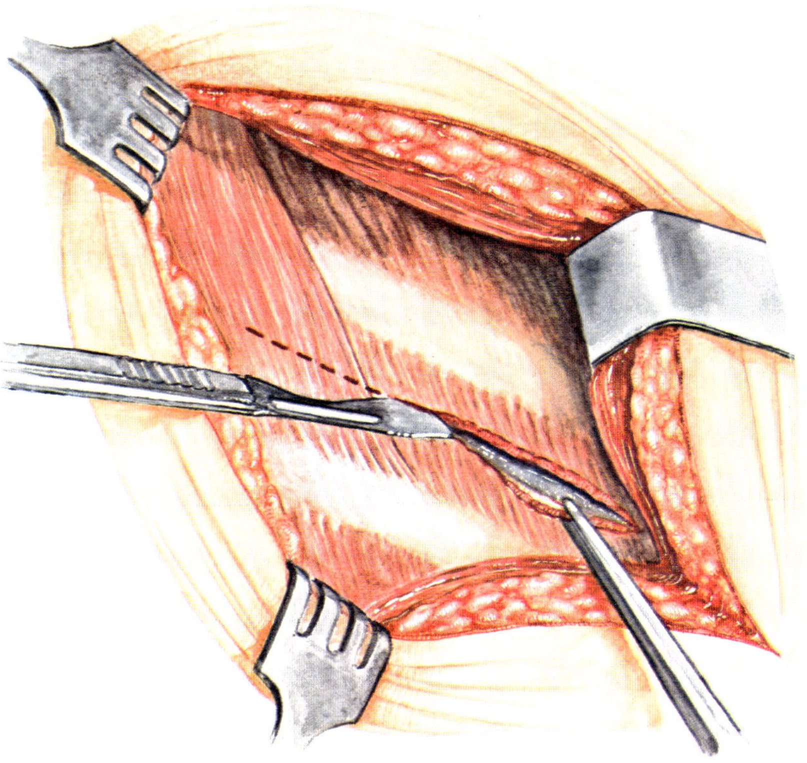

FIG. 4-18.

is done, an additional centimeter of cartilage should be resected just prior to closure, and the anterior end of the rib should be stabilized by a suture through the rib and the sternum.

The insertion of one or two intercostal suction catheters and the closure of the incision is similar to the closure of an intercostal posterior lateral incision; however, creating an air-tight seal of the anterior portion may be difficult in old or debilitated patients because of the sparsity of intercostal muscles. In such patients, after the pericostal sutures approximating the ribs have been tied, the fibers of the pectoralis major may be imbricated with the intercostal muscles to close the interspace. Generally, however, to prevent a cosmetic deformity, the approximation of each muscle should be anatomically accurate.

Thoracoabdominal Incision

A thoracoabdominal incision, if used at all, is employed by thoracic surgeons primarily for operations on the esophagus or cardioesophageal junction, but it may be used also for operative procedures on any of the upper abdominal viscera or blood vessels. A left thoracoabdominal incision gives excellent exposure of the upper abdomen, but results in relatively poor exposure of the thoracic esophagus above the level of the inferior pulmonary vein and very poor exposure medial to and above the aortic arch. It should never be employed for operations on the lung. Compared to other thoracic incisions, it is associated with a higher risk of complications. The risk of atelectasis and pneumonia is greater because coughing is more painful. Because the costal cartilages of two or more lower ribs must be divided, there is a risk of infection of the whole cartilagenous webb, and because the diaphragm must be divided, there is a risk of segmental paralysis from cutting a branch of the phrenic nerve.

For a left thoracoabdominal incision, the patient is positioned with the left side elevated about 45° by sand bags placed under the shoulders and

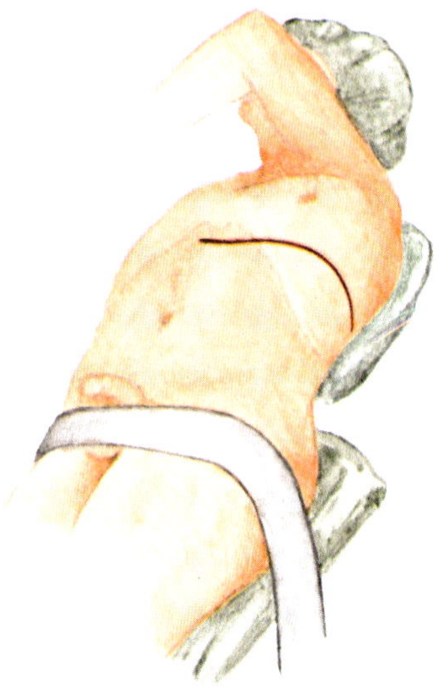

FIG. 4-19.

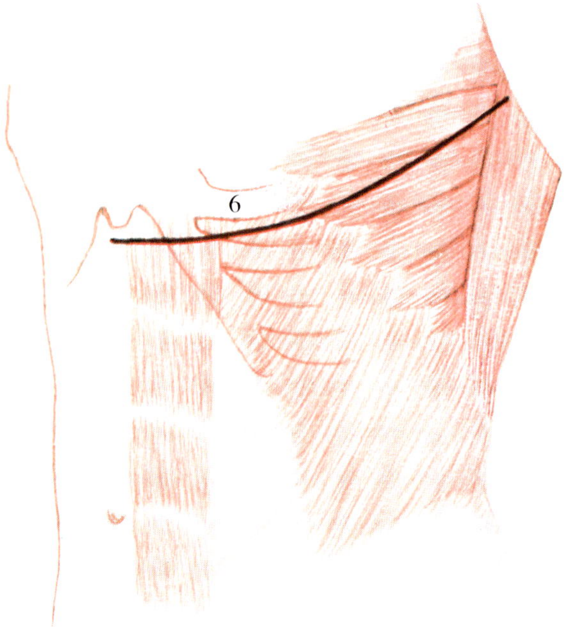

FIG. 4-20.

hips, and the left arm is secured to a support with tape (Fig. 4-19). The posterior part of the chest should be exposed to the right side of the vertebra. For most operations it is advisable to make first the abdominal portion of the incision in order to determine resectability or verify the diagnosis. The abdominal incision is usually made horizontally between the midline and the anterior end of the sixth or seventh intercostal space, although a vertical midline incision can also be extended into the chest in a similar manner by curving the upper part to the left. The anterior rectus fascia, the rectus muscle, and the posterior rectus fascia are divided, the fibers of the external oblique muscle are split, and the other layers of the abdominal wall are divided.

If the operation is to be continued after the abdominal exploration, an incision is made over the sixth interspace from the posterior axillary line to the lateral end of the abdominal incision (Fig. 4-20), taking care not to create an acute angle of skin. The fibers of the serratus anterior may be split, and if necessary, the anterior margin of the latissimus dorsi may be mobilized

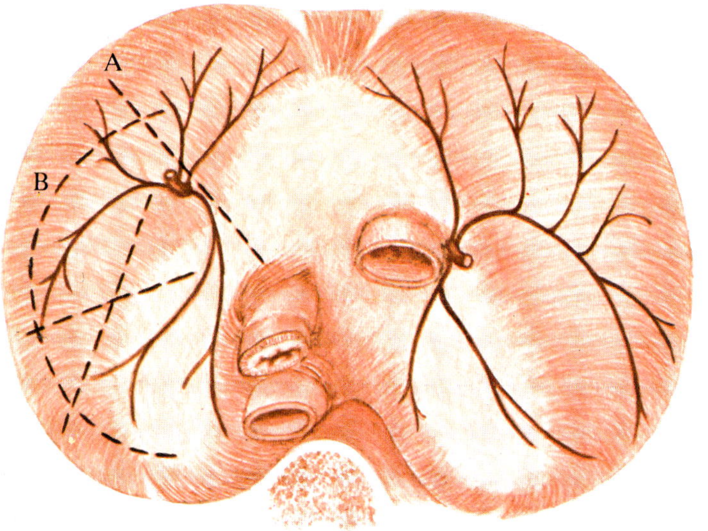

FIG. 4-21.

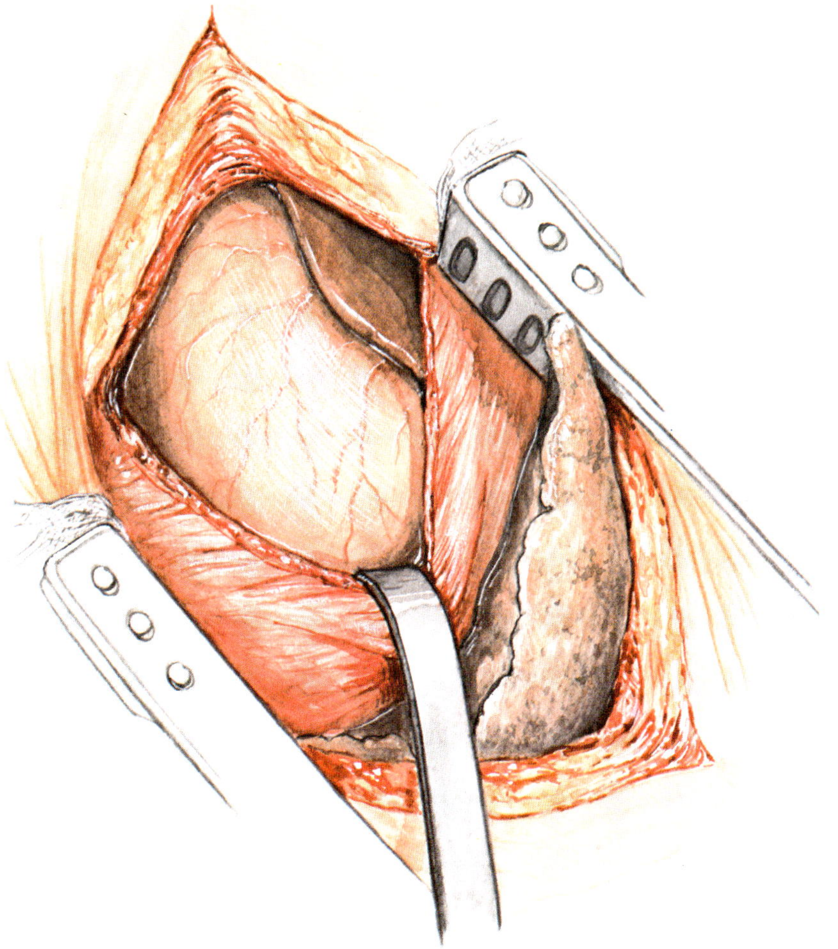

FIG. 4-22.

to expose the interspace. The intercostal muscles are divided, the pleura exposed and incised, and the cartilages between the abdominal incision and the sixth interspace are divided obliquely with a scalpel. Resecting a rib is usually unnecessary in making this incision; an interspace incision is quicker to make, the exposure is as satisfactory, and it is easier to close because the disparity between the costal margin and the chest wall, which results from a rib resection, is not created.

Incising the diaphragm is the most critical part of this incision. The usual pattern of the diaphragmatic branches of the phrenic nerve and the placement of incisions in the diaphragm that have the least effect on diaphragmatic function (5) are shown in Figure 4-21. Dashed lines A and B indicate the two most commonly employed diaphragmatic incisions. Placing the incision so as to divide the anterior–lateral or posterior–lateral branches would incur extensive segmental paralysis of the diaphragm with consequent difficulty in coughing. The edges of the wound and especially the ends of the costal cartilages should be protected from contamination by gastrointestinal contents, because an infection of the cartilaginous web is extremely difficult to control. Notice in Figure 4-22 the excellent exposure of the stomach that can be obtained with this incision after the diaphragm is opened, but also notice the difficulty that might be expected in exposing the middle or upper third of the esophagus.

Prior to closure, an intercostal suction catheter should be inserted, as previously described (Posterior Lateral Thoracotomy). The diaphragm is

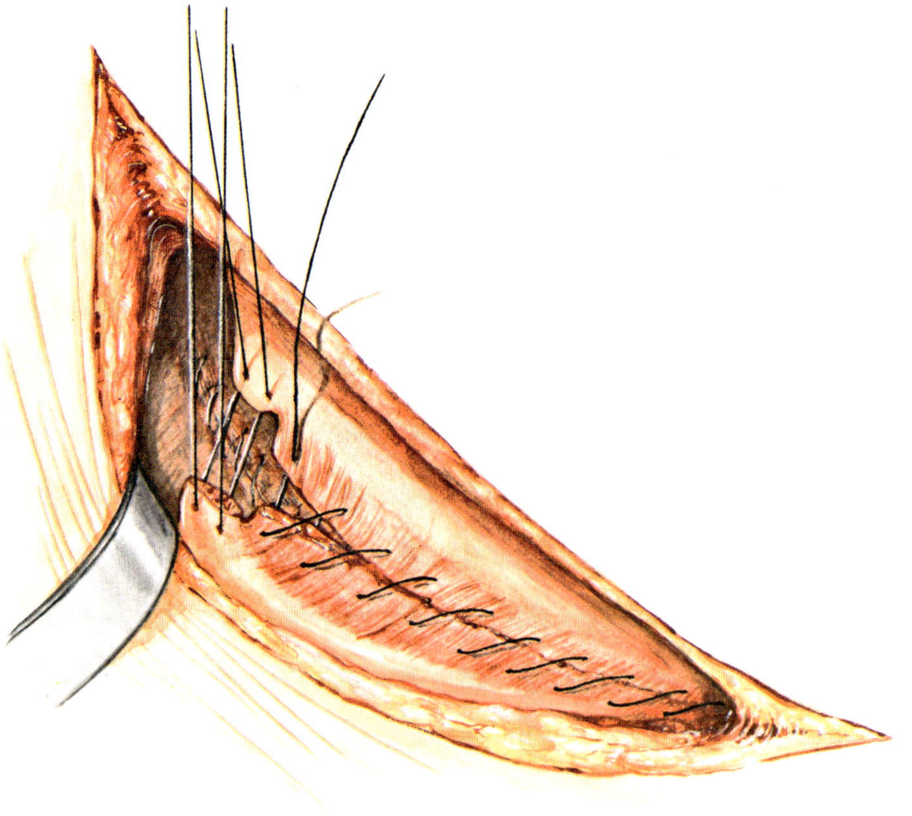

FIG. 4-23.

closed with interrupted mattress sutures of a nonabsorbable material and with a second continuous absorbable 2–0 suture for hemostasis. Close the intercostal portion of the incision (Fig. 4-23) by placing three or four pericostal sutures of #1 chromic gut and loosely lacing the intercostal muscles with a continuous suture of the same material. The ribs are brought together with a Bailey rib approximator, the pericostal sutures are tied, and the intercostal muscle suture is pulled tight. Remove 4–5 mm of the exposed ends of the costal cartilages in case any contamination has occurred, and approximate the beveled ends firmly by one or two nonabsorbable sutures so that no motion is possible (Fig. 4-23). The abdominal incision is closed by layers in the usual manner.

Median Sternotomy

A median sternotomy is the incision most commonly used for cardiac surgery and for operations on the superior mediastinum. It provides excellent exposure of the ascending aorta, the pulmonary artery, and the right side of the heart. The left ventricle may be visualized through this incision by displacing the heart anteriorly. For cardiovascular operations, the skin incision extends in the midline from the suprasternal notch to a point halfway between the xiphoid process and the umbilicus, and the sternum is completely divided longitudinally. The extent and location of this type of sternotomy is delineated in Figure 4-24 by the vertical dotted line in the center of the sternum.

Complete division of the sternum is usually unnecessary for exposure of the anterior–superior mediastinum; adequate exposure for resection of the thymus and most superior mediastinal tumors is obtained by dividing the sternum to the level of the third interspace and joining it to an incision in that interspace (represented by the horizontal line to the right of the sternum in Fig. 4-24). This incision should be used whenever it will provide adequate

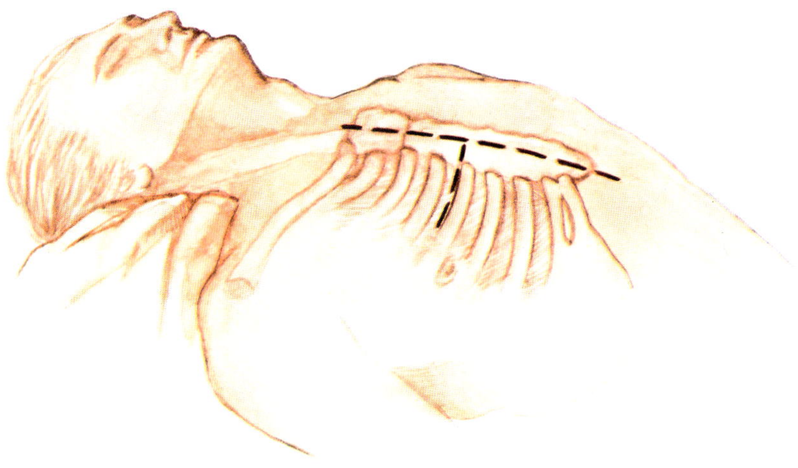

FIG. 4-24.

exposure, because the impairment of respiratory function is less with it than with a lateral thoracotomy; however, if a large anterior carcinoma of the lung is encountered instead of a mediastinal tumor, exposing the posterior aspect of the pulmonary hilus from this anterior approach can be very difficult. Postoperative back pain occurs in a significant fraction of those patients having a sternotomy for a cardiac operation. This may be the result of deforming the costovertebral joints by spreading the sternal incision.

With the patient supine, an incision is made through the subcutaneous fascia to the periosteum over the length of sternum to be divided. With a scissors the cervical fascia is incised for 2–3 cm above the suprasternal notch, and the posterior surface of the manubrium is exposed. During this dissection a small vein, which should be ligated or cauterized, is often found running transversely immediately above the manubrium. When the retrosternal space has been entered, insert a finger behind the sternum and develop this space as far inferiorly as possible.

If a complete sternotomy is to be done, make an incision through the fascia of the linea alba for 7–8 cm below the xiphoid process, but leave the peritoneum intact. With a scissors, divide the slip of the diaphragm that attaches to the posterior surface of the xiphoid, and insert a finger into the retrosternal space. Develop this space superiorly as far as possible, always staying in contact with the posterior periosteum of the sternum. After the retrosternal space has been created from both the superior and inferior ends of the sternum, with the cautery divide the anterior periosteum in the midline of the sternum (Fig. 4-25), but do not strip it from the bone. All bleeding points in the incision should be coagulated; then completely divide the sternum, using a universal air drive with a pleura guard attachment for the sternal blade (Fig. 4-26). The bleeding from the cut edge of this bone may be troublesome and should be stopped by applying bone wax. An Ankeny sternal retractor is inserted, and the incision is gradually widened; however, before the incision can be spread to its full extent, the pericardium must be opened.

If the sternotomy is made to expose the anterior–superior mediastinum, the skin incision should curve from the midline of the superior portion of the sternum to a direction overlying either the left or right third intercostal space, and it should extend laterally 6–8 cm. With either the air-drive sternal blade or a Lebsche knife, the sternum is divided in the midline from the manubrium to the third intercostal space, where the incision is angled off either to the left or right. Take care not to accidentally injure the internal mammary vessels before they are exposed and ligated. If the Lebsche knife is used to divide the sternum, upward traction on it while it is being driven

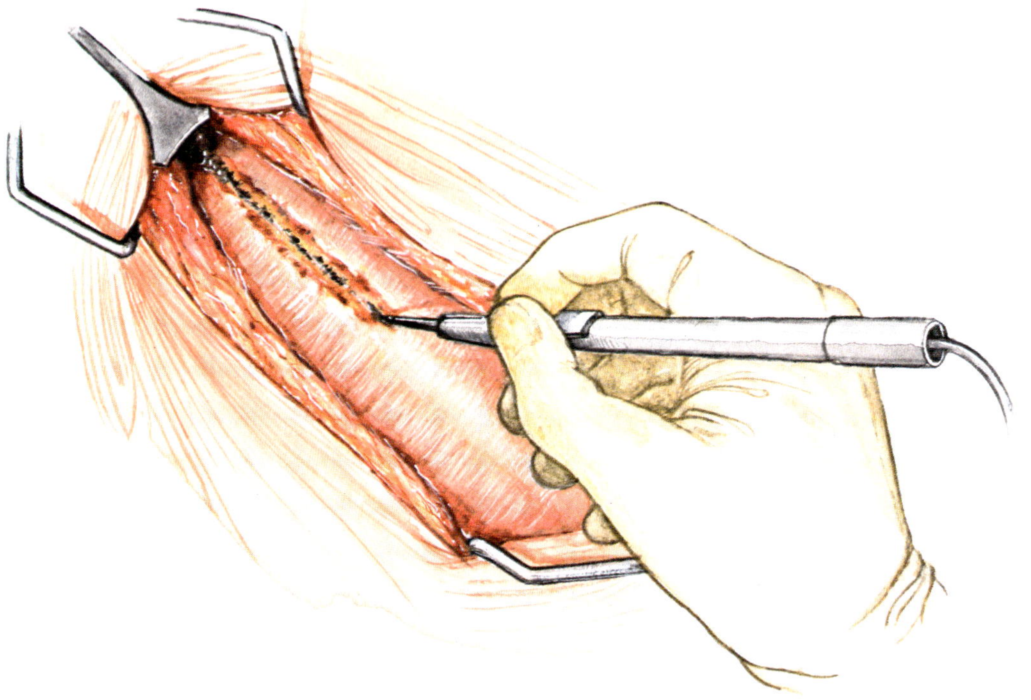

FIG. 4-25.

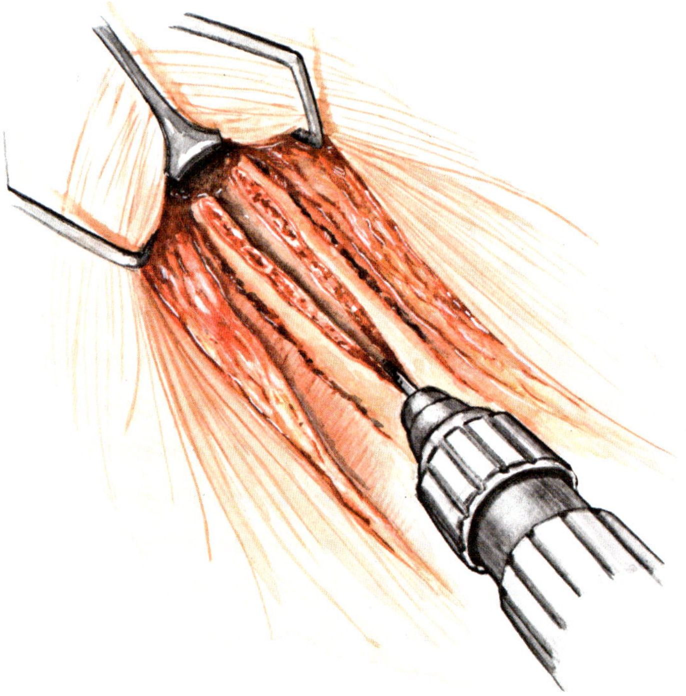

FIG. 4-26.

through the sternum with a hammer will help prevent injury to the underlying mediastinal structures. Divide the intercostal muscles of the interspace, doubly ligate then divide the internal mammary artery and vein lateral to the sternal border. The pleura underlying the interspace may be incised, and as the sternal incision is widened by opening the Himmelstein sternal retractor, the anterior mediastinal reflection of the parietal pleura may also be divided, if necessary.

Before closing a sternotomy incision, the required drainage tube should be placed. The dashed-line portion of the tubes sketched in Figure 4-27 represent the intrapleural placement for operations on the superior mediastinum. Two #24 intercostal catheters are often used, one at the apex of the chest

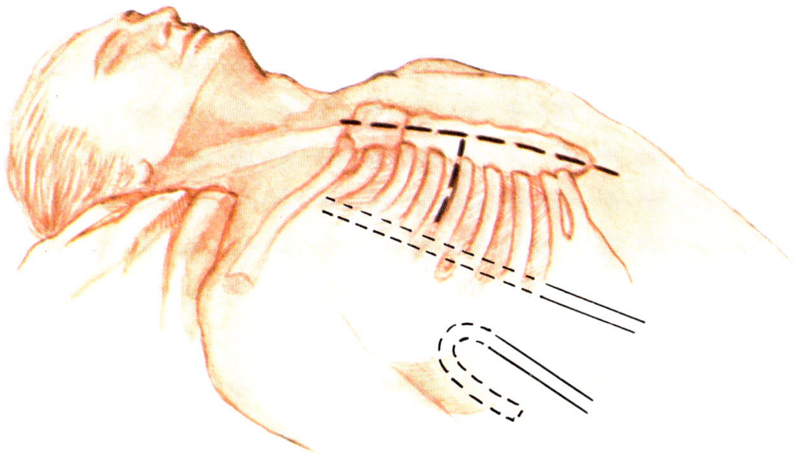

FIG. 4-27.

and one just above the diaphragm if an extensive dissection has been done. Both are fixed to the skin with 2–0 nonabsorbable sutures. A retrosternal catheter is unnecessary in this situation. The placement of drainage tubes for cardiac operations is covered in *Manual of Cardiac Surgery* (3).

After hemostasis is complete, the sternum is reapproximated with interrupted 22- or 24-gauge wire placed 3–4 cm apart with an awl or by forcing a sternal needle swaged to the wire through the sternum (Fig. 4-28). As an assistant approximates the two halves of the sternum by crossing and pulling on adjacent sutures, the surgeon twists the wire together and, after cutting off the excess, buries the ends into the sternum.

To close a partial sternotomy accompanying an interspace incision, the sternum is reapproximated as described above. The interspace incision is then closed by placing three pericostal sutures of doubled #1 chromic gut and

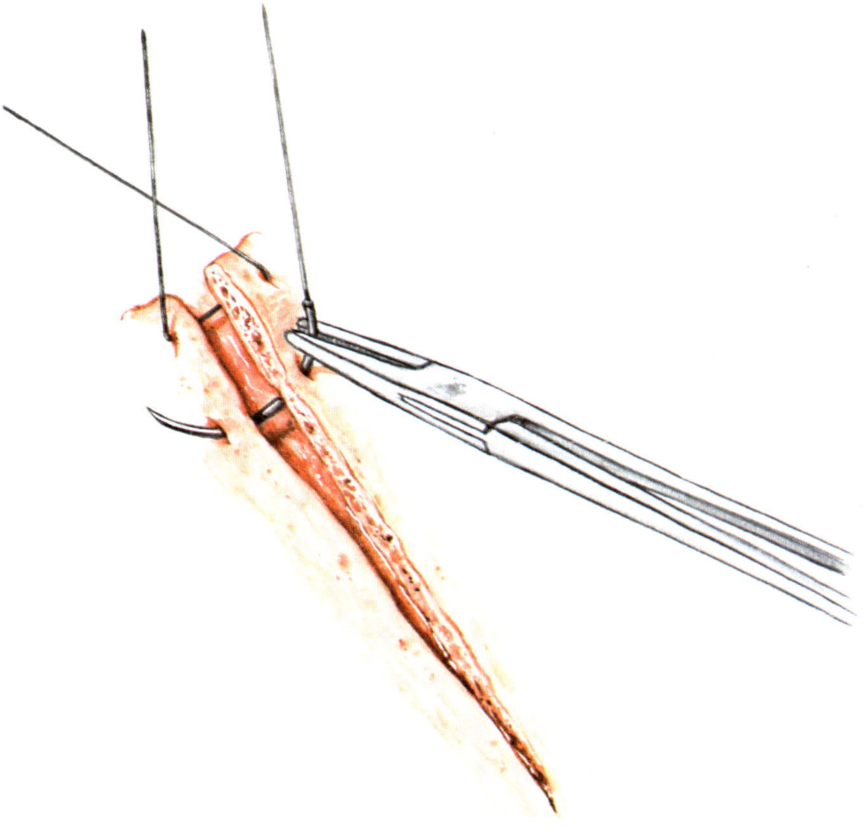

FIG. 4-28.

loosely lacing the intercostal muscles with a running suture of #1 chromic gut. The ribs are brought together with a Bailey rib approximator, the intercostal muscle suture is pulled tight, and the pericostal sutures are tied. Intercostal spaces are usually widest near the sternum, so do not force the ribs more closely together than they normally are. The fascia of the shoulder girdle muscles are approximated with interrupted 3–0 nonabsorbable sutures, as previously described.

General Principles of Thoracic Surgical Techniques

Most resections performed for cancer involve few difficult technical problems. Those performed for inflammatory conditions, however, may be arduous, with the planes of dissection obliterated and the vessel walls softened. The pulmonary arteries often tear more easily than do the adhesions to the surrounding lung tissue. Resections on patients with numerous calcified lymph nodes in the hilus of the lung may also present difficulties, because a ligature tied around a branch of the pulmonary artery near such a node may tear the artery rather than occlude it.

Division of Pleural Adhesions

Of adult patients undergoing a thoracotomy, 25%–35% will have adhesions between the parietal and visceral pleura (such as those illustrated in Fig. 4-29). These adhesions vary from a few filmy bands to a complete obliteration of the pleural space. Before placing the intercostal retractor, a large enough area of these adhesions must be divided to prevent the lung from being torn when the ribs are spread. In addition, the adhesions over the region of the lung to be removed, the portion of the hilus to be exposed, and any lobe of the lung that must ascend to fill the resulting intrathoracic space should also be divided. This implies that prior to a pneumonectomy or an upper lobectomy, all pleural adhesions must be divided, but in the course of a lower lobectomy,

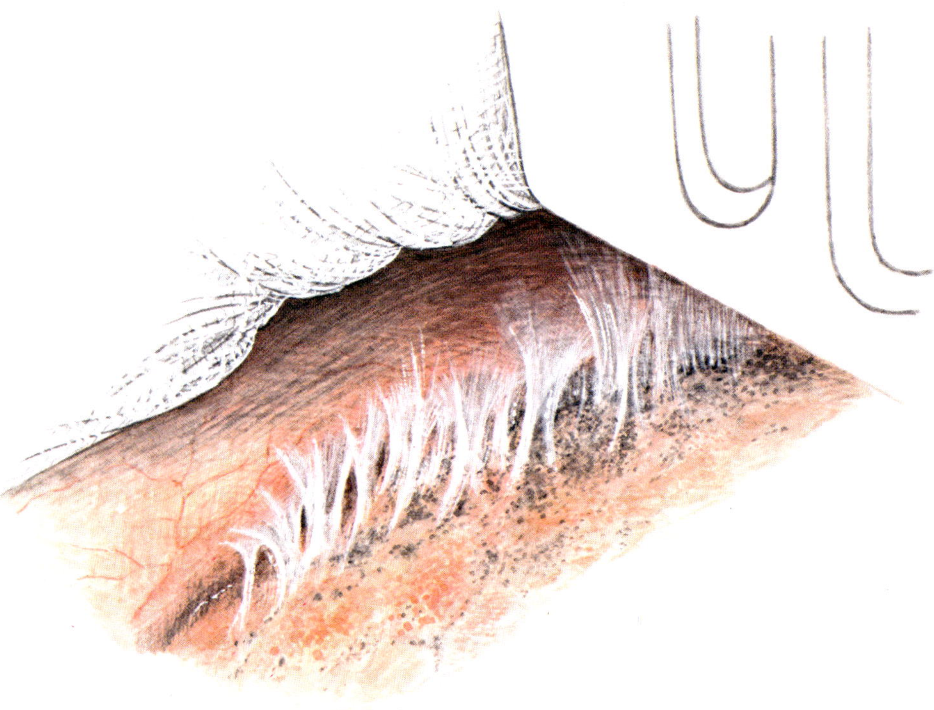

FIG. 4-29.

adhesions to the apex of the upper lobe should not be divided because they can prevent the formation of an apical pleural pocket after the lobectomy. An exception to this rule is that during a lobectomy for a superior sulcus tumor, the hilar structures should be divided prior to resecting the region of chest wall invasion.

Division of filmy adhesions (such as those illustrated in Fig. 4-29) is uncomplicated, but long-standing dense adhesions, particularly those associated with a chronic inflammatory disease such as tuberculosis, often contain relatively large systemic arteries; division of these will result in considerable blood loss unless the vessels are coagulated. Occasionally pleural adhesions may be so dense and extensive that an attempt to divide them intrapleurally would cause significant damage to the lung parenchyma. In this situation, the dissection is quicker and easier if done outside the parietal pleura in the plane of the endothoracic fascia.

Exploration of the Thorax

The surgeon should establish a routine of careful preresectional exploration of the entire thoracic cavity. After the intercostal retractor has been positioned, the whole lung, both parenchyma and bronchi, should be palpated bimanually, and the mediastinum should be examined for abnormal lymph nodes. On the right side, this includes the regions between the trachea and superior vena cava, below the carina, along the esophagus, below the inferior pulmonary vein, and along the internal mammary vessels. On the left side, in addition to the subcarinal region, the lymph nodes in the aortic window, above the aortic arch, and in the anterior mediastinum should be examined. The parietal pleura, pericardium, and diaphragm should be inspected for small nodular implants of carcinoma, and on the right side, the right lobe of the liver should be palpated through the diaphragm. If an abnormality suggesting a hepatic metastasis is felt, open the diaphragm and biopsy the lesion.

The heart should be palpated for thrills, and the great vessels should be examined. With practice, the presence of pulmonary hypertension can be quite accurately detected by palpating the tension in the pulmonary artery. Before an unknown abnormality of either lower lobe is removed, the region of the pulmonary ligament should be examined for abnormal systemic arteries branching directly from the aorta or coming through the diaphragm. Finally, because carcinoma of the esophagus, as well as carcinoma of the lung, is related to cigarette smoking, the esophagus should be palpated throughout its length.

Dissection and Ligation of the Pulmonary Vasculature

Great care must be taken in handling and isolating branches of the pulmonary artery, because these vessels have very little tensile strength. The dissection around these arteries should never be done by spreading tissues with a hemostat or a scissors, because inflamed or calcified lymph nodes in the hilus, firmly attached to these vessels, may be present. Any attempt to spread the tissue of the hilus may cause the pulmonary artery to tear before the adhesions binding the lymph node to the vessel tear. For the same reason, the proximal ligature on a branch of the pulmonary artery should be placed far enough from a main pulmonary artery that has an adherent node to prevent the branch from partially being avulsed by the ligature. Additionally, all tension on the artery should be relieved before the knot is snugged down. Branches of the pulmonary artery should never be clamped and divided prior to ligation.

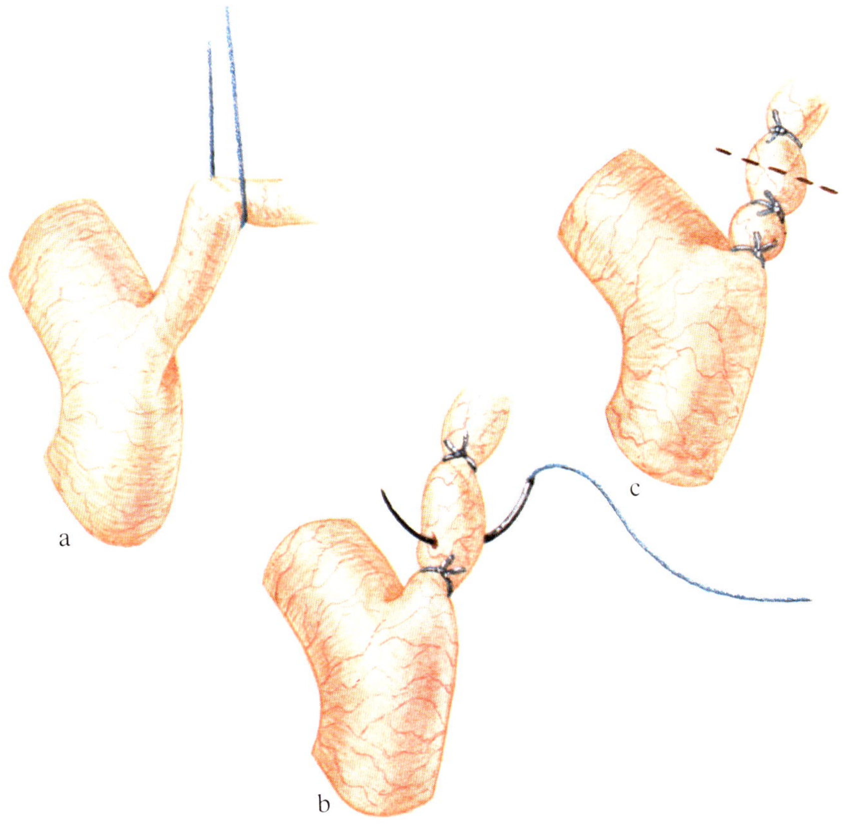

FIG. 4-30A–C.

Instead, the arteries should be ligated in situ, then divided (Fig. 4-30A–C) using a proximal and distal 2–0 nonabsorbable ligature and a proximal 3–0 suture ligature.

When one of the main pulmonary arteries must be divided, first clamp the artery with two curved or right angle vascular clamps, such as the curved Glover clamp, placed 10–15 mm apart (Fig. 4-31A and B). Place and tie a 4–0 nonabsorbable cardiovascular suture on each corner of the artery just distal to the proximal clamp; then divide the artery just proximal to the distal clamp. Each suture is used in turn in the continuous over and over fashion (Fig. 4-31A) to close the proximal stump of the pulmonary artery. The use of a suture ligature to close the distal end of the artery attached to

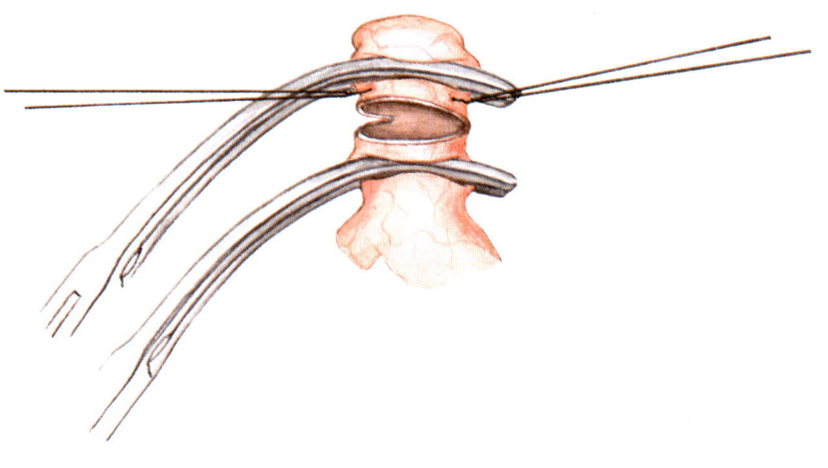

FIG. 4-31A.

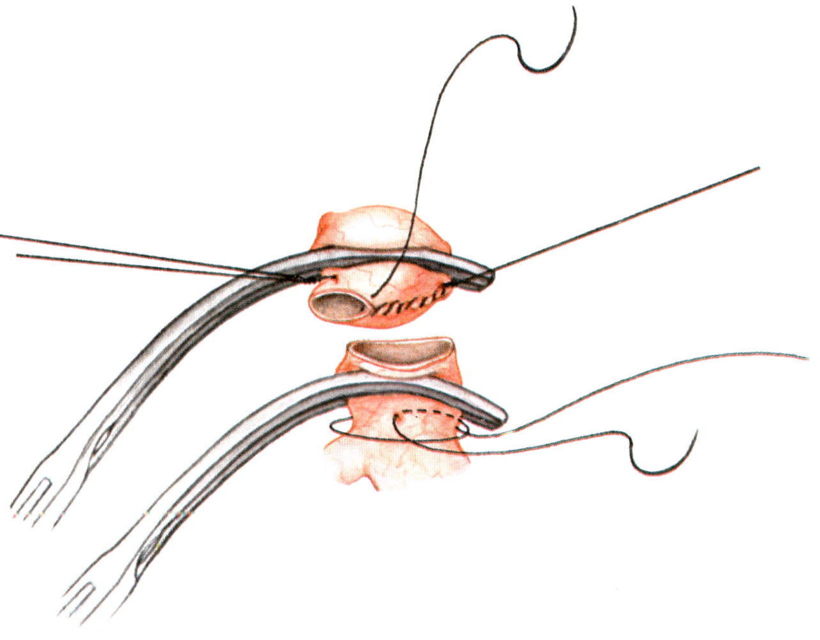

FIG. 4-31B.

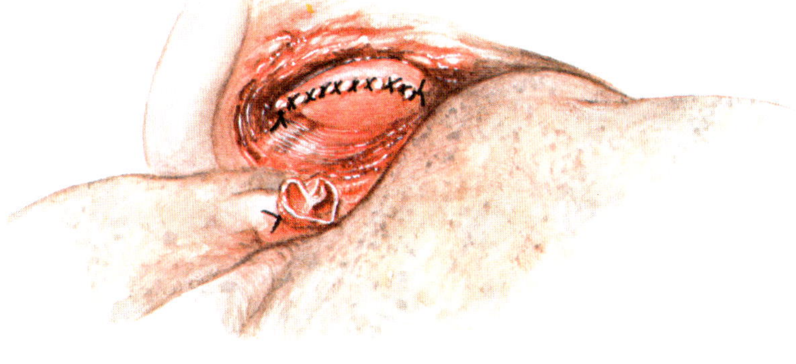

FIG. 4-32.

the lung being resected is also illustrated in Figure 4-31B. The arterial stump after closing appears similar to Figure 4-32, which depicts the divided right pulmonary artery with the two superimposed running suture lines. The practice of using two circumferential ligatures or suture ligatures to close the main pulmonary artery has been attended by late hemorrhage due to ligature slippage, and is to be condemned.

The main pulmonary veins may be securely closed with 30-V staples using the TA-30 stapler (Fig. 4-33). It seems unwise to use this method for closing the pulmonary artery because of the resulting crushed region. If control of a branch of the pulmonary artery is lost, instead of attempting to grasp the branch with a hemostatic clamp through a pool of blood, the surgeon should occlude the main right or left pulmonary artery near the heart with his fingers, remove the blood with suction, and visualize the bleeding site. The portion of the adjacent pulmonary artery with the bleeding site should be occluded with a vascular clamp and the bleeding site closed with fine sutures, accurately placed.

If possible, the arterial supply to a lung or lung lobe should be divided prior to interrupting the venous drainage, otherwise the lung becomes so congested with blood that it is difficult to retract.

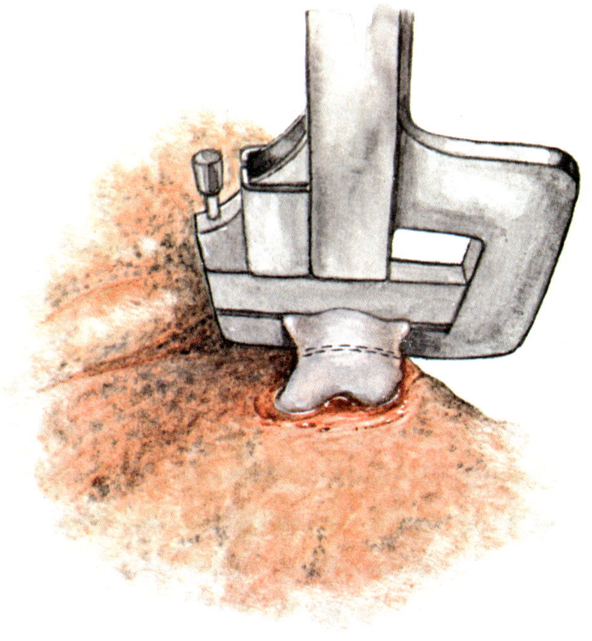

FIG. 4-33.

Division and Closure of Bronchi

A bronchus must never be clamped with a crushing forceps proximal to the site of division, because this will damage the tenuous blood supply and could result in a bronchial stump leak. Because a long bronchial stump will collect secretions and may become the site of recurrent bronchitis, a bronchus should be divided close to its origin, leaving just enough length so the staples or sutures will not impinge on the lumen of the next-larger-order bronchus. The two main bronchi and the lobar bronchi are best closed with the TA-30 stapler, using 3.5-mm staples for lobar bronchi and 4.8-mm staples for the main bronchi. The staple line must be at a right angle to the edge of the bronchus and parallel to the cartilaginous rings so as to oppose the membranous to the cartilaginous portion (Figs. 4-75 and 4-87). This leaves no area with a poor blood supply.

In my experience no bronchopleural fistula has resulted from the use of a staple closure in 15 years, a major improvement over suture closure; however, in certain situations, when a bronchus must be divided very close to its origin, suture closure becomes mandatory. Closure is accomplished using interrupted 4–0 nonabsorbable sutures swaged on a Tapercut™ type needle (Fig. 4-34). These sutures should be placed about 3 mm apart and 3–4 mm from the cut edge of the bronchus (after the manner illustrated in Fig. 4-86). If they are placed too close to the edge, they may tear out, and if too far from the edge, when tied they will lacerate the membranous portion of the bronchus, resulting in air leaks. Segmental bronchi should, by choice, be closed with interrupted 4–0 sutures. Do not permit blood to be aspirated through the open bronchus. Such aspiration may cause significant respiratory insufficiency.

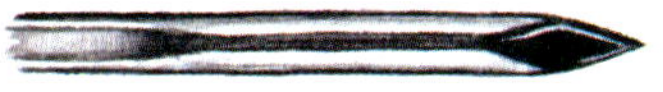

FIG. 4-34.

To determine that a bronchial closure is secure, the stump is covered with warm saline and an airway pressure of 20 cm of water is maintained for several seconds so that any air leaks can be detected and closed. If the closure is airtight, a flap of parietal pleura, pericardium, or pericardial fat is developed and sutured over the cut end of the bronchial stump (as illustrated for the right upper lobe in Fig. 4-77). It is a clinical impression that this covering decreases the risk of a bronchial leak.

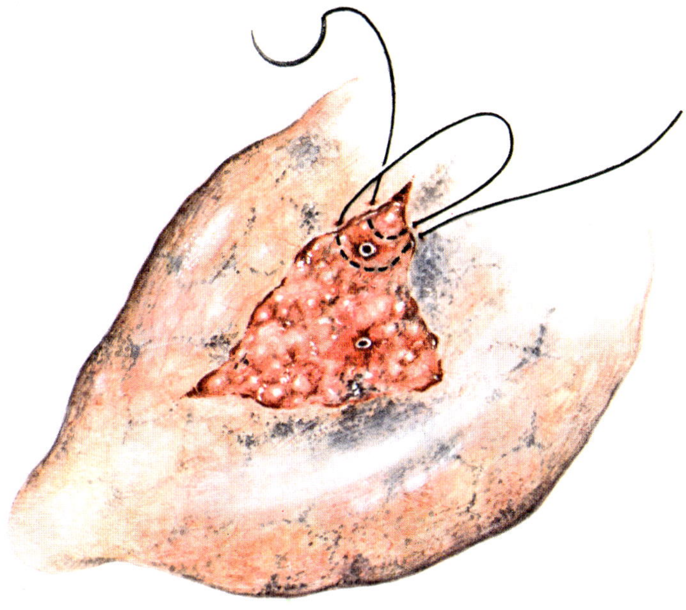

FIG. 4-35.

Air Leaks and Residual Intrathoracic Space

If a large, raw area of lung parenchyma is present after a resection, the surgeon will be faced with innumerable small air leaks. All of these need not and cannot be closed, but the larger ones should be stopped by suture ligatures of 3–0 Dexon or its equivalent (Fig. 4-35). The ligatures should be tied only tightly enough to stop the air leak; too much tension will tear the parenchyma of a lung with emphysematous disease, causing additional air leaks. These raw areas should never be closed by approximating the visceral pleural edges, which may leave an intrapulmonary pocket that will accumulate fluid. Such a pocket of serum will become infected and virtually assure the development of prolonged air leaks and pleural space problems. If the large leaks are closed and the raw area is permitted to seal itself against the parietal pleura, the smaller leaks will stop quickly.

After an upper lobectomy, the pulmonary ligament should be divided to permit the remaining lung to rise in the chest and decrease the likelihood of an apical air space developing. During this division (Fig. 4-36), care must be taken not to injure the inferior pulmonary vein, which forms the superior margin of this ligament, nor to overlook the several small blood vessels that must be divided and can be the source of considerable postoperative bleeding. It is unwise either to crush the phrenic nerve or to perform a so-called tailoring thoracoplasty at the time of a lobectomy in order to obliterate a pleural space; both result in marked interference with the patient's ability to cough and frequently lead to postoperative atelectasis.

If in the surgeon's opinion, the remaining lung will not fill the hemithorax, the residual space is preferably made extrapleural by freeing the parietal pleura over the apex of the chest, using the method shown in Figure 4-37. Leave the pleura attached over the mediastinum and drop it over the remaining lung like a tent. The intrapleural suction catheters are positioned inside this pleural tent. If the surgeon believes preoperatively that the lung remaining after a given resection will not fill the hemithorax, a thoracoplasty of the first three ribs may be done two to three weeks prior to the resection and the fourth rib removed at the time of the resection. Such a four rib thoracoplasty results in little cosmetic deformity; yet together with the usual postoperative shift in the mediastinum and diaphragm, it will usually reduce the pleural space to a size that can be filled by only the basilar segments of the lower lobe.

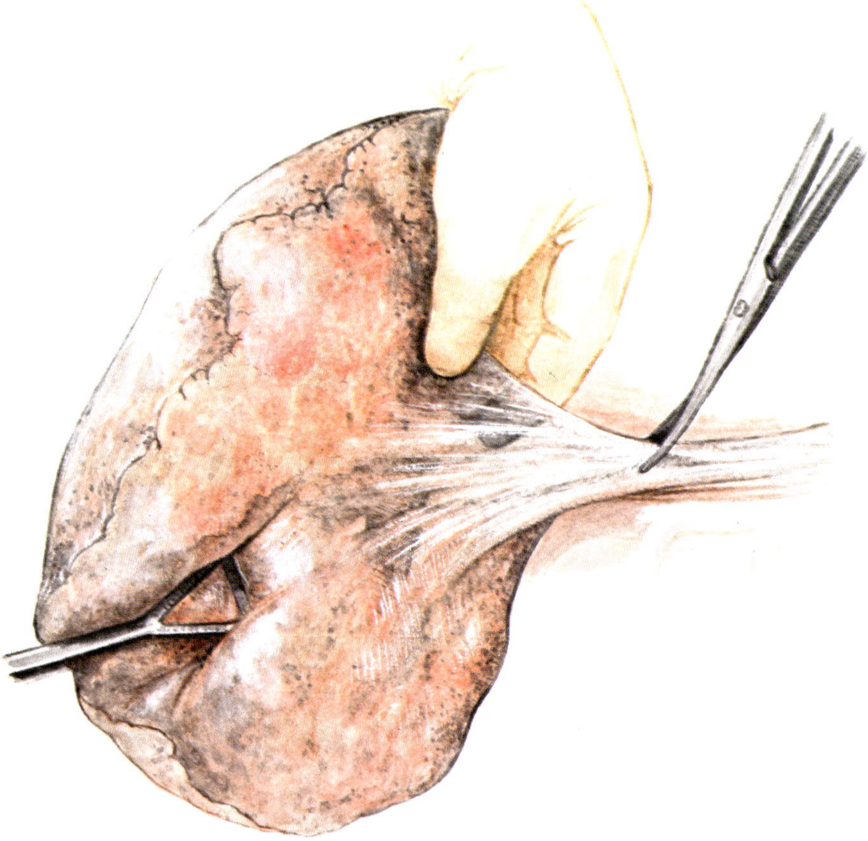

FIG. 4-36.

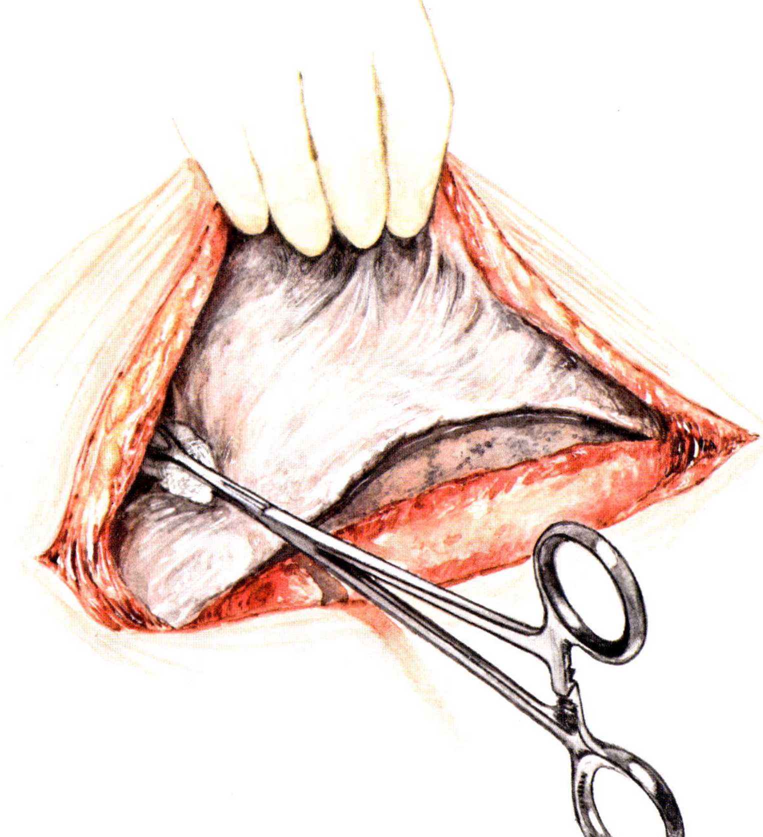

FIG. 4-37.

Following any pulmonary resection other than a pneumonectomy, intercostal catheters are used to evacuate air and blood from the pleural cavity, one placed just above the diaphragm, one running posterior to the hilus up to the apex of the chest and one anterior to the hilus about two-thirds of the distance to the apex (Fig. 4-38). Because the principal function of these catheters is to evacuate air, not blood, cutting extra holes in them is unnecessary and should not be done. Patients with chronic obstructive lung disease have fragile lungs that are easily eroded by catheters. If erosion occurs, it is helpful to advance the catheters slowly, over a period of days, to permit the parietal and visceral pleura to adhere to each other behind the catheter and obliterate the tube track and the air leak. With extra holes in the catheter, advancement cannot be done because some holes will then be positioned outside the pleural cavity.

Following a pneumonectomy, no drainage catheters are placed in the pleural cavity. Instead, after the thoracic incision has been closed and the patient is supine and breathing without a respirator, a volume of air adequate to reduce the expiratory pressure in the pleural space to zero should be removed by thoracentesis. Within an hour after surgery, the position of the mediastinum should be verified by a chest radiogram. If the position is unsatisfactory, an additional volume of air should either be removed from or injected into the pleural space on the side of the pneumonectomy in order to position the mediastinum 1–2 cm toward the side of the pneumonectomy. The mediastinum can usually be moved by this maneuver for the first 72 hours after surgery, but after that, the mediastinum becomes fixed and relatively immobile.

Segmental Resection

A segmentectomy became possible with the definition, by Churchill and Belsey, (2) of the bronchopulmonary segment as the surgical unit of the lung. The two segments of the middle lobe, the two segments of the lingula, and

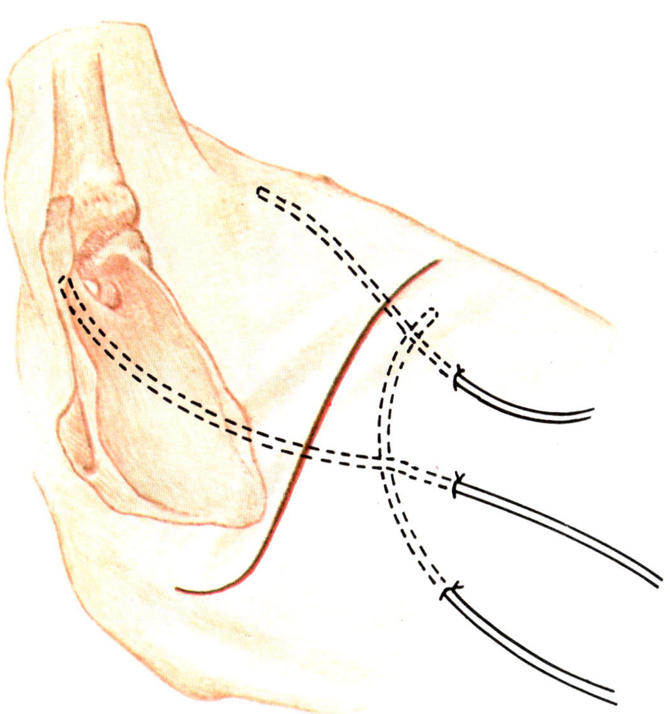

FIG. 4-38.

the four basilar segments of the lower lobes are removed usually as a unit, but the individual segments of the right upper lobe, of the upper division of the left upper lobe, and the superior segments of each lower lobe may be removed separately. Segmentectomy had its greatest use in the removal of bronchiectatic areas or the residuals of tuberculosis. With the decline of such surgery and with the development of the various stapling devices, formal segmentectomy has become a relatively infrequent operation. Its advantage is the conserving of as much functioning lung mass as possible, but in exchange, its disadvantages are increased risks of postoperative complications and of the spreading of the disease caused by dissecting into the diseased tissue rather than through normal tissue.

In the ensuing discussion, except when noted, all anatomic nomenclature and frequencies of anatomic variations are taken from Professor Edward Boyden's book, *Segmental Anatomy Of The Lungs* (1), a classic for any surgeon interested in the lung. Figures 4-41, 4-47, 4-48, 4-56, and 4-60 are modified from that book. The procedures described are for the usual architecture and the common variations. For each operation it is imperative that the surgeon confirms that the selected segmental bronchus and vasculature actually are distributed to the parenchymal region to be removed.

Segmental Resections of the Right Upper Lobe

The segments of the right lung and the right bronchial tree are shown in Figure 4-39. These segments are identified in the corresponding diagramatic Figure 4-40. Each bronchus takes the name of the pulmonary segment it supplies. The right upper lobe has three segments: apical, anterior, and posterior. The resection of each of the segments begins similarly.

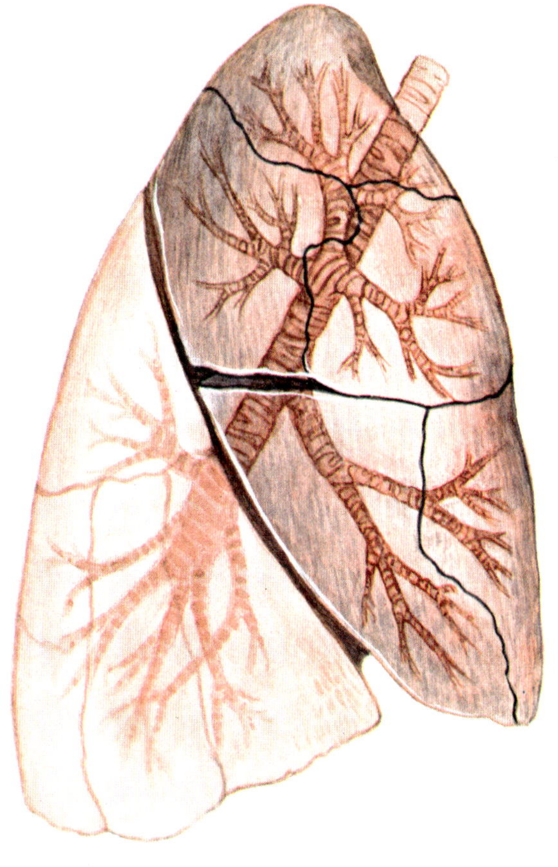

FIG. 4-39.

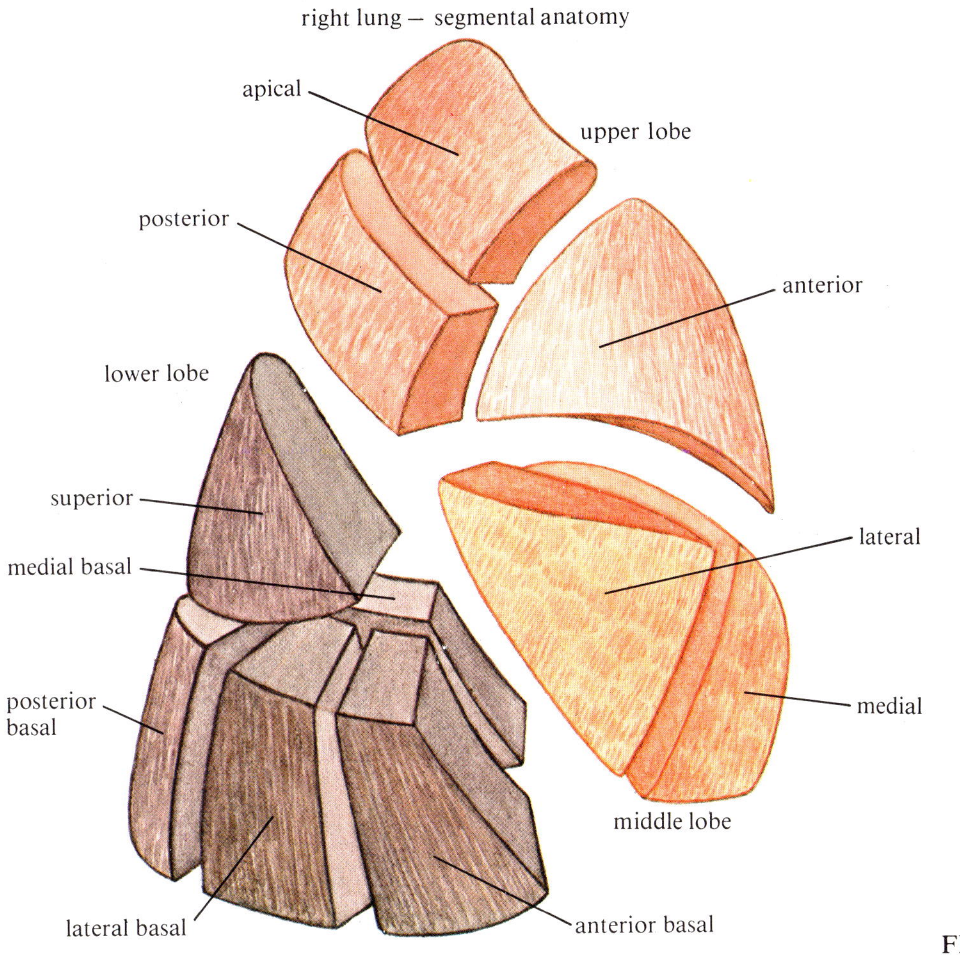

FIG. 4-40.

On the posterior superior aspect of the hilum, the division of the right main bronchus into the upper lobe and the bronchus intermedius may be palpated. The pleura is incised from this point superiorly, then down the anterior surface of the hilum to the inferior border of the superior pulmonary vein. The dashed line in Figure 4-65 shows the site of this incision beginning at the anterior limit of the superior pulmonary vein. The truncus anterior of the right pulmonary artery and the upper lobe division of the superior pulmonary vein, which may cover the artery anteriorly, should be exposed on the mediastinal surface of the lobe. This dissection can be seen in Figure 4-66, in which the truncus anterior has been dissected out and is looped by a ligature. If no significant inflammation is present, much of the dissection can be done bluntly using the closed scissors or a Küttner dissector.

With the major vessels identified, the branches of the truncus anterior should be isolated and tentatively identified. Figure 4-41 shows the most common distribution of the upper lobe vasculature. Usually (68%), the truncus consists of a single stem which bifurcates into a superior and an inferior division. The inferior division usually supplies the anterior segment only, but the upper division is quite variable. It supplies the apical segment and, in over half the cases, a portion of the posterior segment by a recurrent artery that crosses the superior surface of the apical bronchus (Fig. 4-41). According to Boyden, in 14% of lungs, these two divisions take origin from the pulmonary artery separately rather than as a single trunk.

Subsequently, the venous tributaries from the upper lobe segments should be isolated and tentatively identified. Usually three segmental veins from the

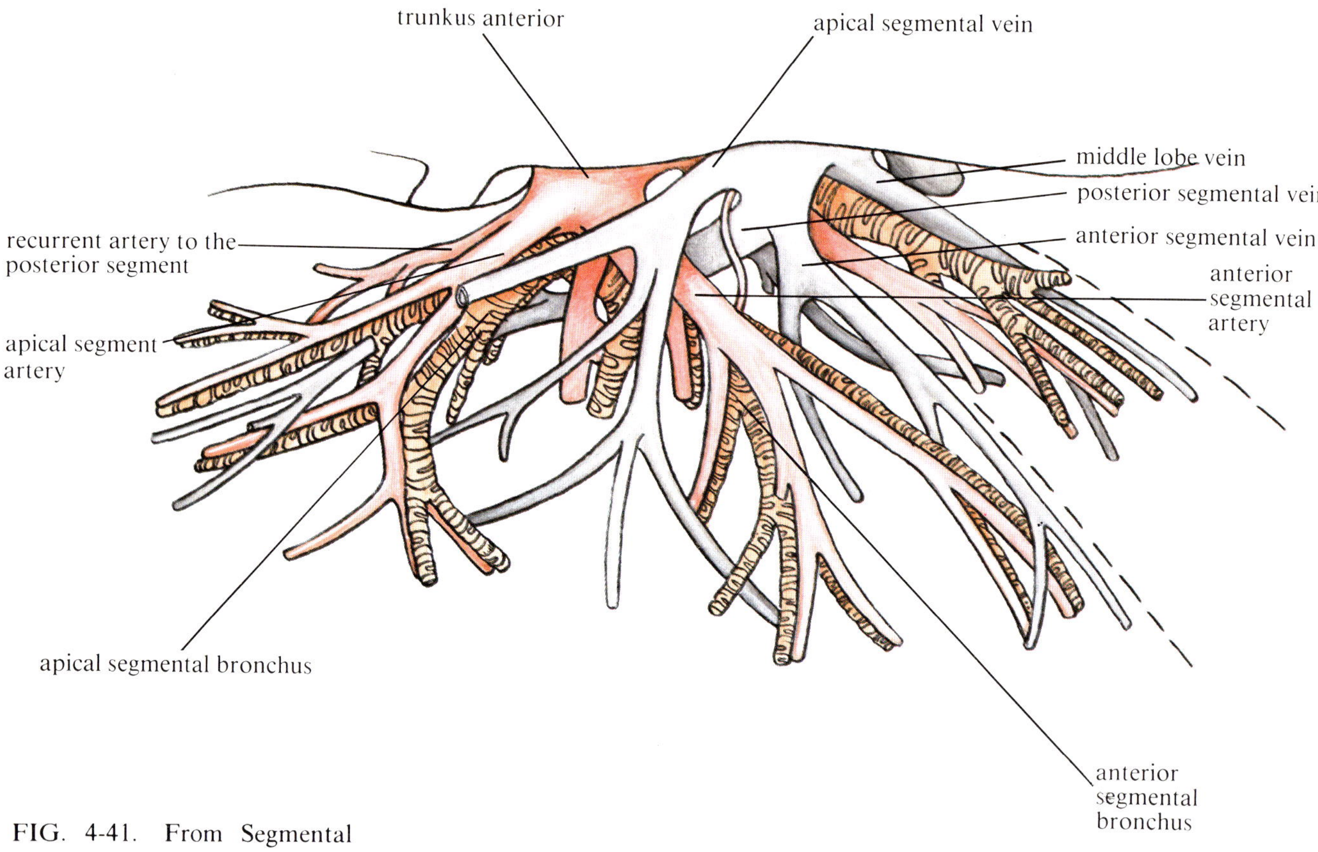

FIG. 4-41. From Segmental Anatomy of the Lung by Boyden EA. Copyright © 1955. Used with the permission of the McGraw-Hill Book Company.

upper lobe are found. These three veins, isolated by a clamp, are shown in Figure 4-67. The apical vein is at the left, looped by a ligature, the posterior vein is in the center, and the anterior vein is on the right. The middle lobe vein can be seen at the top of the figure running into the middle lobe on the right. This distribution of veins is illustrated graphically in Figure 4-41. As suggested by Overholt et al. (6), each vein has intrasegmental and intersegmental branches. Such an arrangement is of great convenience in the surgical separation of segments, because the dissection can follow the course of the intersegmental veins.

In the ensuing discussion, the described course of a vein is that followed by the surgeon during the dissection, not that corresponding to the blood flow; the discussion may be followed in Figures 4-41 and 4-47. The apical vein usually drains the apical segment and the intersegmental region of the apical and anterior segments. It ascends beneath the pleura of the mediastinal surface and crosses the inferior division of the truncus anterior. The anterior vein usually drains the anterior segment and the interlobar region of the anterior segment and the middle lobe when, as is common, the horizontal fissure is incomplete. At its junction with the pulmonary vein, this vein is in the same superficial plane as is the apical vein, but inferior to it. In approximately 30% of patients, the two branches of the anterior vein empty separately into one of the other tributaries of the superior pulmonary vein and no distinct anterior vein occurs. The posterior vein, largest of the upper lobe veins, usually drains the posterior segment, a portion of the anterior segment, the intersegmental region of the apical and posterior segments, the intersegmental region of the anterior and posterior segments, and the interlobar region between the posterior segment and the lower lobe. From the mediastinal approach, at its confluence with the pulmonary vein, the posterior vein is deep to the apical and anterior veins and superficial to the interlobar portion of the pulmonary artery (note this arrangement in Fig. 4-47 and 4-67). The posterior vein is closely applied to the surfaces of both the pulmonary artery and the other segmental veins, so blindly forcing an instrument behind the two superficial veins or behind the posterior vein may injure the adjacent vessel. From this point, the posterior vein courses behind the segmental bronchi of the anterior segment.

During this initial part of the dissection, the segmental arteries and veins on the mediastinal aspect of the hilum should be freed over a distance of 1–2 cm; then the bronchus to the segment to be resected should be isolated. The bronchus to the apical segment is approached from the superior aspect of the hilus, while the bronchi to the posterior or anterior segments are approached posteriorly or from the interlobar aspect. Because the right upper lobe bronchus divides by trifurcation in only half the patients, it is important that the identity of the bronchus to be divided is established beyond question. Identification can usually be made by palpation; however, if there is doubt, the upper lobe should be deflated, the bronchus in question occluded, and the lobe reinflated. Although the segmental region supplied by the occluded bronchus will inflate in time due to the collateral ventilation in the human lung, it inflates more slowly than does the lung tissue ventilated by open bronchi. It can be readily identified.

If the apical segment is to be resected, the apical bronchus is clamped, then divided proximal to the clamp 3–4 mm from its origin with the lobar bronchus, and the proximal stump is closed with interrupted 4–0 nonabsorbable sutures. With some tension on the lesion or on the lung segment itself, the blood vessels supplying this segment are identified again, and they are ligated and divided, the artery usually at its origin from the superior division of the trunkus anterior and the vein at its junction with the other upper lobe veins. Figure 4-42 shows the exposed trifurcation of the right upper lobe bronchus and the clamped and divided apical segmental bronchus. The

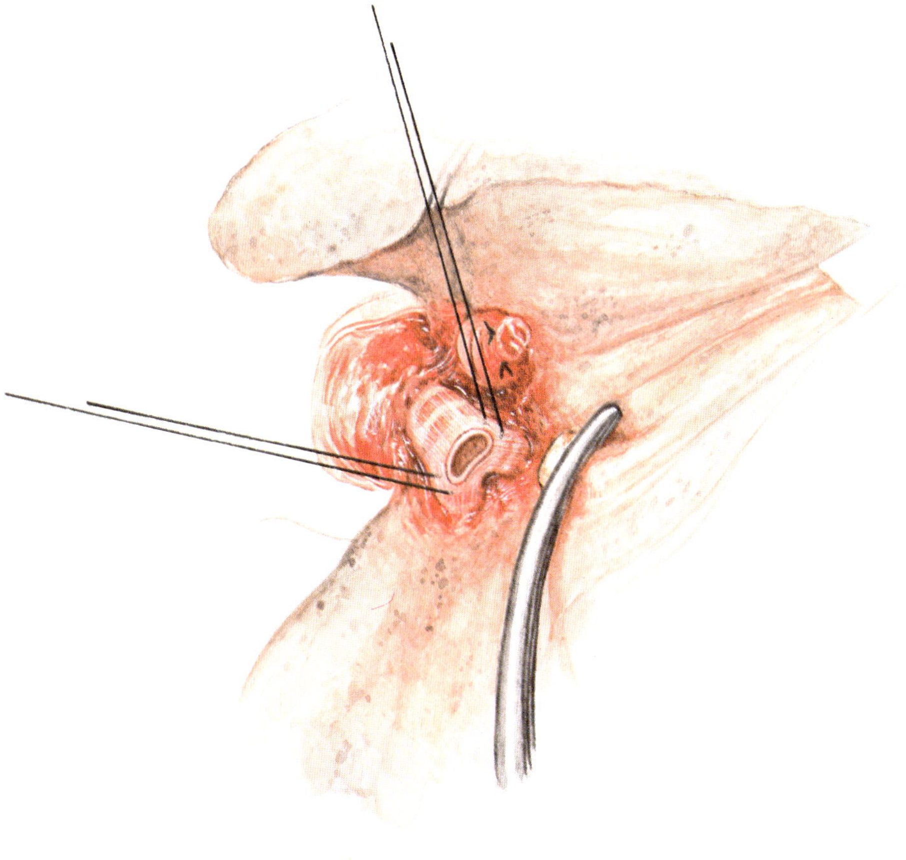

FIG. 4-42.

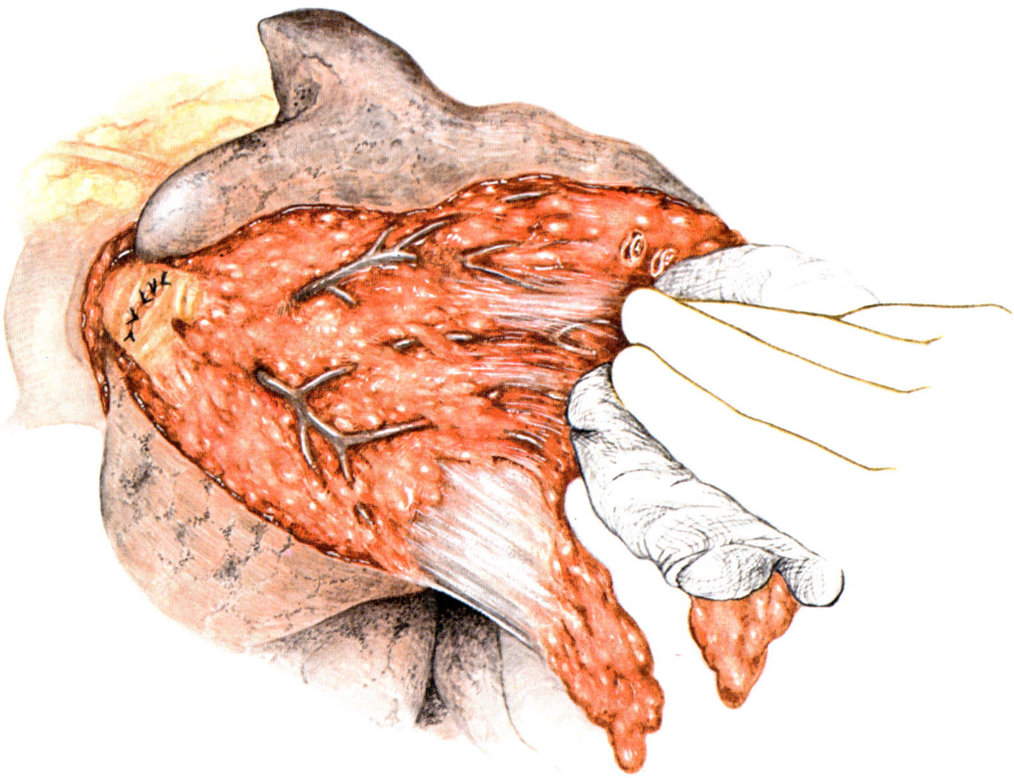

FIG. 4-43.

two stay sutures are on the stump of the apical bronchus. Superior to the upper lobe bronchus, the artery to the apical segment has been ligated and divided. There was no recurrent artery to the posterior segment in this patient.

If the surgeon is right-handed, the apical segment is grasped with the left hand, the fingers marking the approximate junction with the rest of the lobe. Using dry gauze in the right hand, (Fig. 4-43), the apical segment is wiped off the rest of the lobe following the plane of the intersegmental veins, which are exposed in the illustration. Any small vessels encountered crossing the intersegmental plane should be divided and ligated. An alternative method is to dissect the segment along the intersegmental veins just far enough to establish their course, then complete the parenchymal division with the GIA stapler.

To resect the posterior segment, the lymph node found just inferior to the right upper lobe bronchus near its posterior aspect should be removed. Notice in Figure 4-44 that the node has been dissected out and turned up behind the upper lobe bronchus. This node sits in a pocket, the inferior wall of which is the artery to the superior segment of the lower lobe, seen running under the fold of tissue held by the forceps; the posterior wall is the bronchus intermedius, the superior wall is the upper lobe bronchus, and the deep wall is the ascending artery to the upper lobe, seen running deep to the upper lobe bronchus.

With this lymph node removed, a finger should be placed in the pocket, then exposed through the oblique fissure at its junction with the horizontal fissure (Fig. 4-45). The location of the pulmonary artery in this dissection is shown in the figure: the artery to the middle lobe goes to the right, the artery to the superior segment of the lower lobe runs to the left under the finger, and the basilar artery extends down and to the left. The opening in the depth of the fissure created by this maneuver permits the identification of the interlobar portion of the pulmonary artery with its ascending branch(es),

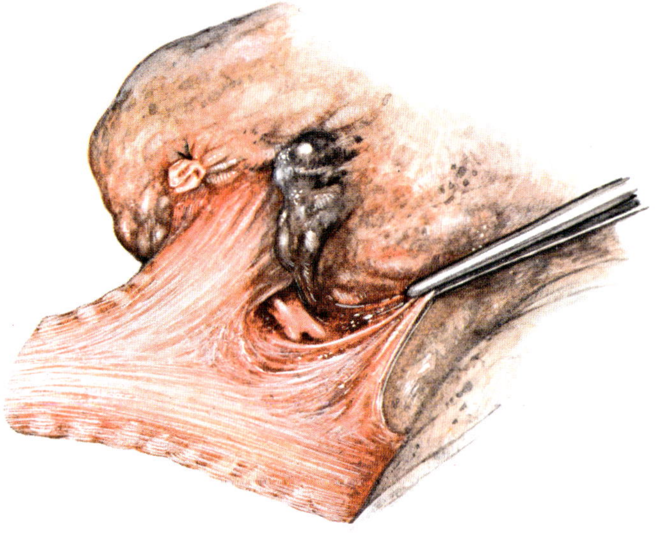

FIG. 4-44.

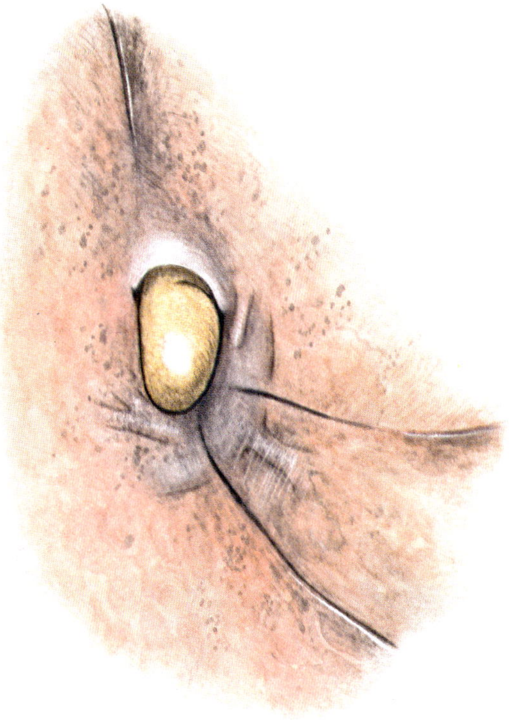

FIG. 4-45.

the branch to the superior segment of the lower lobe, and the main trunk of the posterior vein. With these structures protected, the parenchyma of the posterior segment is separated from the superior segment of the lower lobe with a GIA stapler or with the TA-55 stapler (Fig. 4-46). In this figure, the middle lobe is being held by the lung grasping clamp. In over 80% of patients, the posterior segment will receive some blood supply from an ascending artery taking origin from the interlobar portion of the pulmonary artery or occasionally from the artery to the superior segment of the lower lobe. The ascending artery is shown graphically in Figure 4-47. In Fig. 4-78, it is illustrated as seen from the oblique fissure, running superior and slightly anterior. In Figure 4-70, from the anterior aspect of the lobe, the ascending artery is pictured with the ligatures extending from it. The ascending artery must be ligated and divided. After final identification, the recurrent artery to the posterior segment should be ligated and divided at its origin from the superior division of the trunkus anterior (Fig. 4-41). The posterior vein is ligated in the depths of the oblique fissure where it was exposed. The location of this vein in the fissure can be seen in Figure 4-47. The posterior segmental bronchus is isolated deep to the ascending artery through the horizontal fissure, or

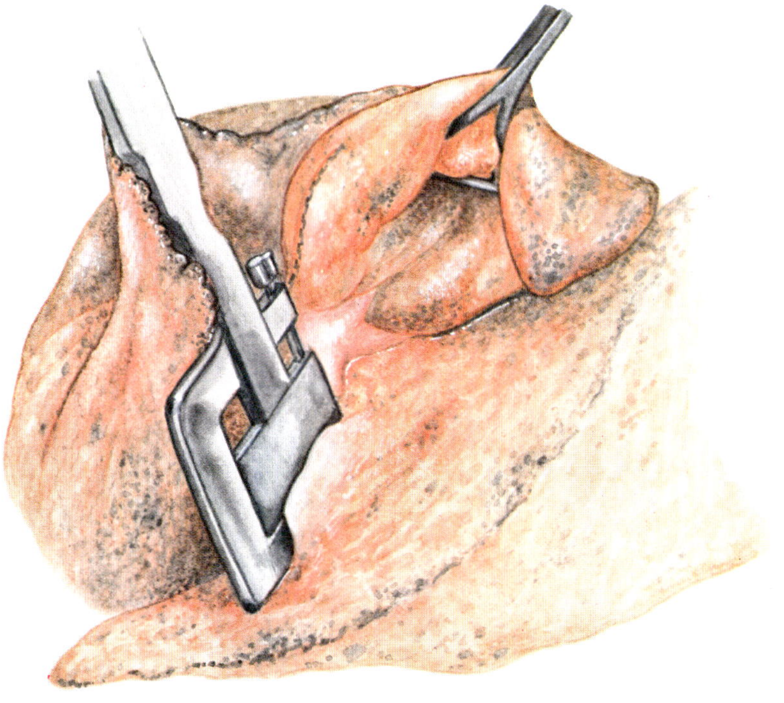

FIG. 4-46.

from the posterior aspect of the hilus. It should be clamped and divided proximal to the clamp. The stump is sutured closed and the segment is separated from the rest of the lobe, as previously described.

The resection of the anterior segment, after the initial exposure of the truncus anterior and the upper lobe pulmonary veins, is continued by dissecting along the anterior vein for 2–3 cm to determine whether a middle lobe vein

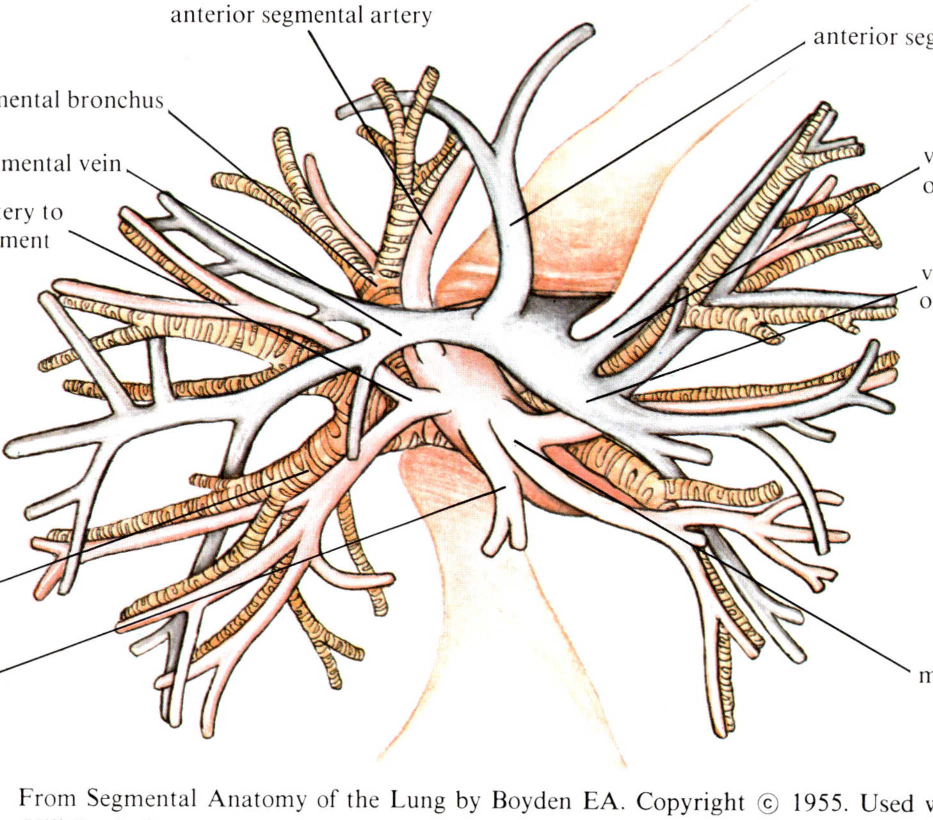

FIG. 4-47. From Segmental Anatomy of the Lung by Boyden EA. Copyright © 1955. Used with the permission of the McGraw-Hill Book Company.

drains into it or it drains into a middle lobe vein. The anterior vein should then be ligated at a location that does not interfere with middle lobe venous drainage. If these frequently occurring anomalies are overlooked, the result may be edema of the middle lobe. The dissection is continued along the interlobar portion of the pulmonary artery until an ascending branch is encountered. In 40% of patients, there will be an ascending artery at least partially supplying the anterior segment. In the lung illustrated in Figure 4-47, the ascending artery divides and sends one branch to the posterior segment and one to the anterior segment. In 20%–30% of patients, two ascending arteries are present, usually one to the anterior and one to the posterior segment, (Fig. 4-49).

From the anterior side of the hilus, a finger is placed along the lateral surface of the interlobar portion of the pulmonary artery, and the finger is exposed by dissecting in the depths of the oblique fissure at its junction with the horizontal fissure, as previously described for a similar maneuver from the posterior aspect of the hilus. Using this opening and the mediastinal area of dissection, the following structures should be visualized: the middle lobe veins and artery, the ascending arteries, the vein to the posterior segment, and the artery to the superior segment of the lower lobe (Figs. 4-47, 4-67, and 4-78). If the horizontal fissure is incomplete, as is usually the case, the middle lobe should be separated from the anterior segment of the upper lobe with the GIA stapler (Figs. 4-71 and 4-72). After final identification, the artery to the anterior segment from the truncus anterior and any ascending arteries to the anterior segment are ligated and divided. The bronchus to the anterior segment is found anterior to the posterior segmental bronchus on the fissural aspect of the upper lobe bronchus (Fig. 4-47). This bronchus is clamped and divided proximal to the clamp; the stump is closed, and the segment is separated from the rest of the lobe along the plane of the intersegmental veins.

Segmental Resections of the Right Lower Lobe

As depicted in Figure 4-48 (mediastinal and lateral views of the right lower lobe), the lobe is composed of five, often six segments: the superior segment,

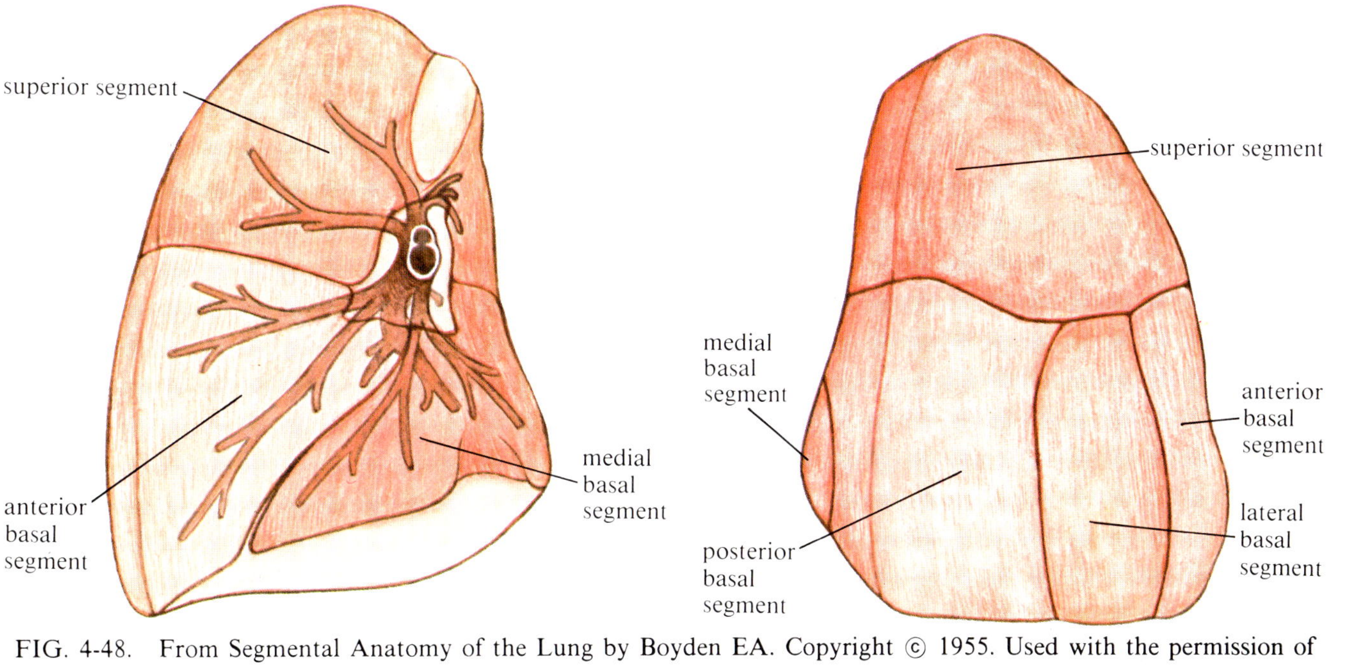

FIG. 4-48. From Segmental Anatomy of the Lung by Boyden EA. Copyright © 1955. Used with the permission of the McGraw-Hill Book Company.

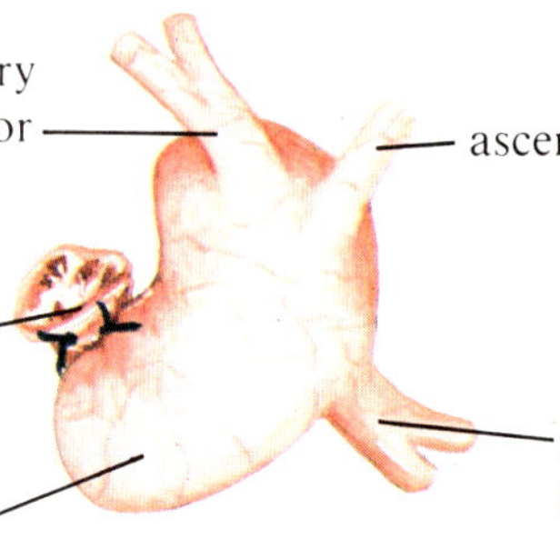

FIG. 4-49.

the medial basal, anterior basal, lateral basal, and posterior basal segments, and in some patients, a subsuperior segment. The superior segment commonly occupies the upper half of the lower lobe, and in common with the superior segment of the left lung, it is the largest of the lung segments. The two types of segmental resections of the right lower lobe are a superior segmentectomy, sparing the basilar segments, and a basilar segmentectomy, sparing the superior segment. Although the individual basilar segments can be resected, such an operation is rarely performed because first, most disease of the basilar segments involves all of the segments and second, because the anatomy of the basilar segments is quite variable.

The resection of either the superior segment or the basilar segments begins by dividing the pulmonary ligament from the diaphragm to the inferior pulmonary vein and continuing the pleural incision along the junction of the lower lobe with the posterior mediastinum. In the course of this dissection, expose the posterior surface of the inferior pulmonary vein and the posterior surface of the bronchus intermedius at its junction with the upper lobe bronchus. Divide the pleura in the depths of the oblique fissure and dissect the central portion of the fissure between the middle and the lower lobes until the lateral surface of the interlobar pulmonary artery is exposed. This portion of the pulmonary artery lies lateral and superficial to the bronchus and is usually covered by lymph nodes near the posterior limit of the middle lobe. Remove these nodes with care, because if inflamed they may be densely adherent to the artery. When this portion of the pulmonary artery has been exposed, the middle lobe artery will be found near the junction of the horizontal and oblique fissures, taking origin from the anterior surface; the artery to the superior segment will be found at or slightly distal to this level, taking origin from the posterior surface (Fig. 4-78).

If the superior segment is to be removed, first isolate and divide the pulmonary arterial branches to that segment. Figure 4-49 depicts the superior segmental artery ligated and divided in a patient with two ascending arteries to the upper lobe. According to Boyden, 80% of patients will have one artery to the superior segment, 16% will have two arteries, and 4% will have three. If more than one branch exists, the superior branch may arise from the pulmonary artery very close to the ascending artery to the upper lobe, and this latter branch may be accidentally divided or lacerated unless the identity of each branch is determined prior to its ligation. This juxtaposition may be seen in Figure 4-82.

After the arterial branches to the superior segment have been divided, the bronchus to that segment will be exposed lying just medial to the artery, taking origin from the dorsal side of the lower lobe bronchus. Isolate about 1 cm of the superior segmental bronchus, and occlude it distally with a right

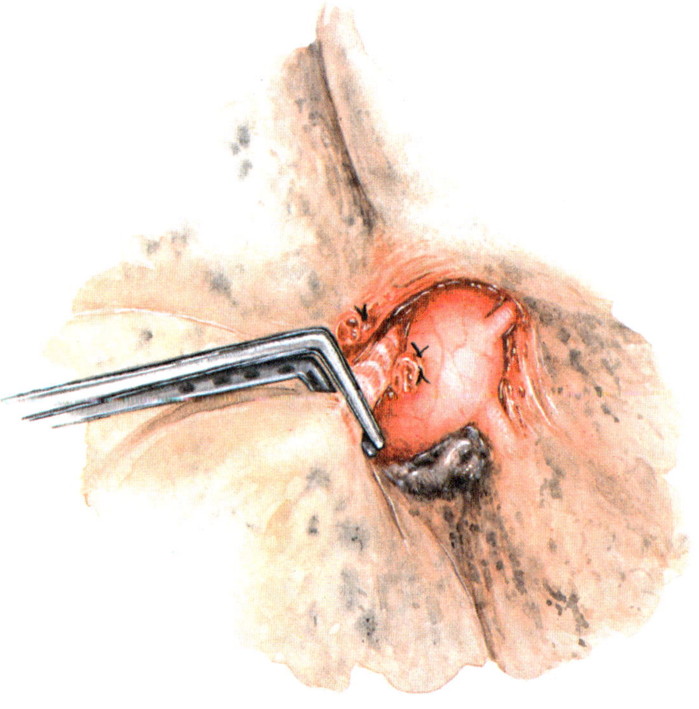

FIG. 4-50.

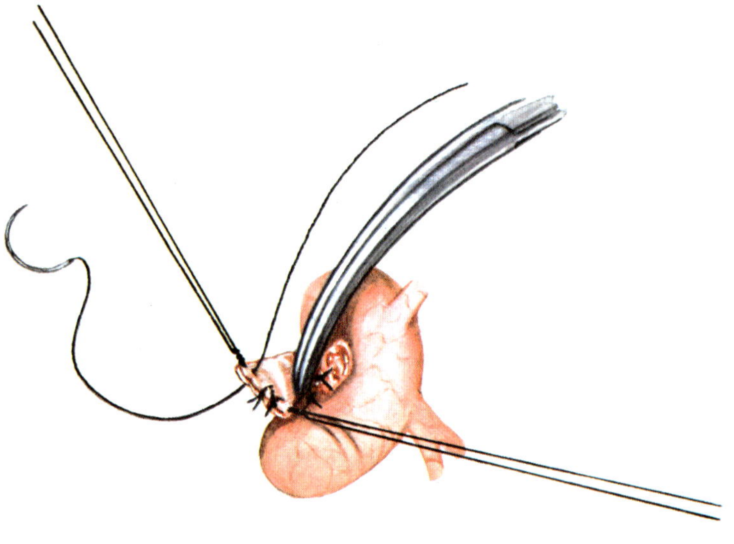

FIG. 4-51.

angle clamp (Fig. 4-50). Divide it 4 mm from the lower lobe bronchus. Close the stump with three or four interrupted 4–0 nonabsorbable sutures (Fig. 4-51).

Grasp the superior segment in the left hand with one finger on the bronchus intermedius distal to the upper lobe bronchus; from the fissure, dissect posteriorly on the bronchus intermedius until an opening is made between the fissure and the posterior area of dissection marked by the finger. The superior segment will now be connected to the upper lobe by a small zone of parenchymal fusion, which should be divided with the GIA stapler. Approximately 50% of patients will have a small venous tributary between the superior segment and the upper lobe, which usually does not require isolation if the stapler is used.

The vein draining the superior segment runs posterior to the lower lobe bronchus; although it can be exposed and divided through the oblique fissure after the superior segmental bronchus has been divided, I have found it easiest

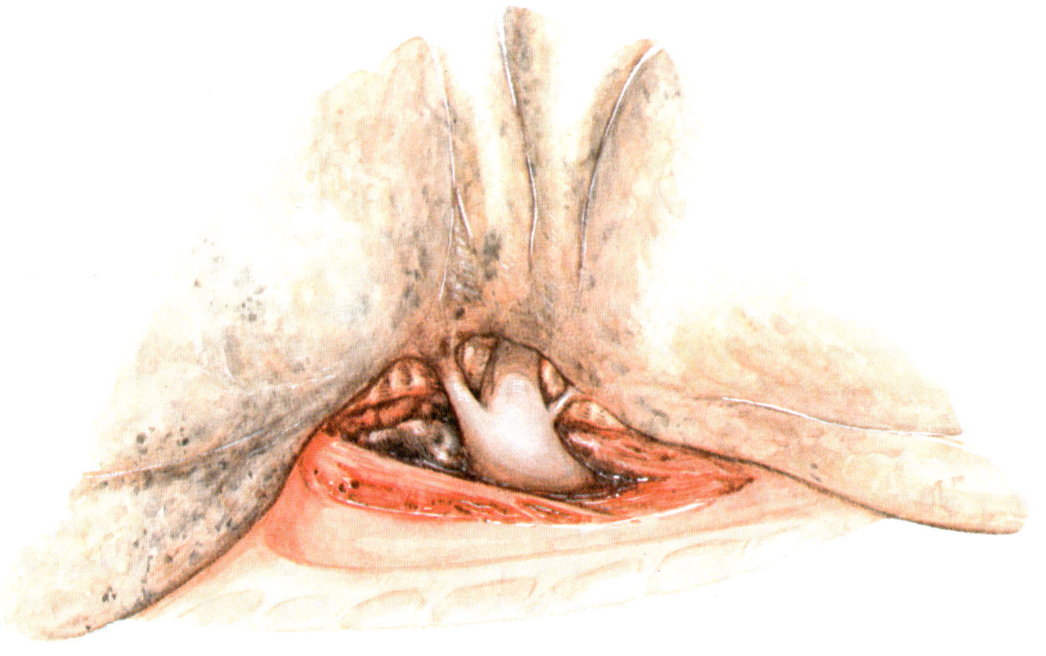

FIG. 4-52.

to approach the vein posteriorly. The inferior pulmonary vein commonly has two divisions (illustrated from the posterior in Fig. 4-52): a superior vein, which drains the superior segment (the smaller vein ascending on the left in Fig. 4-52), and a common basal vein, which drains all of the basal segments. A single superior segmental vein is the most constant anatomic feature of the inferior pulmonary vein. During the exposure of the inferior pulmonary vein from the posterior aspect of the hilus, the superior segmental vein will usually be the first vein encountered ascending posterior to the lower lobe bronchus. Rarely, however, the vein draining the posterior segment of the upper lobe will descend posterior to the lower lobe bronchus and empty into the inferior pulmonary vein. If the division of the upper lobe from the superior segment of the lower lobe has been completed prior to division of the segmental veins, the identity of such a vein should be apparent. Ligate and divide the superior segmental vein; then begin the dissection of the intersegmental plane along the superior segmental vein tributaries. After this plane has been established over a length of 2–3 cm, use the GIA stapler to complete the separation of the superior segment from the basal segments.

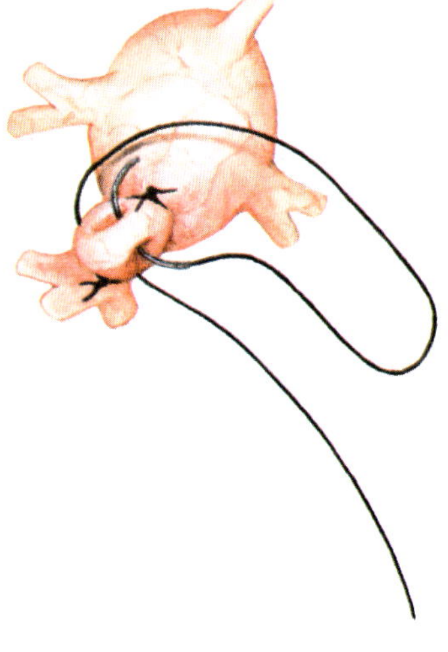

FIG. 4-53.

If the basilar segments are to be removed, identify all arterial branches to the middle lobe and to the superior segment; then ligate and divide the basal portion of the pulmonary artery distal to the above branches. In Figure 4-53, the basilar artery has been doubly ligated and a proximal suture ligature is being placed. The superior segmental artery is the branch on the left, the middle lobe artery is on the right, and the ascending artery to the upper lobe is the uppermost branch. The common basal bronchus is located just medial to the site of division of this artery. This bronchus should be isolated for 1–2 cm distal to the keels of the superior segmental and middle lobe bronchi; identification of these bronchi may require freeing the pulmonary artery proximal to the level of its division for 1–2 cm. Close the stump of the common basal bronchus with 3.5-mm staples in the TA-30 stapler placed 2–3 mm below the next higher branch (Fig. 4-54).

The venous drainage from the basal segments is more variable than is that from the superior segment. It is hazardous to assume that the arrangement

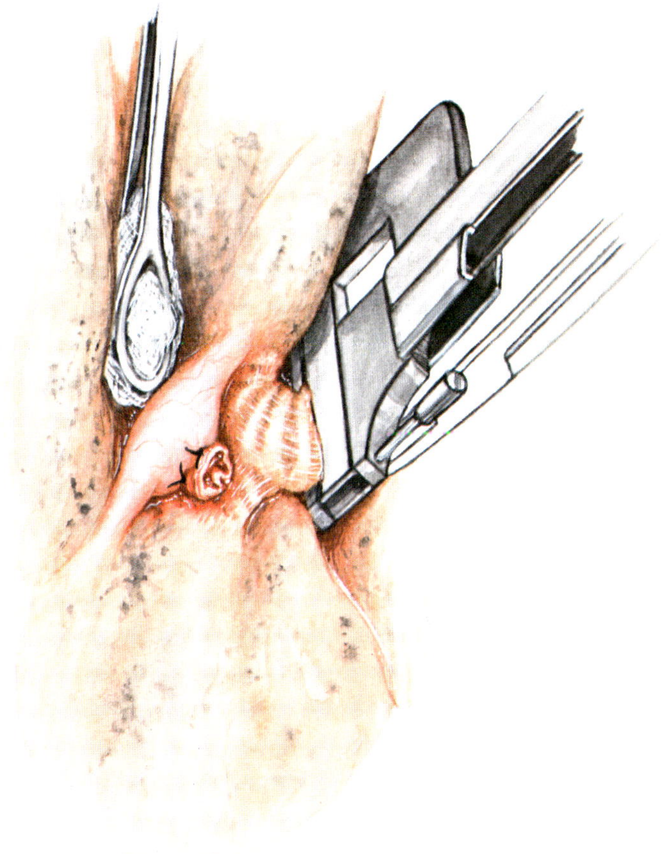

FIG. 4-54.

is always similar to that shown in Figure 4-52, in which all tributaries to the inferior pulmonary vein other than that from the superior segment are from the basal segments. As described previously, there may be a tributary from the posterior segment of the upper lobe, and according to Boyden, the inferior pulmonary vein will receive tributaries from the middle lobe in 10% of patients. The inferior pulmonary vein should be exposed on both its anterior and posterior surfaces as far as its division into principal tributaries. After the above anomalies have been identified or excluded, all other tributaries, exclusive of the vein from the superior segment, should be ligated and divided. Finally the basal segments are removed by dissecting along the intersegmental veins between the superior and basal segments.

Segmental Resections of the Left Upper Lobe

The parenchymal regions occupied by the segments of the left upper lobe and the bronchi supplying them are shown in Figure 4-55. The apical and posterior regions are in actuality subsegments, because the apical and posterior bronchi branch from the left upper lobe bronchus by a single stem that immediately divides. The apical–posterior segment is considered one surgical unit, and usually the two segments of the lingula are also treated surgically as a single unit. Begin any segmental resection of this lobe by incising the pleura overlying the pulmonary artery on the superior aspect of the hilus (Fig. 4-89). Extend this incision anteriorly to the tip of the lingula and posteriorly for several centimeters below the apex of the superior segment of the lower lobe. Both the phrenic nerve and the vagus nerve must be identified and protected. The anterior aspect of the left hilus is illustrated in Figure 4-90.

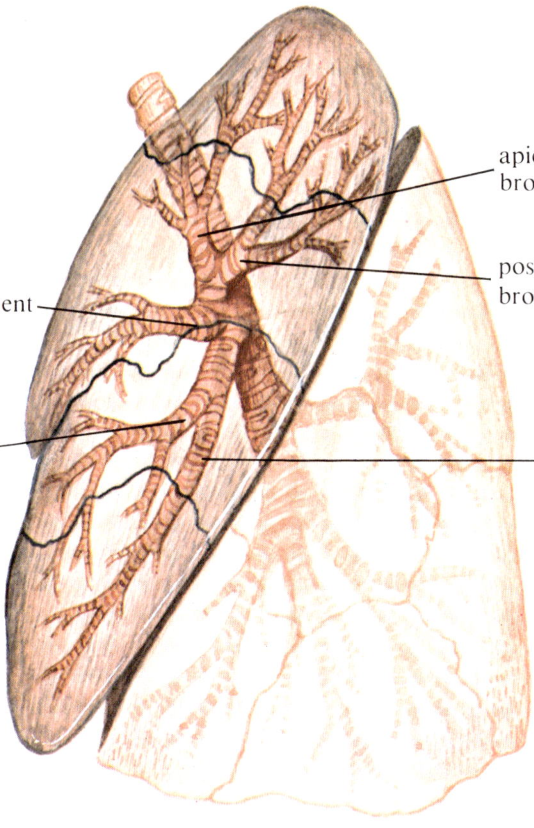

FIG. 4-55.

The phrenic nerve is on the pericardium at the top of the illustration. The left vagus nerve can be seen at the right as it courses over the arch of the aorta, gives off the recurrent laryngeal nerve, and then disappears behind the hilus.

Expose the left pulmonary artery from the pericardium to its entry into the fissure. The lymph nodes above the pulmonary artery and under the arch of the aorta are usually not removed during a segmentectomy, so the dissection of this portion of the artery should be confined to its lateral and inferior aspects in order to protect the recurrent laryngeal nerve from damage. Because the origin of the arteries to the segments of the left upper lobe is less constant than is that of the right upper lobe, all arteries to the left upper lobe must be identified. Figure 4-56 is a sketch of the most commonly found arrangement. In general, the first arterial branch of the left pulmonary artery is to the anterior segment, and occasionally both branches to the anterior segment will arise from this anterior zone, either together or in close proximity. In 20%–30% of patients, an artery to the lingula will be found arising at this level, usually deep (inferior) to the anterior segmental arteries. This lingular artery runs anterior to the upper lobe bronchus and is covered by the apical–posterior vein. In Figure 4-92 the hemostat is retracting the superior pulmonary vein so that the two arteries to the lingula may be seen. The ligated arteries in the figure are those to the anterior segment and to the apical subsegment.

The next group of arteries are those to the apical–posterior segment. These may either arise together (Fig. 4-57) or more commonly as two or three separate arteries. The other branch of the pulmonary artery that can be seen at the level of the fissure in Figure 4-57 is to the anterior segment. Occasionally, one of the posterior segmental arteries may arise as a branch of the artery to the superior segment of the lower lobe (Fig. 4-100d). Just after the left pulmonary artery has descended into the fissure, it commonly gives off the second artery to the anterior segment (Fig. 4-93). In 18% of

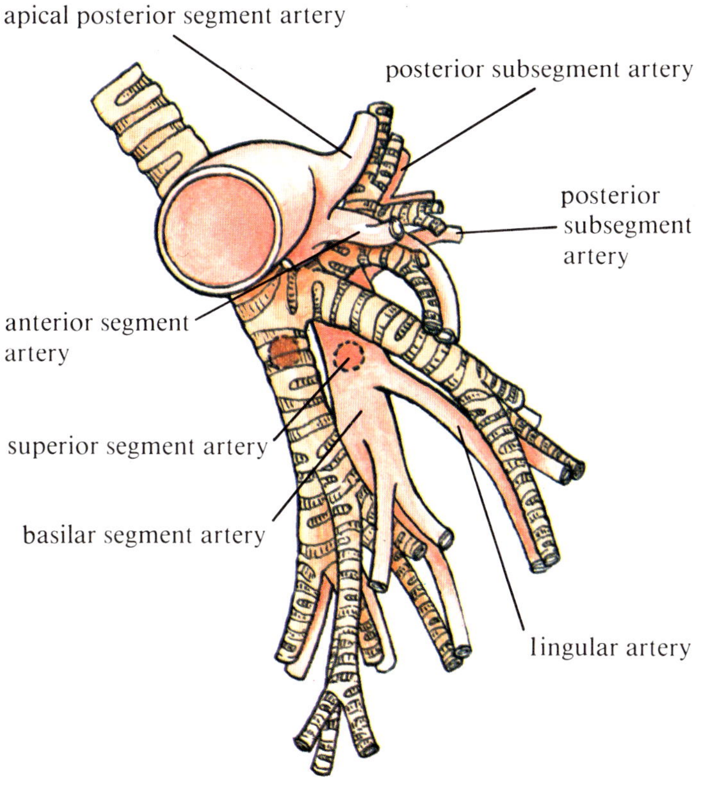

FIG. 4-56. From Segmental Anatomy of the Lung by Boyden EA. Copyright © 1955. Used with the permission of the McGraw-Hill Book Company.

patients, this anterior segmental artery will arise jointly with the lingular arteries. Except in the 8% of patients in whom the total blood supply of the lingula arises from the first or anterior zone of the left pulmonary artery, one or two arteries will ascend to the lingula from the interlobar zone of the pulmonary artery distal to the origin of the artery to the superior segment of the lower lobe (Fig. 4-93).

If the apical–posterior segment is to be resected, ligate and divide the arteries to this segment. In one-third of patients this will require the prior

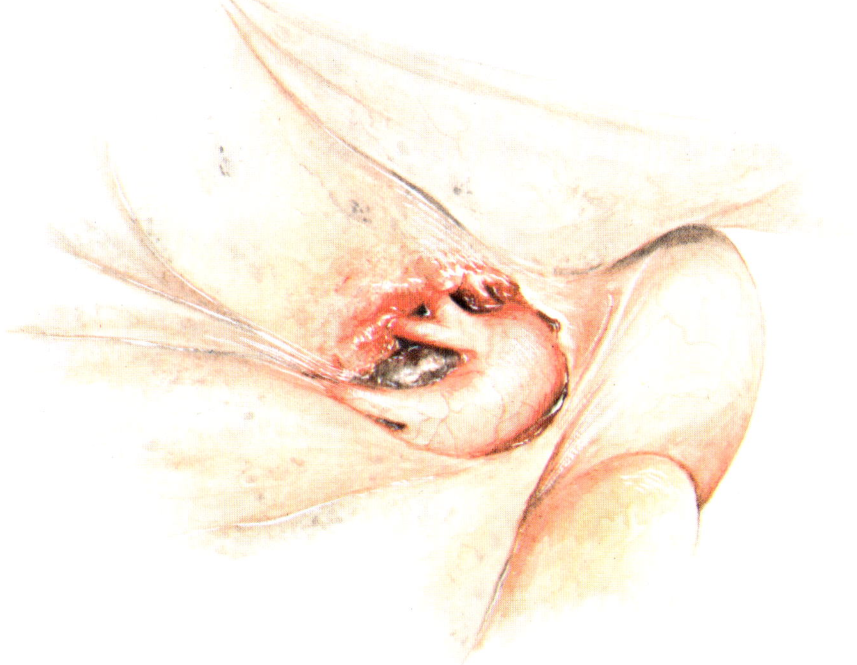

FIG. 4-57.

ligation and division of the superior hilar vein, (Fig. 4-60). The bronchus to the apical–posterior segment will be exposed just inferior to the arteries to that segment (Fig. 4-58). This bronchus is one of the two branches of the superior division of the upper lobe bronchus. To confirm that this bronchus supplies the parenchymal region to be resected, pull slightly on the bronchus or the parenchyma. Place a stay suture on each side of the bronchus (Fig. 4-59). Clamp the bronchus distal to the sutures, divide it, and close the stump with three or four interrupted nonabsorbable sutures.

The left superior pulmonary vein and its principal tributaries must be exposed and identified. The tributaries of this vein are illustrated and labelled in Figure 4-60. Usually three groups of tributaries are found: a superior group draining the apical–posterior segment, a middle group draining the anterior segment, and an inferior group draining the lingula. The superior group may exist either as a single apical–posterior trunk or as two or three separate

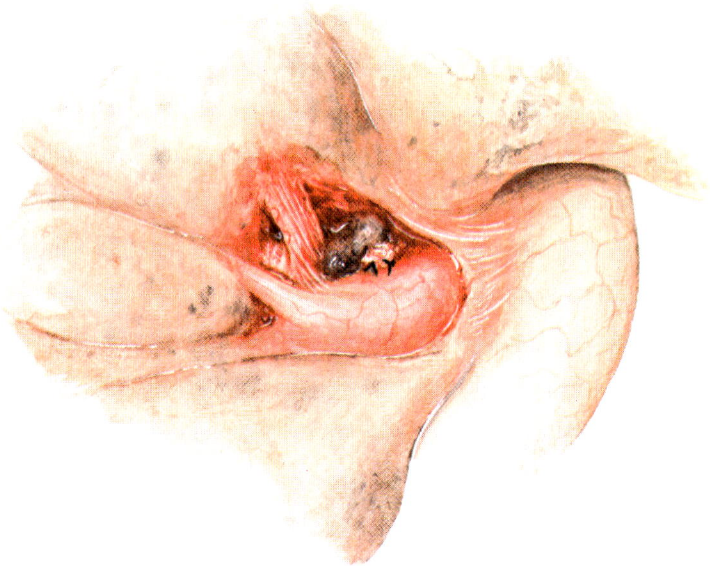

FIG. 4-58.

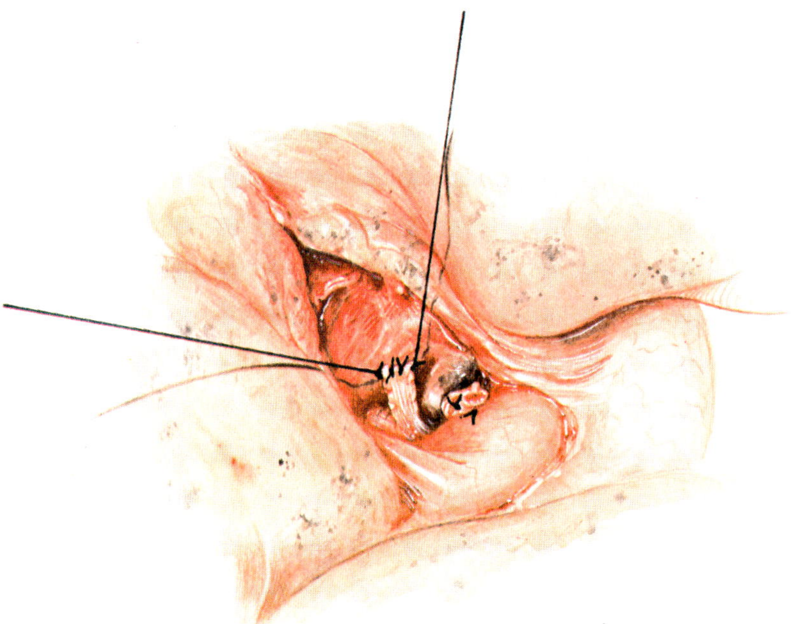

FIG. 4-59.

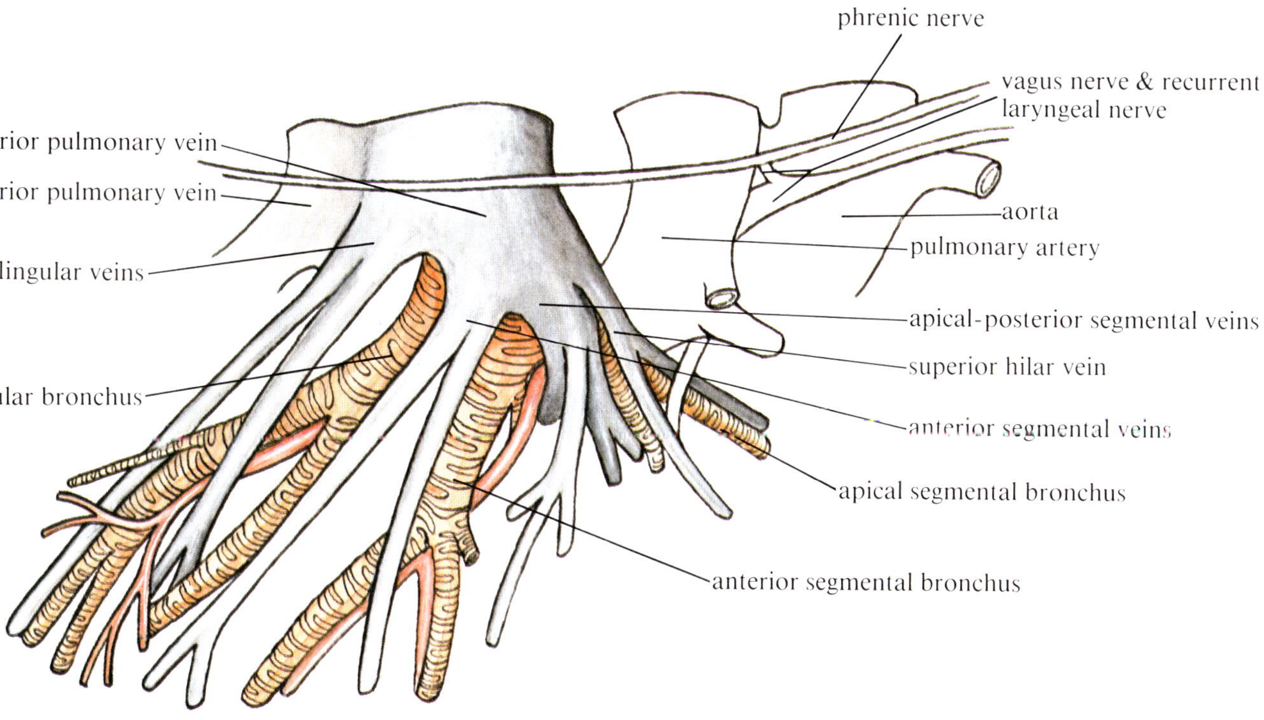

FIG. 4-60. From Segmental Anatomy of the Lung by Boyden EA. Copyright © 1955. Used with the permission of the McGraw-Hill Book Company.

veins draining into the superior pulmonary vein (Fig. 4-60). Ligate and divide those veins from the apical–posterior segment and dissect along the intersegmental tributaries for 2–3 cm until the intersegmental plane is well established and the separation and removal of the segment may be completed with the GIA stapler.

To resect the anterior segment, expose and identify the segmental arterial branches from the anterior and superior part of the pulmonary artery (Fig. 4-56). Expose the interlobar pulmonary artery by identifying the artery in the posterior half of the interlobar fissure and dissecting along the lateral surface of the artery until the fissure communicates with the dissection on the superior part of the artery. Usually the superior segment of the lower lobe can be easily separated from the posterior segment of the upper lobe, but if a significant area of fusion is present, separation may be done with the GIA stapler. As described, there are usually two arteries to the anterior segment, one from the anterior zone of the pulmonary artery and one from the interlobar zone. Ligate and divide both of these segmental arteries. The ligation of the interlobar branch to the anterior segment is shown in Figure 4-61, after the fissure has been dissected down to the artery.

The anterior segmental bronchus is a branch of the superior division of the upper lobe bronchus; it is usually found superior to the location of the interlobar anterior segmental artery. Grasp the hilus of the left upper lobe with one hand and locate the anterior segmental bronchus by palpation. Use a fine hemostatic forceps to dissect this bronchus free of the surrounding lung tissue over a length of 1–2 cm. After confirming that this bronchus supplies the parenchymal region to be resected, divide and close it as described for the apical–posterior segment.

The vein draining the anterior segment may either enter the superior pulmonary vein separately or join the apical–posterior or lingular group of veins. In more than 50% of patients, two or more veins from the anterior segment will be found. In Figure 4-62, the veins to the anterior segment are looped with a ligature. The veins on the right are from the apical–posterior segment and those on the left are from the lingula. Ligate and divide the

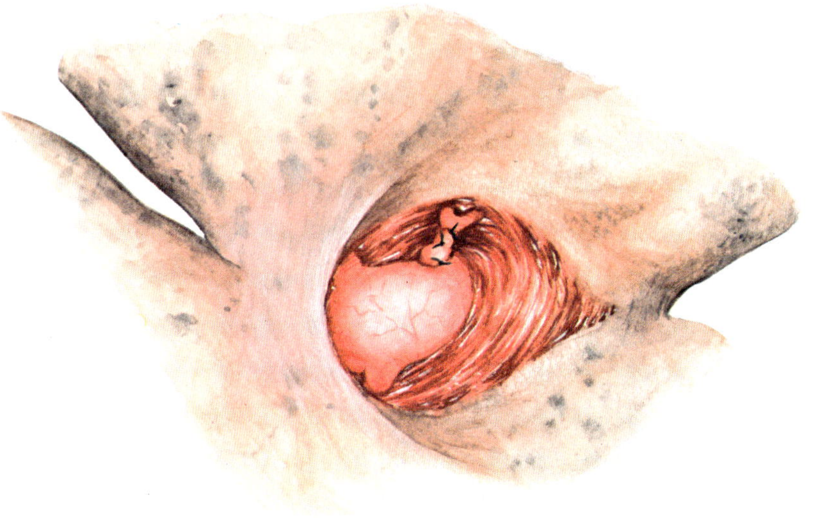

FIG. 4-61.

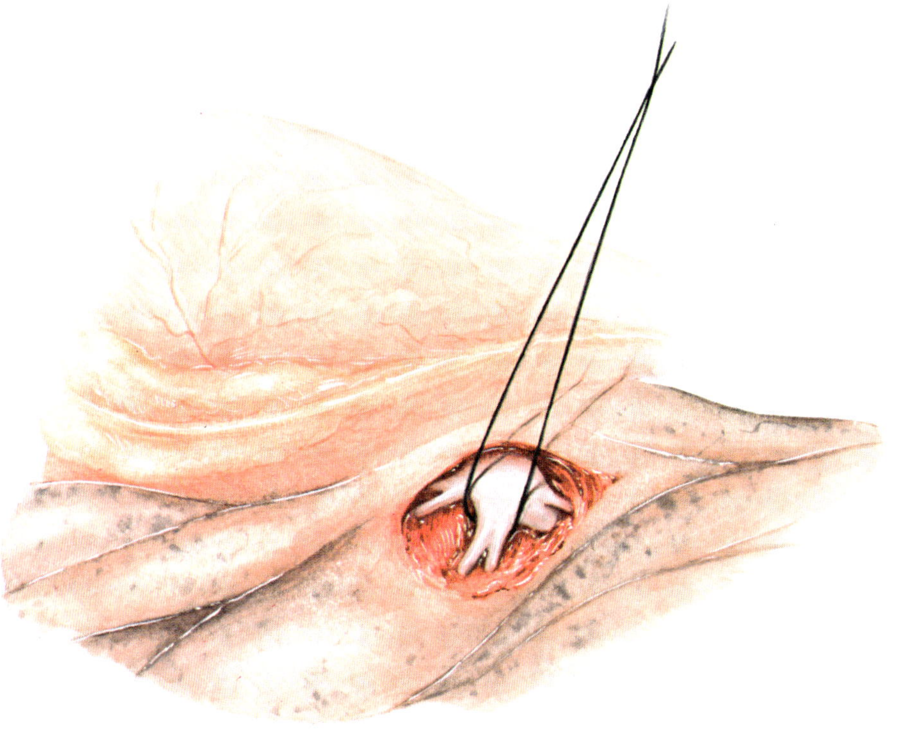

FIG. 4-62.

veins draining the anterior segment and dissect along these veins in the two intersegmental planes for 2–3 cm until the location of each plane is well established. Complete the division of the anterior segment from the lingula and from the apical–posterior segment with the GIA stapler. The removal of the anterior segment will leave the lingula almost completely separated from the apical–posterior segment (Fig. 4-63). Do not attempt to suture these two segments together and so leave a pocket in which blood or serum may collect. Such a pocket, which will also communicate with small bronchi, will most certainly become infected.

The resection of the lingula proceeds by exposing the pulmonary artery in the depths of the interlobar fissure and identifying the arteries ascending to the lingula (Fig. 4-93). Separate the lingula from its attachments with the mediastinum and the left lower lobe. After identifying and protecting

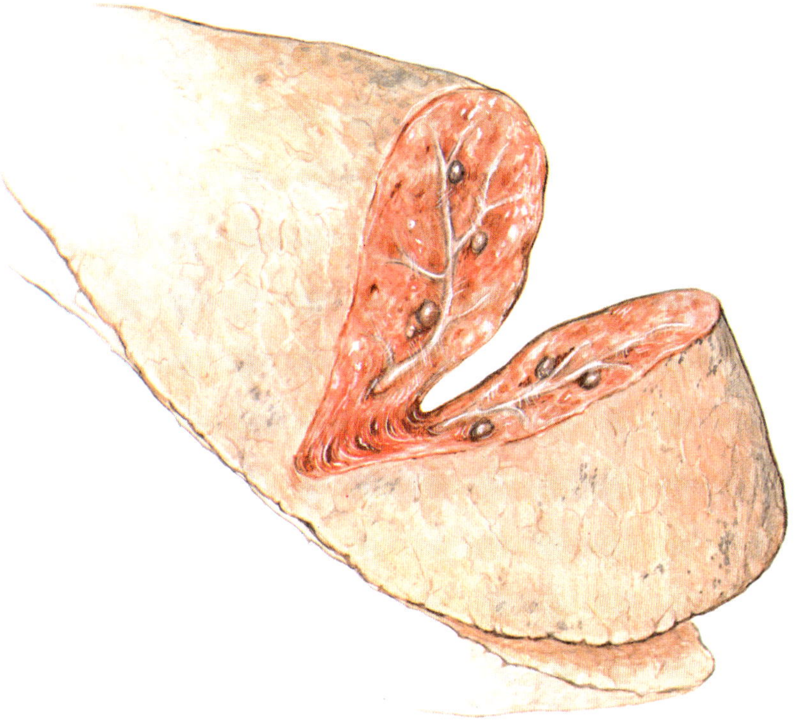

FIG. 4-63.

any arterial branches to the anterior segment, ligate and divide the interlobar lingular arteries. The inferior or lingular division of the upper lobe bronchus is located superior to the origin of the interlobar lingular arteries, but a lymph node, which must be removed, is usually located between these two structures. The main lingular bronchus (inferior division of the upper lobe bronchus) divides to supply both the superior and inferior lingular segments; it should be isolated from the surrounding tissue for a length of 1–2 cm. Free its anterior and superior surfaces under direct vision, because if an arterial branch to the lingula from the anterior zone of the pulmonary artery is present, it will course between the lingular bronchi and the superior pulmonary vein and may be lacerated by an instrument forced around the bronchus. Figure 4-64, a view from the interlobar fissure, shows the ligated stump of the lingular artery and just above it, stay sutures in the stump of the lingular bronchus.

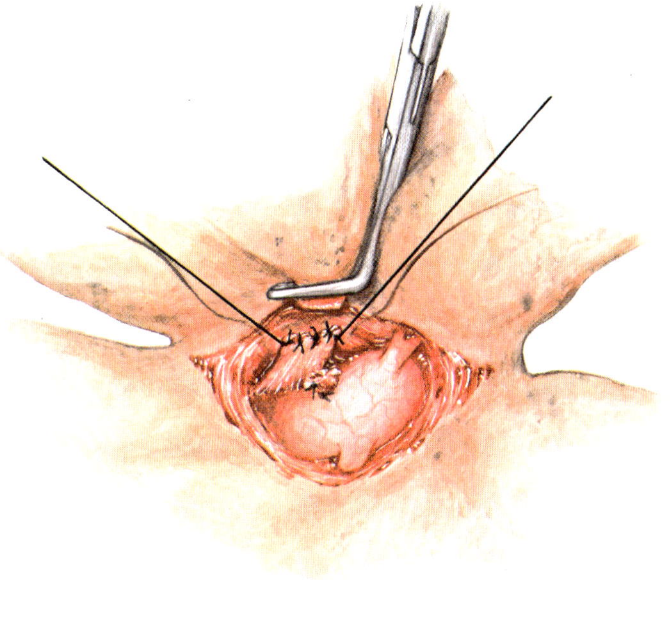

FIG. 4-64.

The distal bronchus is occluded with a right-angle clamp. The segmental artery ascending to the right is an anterior segmental artery to the upper lobe, and the one descending is to the superior segment of the lower lobe.

Approximately 50% of patients will have a single lingular vein that drains into the superior pulmonary vein. The rest have separate veins that drain the superior and inferior lingular segments, usually into the superior pulmonary vein, but in 10% of patients the inferior lingular vein drains into the inferior pulmonary vein. When this latter anomaly occurs, a considerable area of fusion between the upper and lower lobes is usually also present. Ligate and divide the lingular vein, divide the inferior division of the upper lobe bronchus, and close it as described for the apical–posterior bronchus. Examine this region for an anterior lingular artery; if one is present, ligate and divide it. Dissect along the intersegmental vein between the anterior segment and the superior lingular segment until the position of the plane is well established; then complete the separation of the lingula with the GIA stapler.

Segmental Resections of the Left Lower Lobe

The left lower lobe, like the right lower lobe, is composed of five and often six segments: the superior segment, the medial basal, anterior basal, lateral basal, and posterior basal segments, and in 27% of patients, the subsuperior segment. Unlike the right side, however, the plane between the superior segment and the basal segments is not horizontal, but slants obliquely down from the interlobar fissure towards the costovertebral angle.

Two types of segmental resections are performed both on the left lower lobe and on the right lower lobe: a superior segmentectomy sparing the basal segments and a basilar segmentectomy sparing the superior segment. Start either type of resection by dividing the pulmonary ligament (Fig. 4-98) and the reflections of the pleura from the mediastinum to the lower lobe. Incise the pleura at the bottom of the interlobar fissure and locate the interlobar portion of the pulmonary artery by palpating the floor of the fissure near the junction between its middle and posterior thirds. Expose the artery and all of its interlobar branches to the upper and lower lobes.

If the superior segment is to be resected, complete the separation of the parenchyma at the apex of the superior segment from the upper lobe. Because a congenital fusion of these two parenchymal regions is rarely found, the separation may usually be made with scissors, but if the two regions are fused, an artery to the superior segment from the posterior segmental artery of the upper lobe may be found traversing the area of fusion (Fig. 4-100c). Ligate and divide the arteries to the superior segment. These arteries usually arise from the inferior surface of the interlobar portion of the pulmonary artery proximal to the level of the lingular artery. This is illustrated in Figure 4.101 where the artery to the superior segment has been ligated and divided, and a ligature is looped around the basilar artery. Approximately two-thirds of patients will have one superior segmental artery and one-third will have two.

Expose the inferior pulmonary vein from the posterior aspect of the hilus. This vein is commonly formed by the confluence of two trunks: the superior trunk, which drains the superior segment, and the common basal trunk, which drains the basal segments. The superior trunk is the most constant feature of the inferior pulmonary vein; it courses posterior to the lower lobe bronchus at the level of the upper lobe bronchus or superior segmental bronchus. After identifying the principal tributaries of the inferior pulmonary vein, ligate and divide the superior trunk. With both the arteries and the vein to the superior segment divided, the bronchus to this segment can be palpated just anterior to the site of the superior venous trunk or posterior to the superior segmental artery, taking origin from the dorsal side of the lower lobe bronchus. The bronchi to the lower lobe are shown in Figure 4-103; the bronchus to the superior segment is the one descending on the right. Expose the segmental bronchus at its junction with the lower lobe bronchus and isolate a 1–2 cm length. Occlude the bronchus distally with a right-angle clamp; divide it 4 mm from the lower lobe bronchus, and close the stump with three or four interrupted 4–0 nonabsorbable sutures.

Begin the development of the intersegmental plane between the superior and basilar segments by dissecting for 2–3 cm along the tributaries of the superior venous trunk that course in this plane. After the position of the plane has been established, complete the division with the GIA stapler.

The basilar segments are resected by first identifying all of the interlobar branches of the pulmonary artery. Isolate a 1.5-cm length of the common basal artery distal to the origin of the lingular arteries or to the most distal artery to the superior segment if one anomalously arises distal to the lingular arteries; then ligate and divide the basal artery. All tributaries of the inferior pulmonary vein must be identified. Because the superior venous trunk of the inferior vein courses posterior to the lower lobe bronchus, and the basal venous trunk forms inferior or even anterior to the basal bronchi, the anterior, posterior, and inferior surfaces of the inferior pulmonary vein must be exposed. The formation of the left inferior pulmonary vein is less variable than is that of the right, so after the veins draining the superior segment have been identified, the remaining tributaries of the inferior pulmonary vein may be ligated and divided.

The lingula must be separated from the anterior basal segment along the interlobar fissure to the level of the basal bronchus. In 15%–20% of patients there will be a significant area of fusion between these two segments, and the separation will most easily be accomplished with the GIA stapler; otherwise it may be done with blunt dissection. The common basal bronchus and the bronchus to the superior segment should now be easily identified by palpation. The basal bronchus, which lies just medial and slightly anterior to the course of the basal artery, should be isolated for 1–2 cm distal to the origin of the bronchus to the superior segment. Occlude the basal bronchus with a right-angle clamp, divide it 4 mm from the superior segmental bronchus, and close the stump with three or four interrupted 4–0 nonabsorbable sutures.

Dissect for 2–3 cm along the veins marking the intersegmental plane between the superior and basal segments; then complete the separation of the basal segments with the GIA stapler.

Lobectomy

Although the first pulmonary lobectomy has been ascribed to Heidenhain, his was a piecemeal removal of the lower part of a diseased lung. The first reported lobectomy in a human with individual ligation of hilar structures was by H. Morriston Davies, a British surgeon, in 1912.

For many years lobectomy was considered the second choice for resecting a pulmonary carcinoma in a patient who could tolerate a pneumonectomy, but the lack of evidence confirming the superiority of pneumonectomy and the obvious disability resulting from it have caused most surgeons today to use lobectomy as the operation of choice. Because pulmonary resections for tuberculosis are now mostly confined to patients with bacteria resistant to chemotherapy, lobectomy has become the most commonly performed operation for this disease also. In civilian practice, cancer and chronic or uncontrolled infections comprise the most common indications. Bronchiectasis—the condition that provided a principal impetus to the development of segmental and lobar resection—is now rarely seen by the thoracic surgeon.

Right Upper Lobectomy

A moist gauze pack is placed on the lung, and the lung is retracted posteriorly, exposing the hilus and the mediastinum.

The pleura over the anterior portion of the pulmonary hilus is divided between the phrenic nerve and the lung, beginning at the inferior margin of the superior pulmonary vein (the dashed line in Fig. 4-65) and extending superiorly between the azygos vein and the bronchus. The dissection then progresses down the posterior aspect of the hilus past the takeoff of the upper lobe bronchus.

Using mostly blunt dissection, the anterior structures of the hilus are exposed. First, the anterior trunk of the right pulmonary artery is isolated; in Figure 4-66 it is shown looped by a ligature. This artery lies immediately anterior to the upper lobe bronchus and may be covered partially by the apical vein from the right upper lobe.

After the anterior trunk of the pulmonary artery has been ligated and divided, the upper lobe division of the superior pulmonary vein is isolated. The hemostat in Figure 4-67 has isolated the upper lobe tributaries of the superior pulmonary vein, and the ligature is around the vein from the apical segment. The upper division usually consists of three tributaries: the apical vein, running superficially on the mediastinal surface of the lung; the posterior vein, running deep behind the bronchus; and a third, the anterior vein, running between the middle and the upper lobe (Fig. 4-41). The posterior vein is usually covered by the apical and anterior veins from the anterior approach. In Figure 4-67, the inferior division, or middle lobe vein, runs to the right at the top of the figure near the cut edge of the pleura.

If a tumor is close to the junction of these veins, the upper lobe veins may be taken as a whole. Care must be exercised in passing a forceps behind

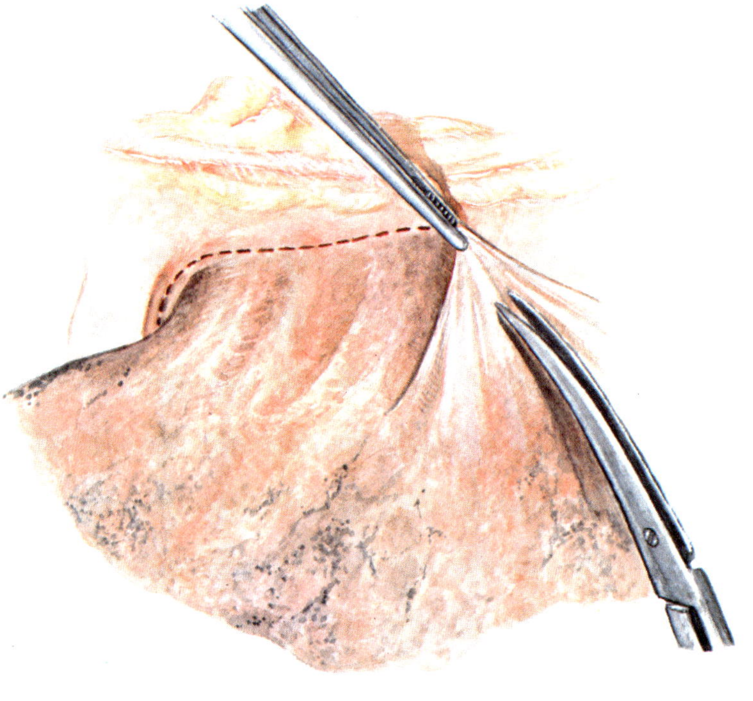

FIG. 4-65.

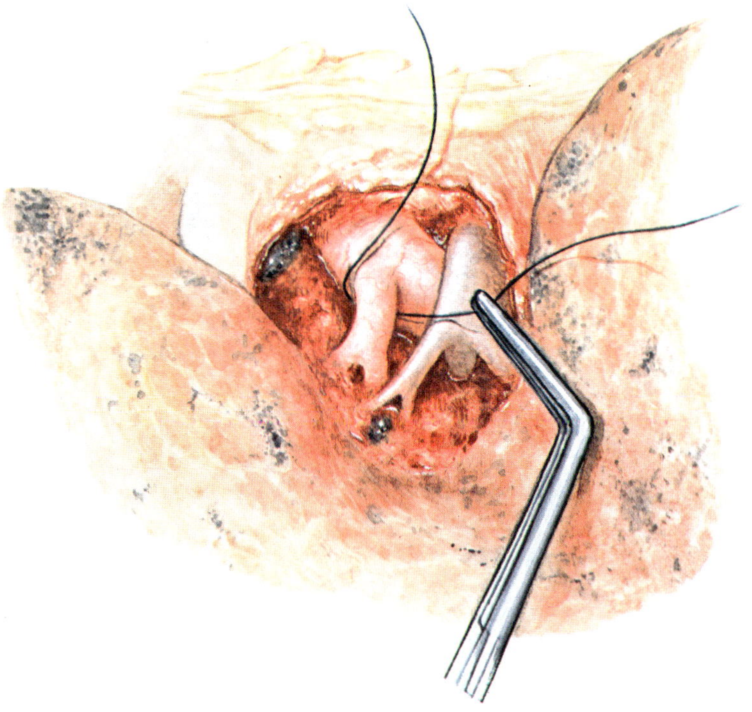

FIG. 4-66.

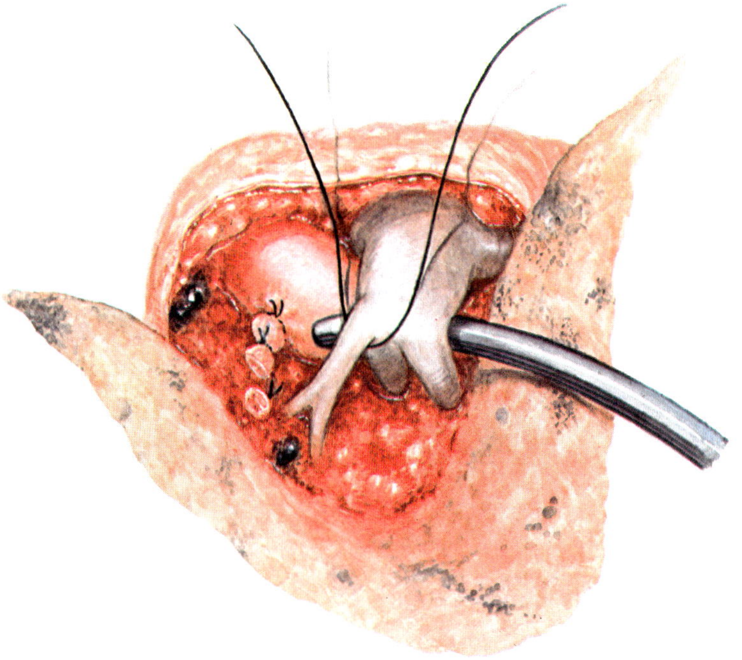

FIG. 4-67.

the whole upper lobe division because often the deep posterior vein does not join in a trifurcation (Fig. 4-67), but rather joins the other two tributaries close to the junction of the upper lobe vein with the middle lobe vein, and the posterior vein may be torn by the forceps if it is forced through the tissue deep to the apical and anterior veins.

If possible, the tributaries of the upper lobe vein should be ligated and divided separately, because 15%–20% of patients have either an anterior vein draining into a middle lobe vein or a middle lobe vein draining into an upper lobe vein. This latter situation is illustrated in Figure 4-68: The ligated stump of the apical vein can be seen; the posterior vein has been ligated and two

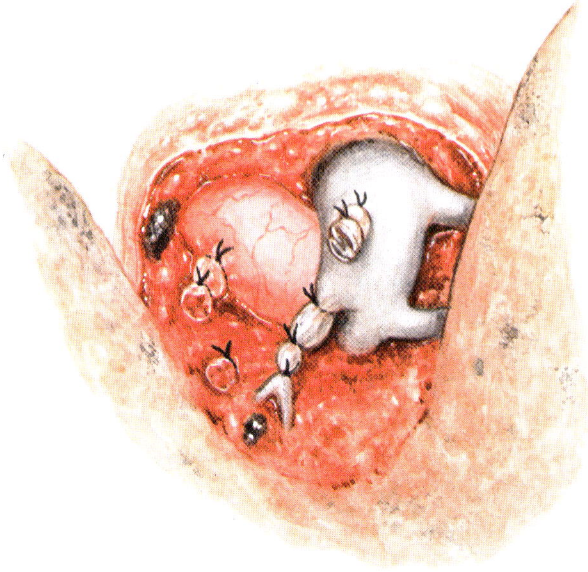

FIG. 4-68.

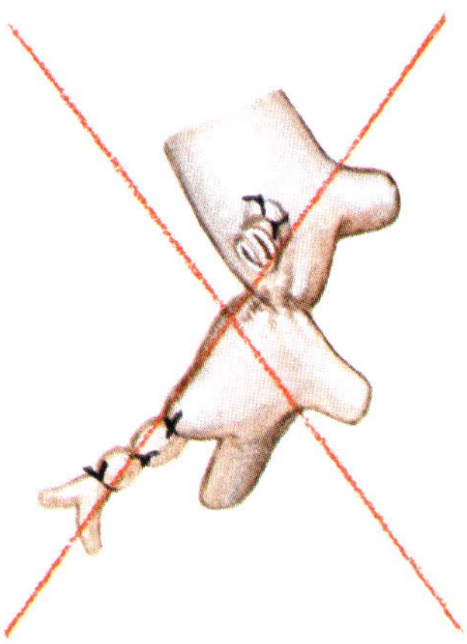

FIG. 4-69.

middle lobe veins have been found running to the right. One of these veins drains into the anterior segment vein. If in patients with this arrangement the upper lobe vein were to be ligated at its junction with the principal middle lobe vein, (Fig. 4-69), the postoperative chest roentgenogram would show diffuse haziness of the middle lobe. This picture is not due to torsion of the lobe, as is often mentioned, but rather to interruption of the venous drainage. The middle lobe may become twisted, but it then infarcts. To preserve venous drainage, the dissection should be continued far enough along the anterior vein to determine whether such connections to the middle lobe exist. If a connection is found, the tributary from the upper lobe is ligated beyond the junction with the middle lobe vein.

After the pulmonary vein tributaries from the right upper lobe have been divided, the interlobar portion of the pulmonary artery should be exposed until the ascending artery to the upper lobe is encountered. With a finger

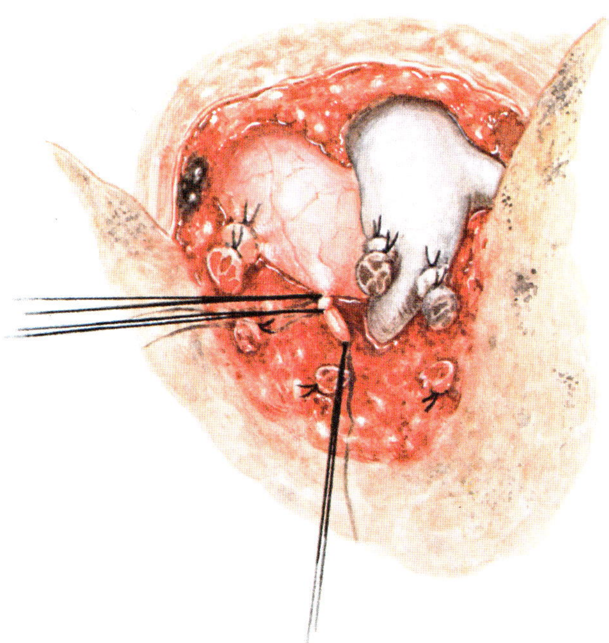

FIG. 4-70.

lying over the interlobar portion of the artery, one can dissect down to the finger at the junction between the major and minor fissures of the right lung. With the interlobar artery exposed, the ascending artery may be safely ligated and divided. Risk of avulsing or cutting the ascending branch exists when dissection is attempted into the fissure before the interlobar portion of the pulmonary artery has been isolated. In Figure 4-70 the ascending artery has been ligated proximally and distally. The ligated stumps of the apical and anterior veins and the truncus anterior are visible. The posterior segmental vein is still intact. In approximately 25% of patients, more than one ascending artery will be found (Fig. 4-49), and on occasion, one ascending artery may take origin from the artery to the superior segment of the lower lobe.

More often than not, the middle lobe is partially or completely fused to the upper lobe. The area of fusion must be divided before the upper lobe is removed. In prior years this division was accomplished by dissecting along the interlobar portion of the pulmonary vein. This dissection was time consuming and sometimes resulted in air leaks. Now a separation is performed by stapling the junction between the middle and upper lobes with the GIA stapler (Fig. 4-71). This stapler places two rows of staples and divides the lung tissue between them (Fig. 4-72). The middle lobe vessels should be protected during this action.

With the upper lobe divided from the middle lobe, the entire interlobar portion of the pulmonary artery is exposed (Fig. 4-73). The ligated stumps of the truncus anterior and the ascending artery to the upper lobe are seen on the main pulmonary artery. In Figure 4-73, the three intact branches of the pulmonary artery extending to the right, from top to bottom, are the middle lobe artery, the basilar artery, and the artery to the superior segment of the lower lobe. The lymph nodes superior to this artery are freed from the pulmonary artery and are kept with the upper lobe bronchus. The hilus of the middle lobe should be dissected as little as possible, because this pedicle is very narrow and may twist postoperatively.

The upper lobe is retracted anteriorly, exposing the posterior portion of the hilus. The bronchus to the upper lobe is freed from its surrounding tissues, and this posterior area of dissection is connected to the interlobar

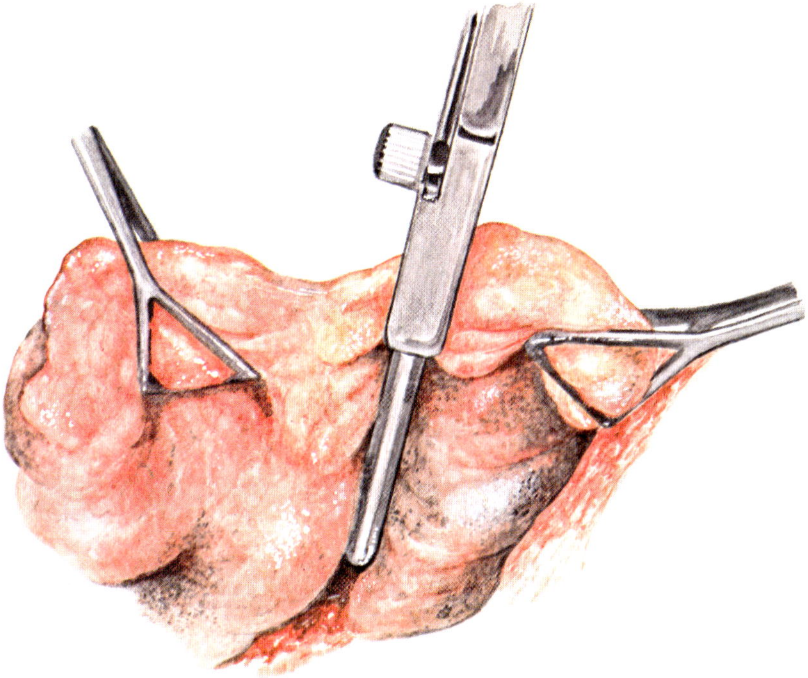

FIG. 4-71.

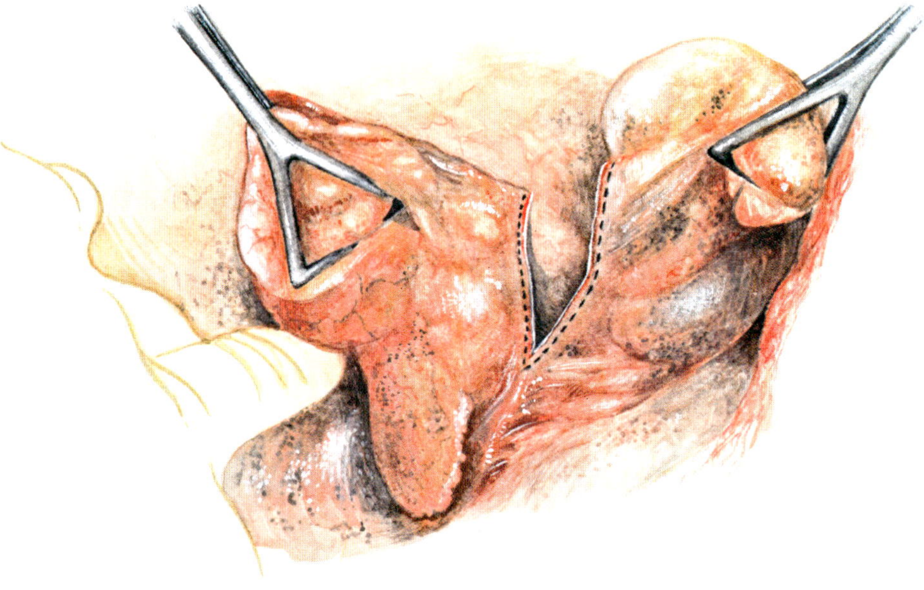

FIG. 4-72.

area of dissection by freeing the region of the bronchus intermedius immediately below the take-off of the upper lobe bronchus (Fig. 4-44). Usually a lymph node that may be calcified and firmly adherent to the bronchus is found in the carina between the upper lobe bronchus and the bronchus intermedius.

Since the superior segment of the lower lobe is often partially fused to the upper lobe, these two regions must be divided in the same manner as that used to separate the upper lobe from the middle lobe. In Figure 4-46, the TA-55 stapler is in position for this division. The artery to the superior segment of the lower lobe lies immediately inferior to the plane of the stapler; it should be seen and protected before staples are placed.

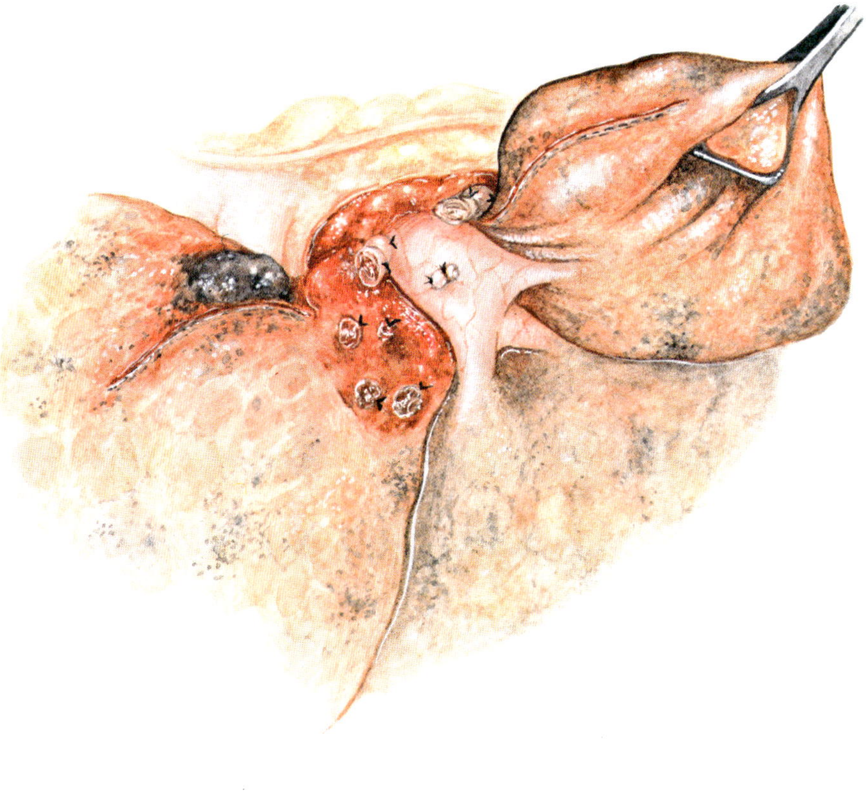

FIG. 4-73.

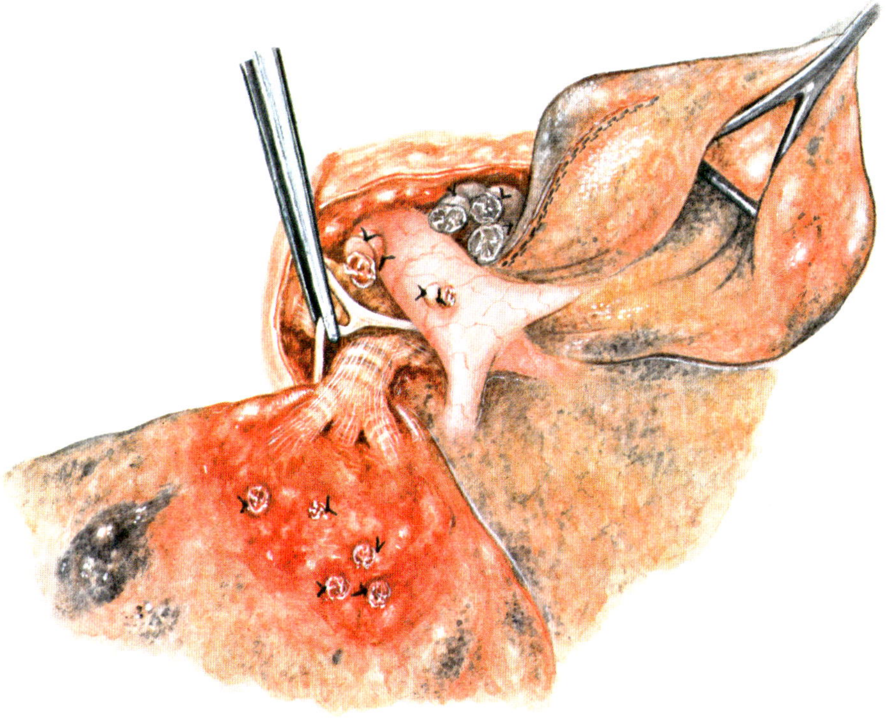

FIG. 4-74.

Figure 4-74 is an anterior view of the hilus after the middle and lower lobes have been separated from the upper lobe, the veins and arteries to the upper lobe have been divided, and the upper lobe bronchus has been exposed. The relationship of the arteries to the middle lobe and the artery to the superior segment of the lower lobe within the interlobar plane is again apparent. In patients with chronic lung disease, there is often a large bronchial artery running over the anterior or posterior aspect of the upper lobe bronchus. In

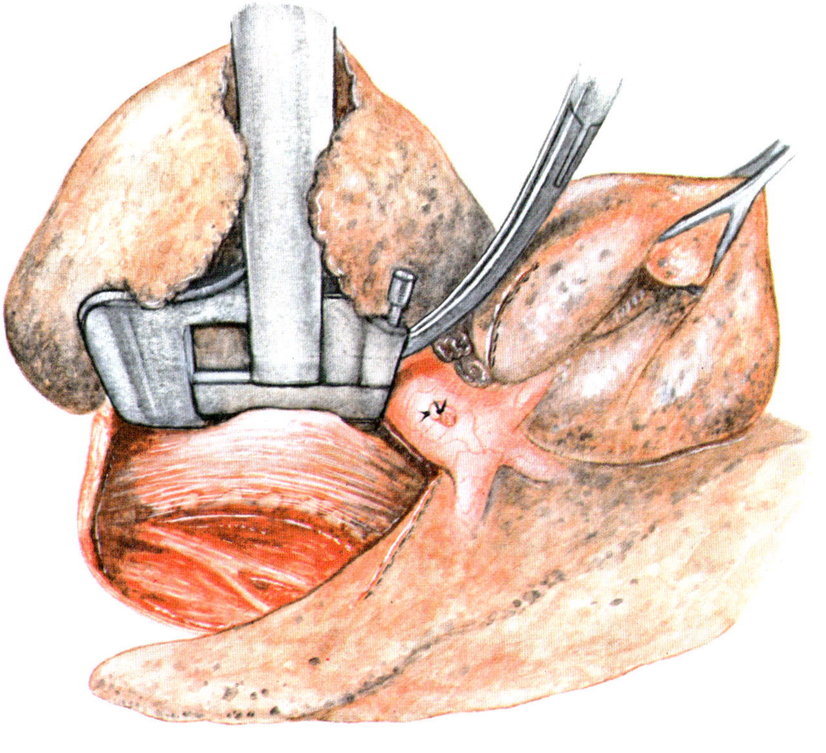

FIG. 4-75.

Figure 4-74, such an artery is being held by the forceps. This artery will be separately ligated and divided before division of the bronchus.

Figure 4-75 is a view from the posterior aspect of the hilus, showing the TA-30 stapler with 3.5-mm staples being used to close the bronchus. After the staple line has been placed, a Sarot bronchus clamp is placed distal to the staples; the bronchus is divided and the lobe removed. Figure 4-76 is a view of the hilus after the upper lobe has been removed. The stapled stump of the upper lobe bronchus may be seen, and just posterior to the right main bronchus, the vagus nerve is visible. The three ligated and divided venous tributaries from the right upper lobe are apparent above the middle lobe artery. The arteries to the superior segment and to the basilar segments extend inferiorly. If the closure is airtight, a flap of pleura is sutured over the cut end of the bronchus (Fig. 4-77).

The pulmonary ligament is divided to permit the lower and middle lobes to rise in the thoracic cavity and thereby decrease the likelihood of an apical air space. Care must be taken not to injure the inferior pulmonary vein, which forms the superior margin of this ligament. There are small troublesome vessels in the pulmonary ligament that may be the source of considerable postoperative bleeding if they are not cauterized or ligated.

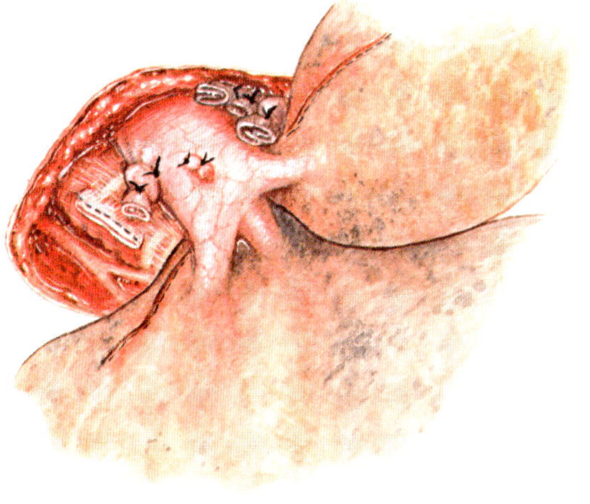

FIG. 4-76.

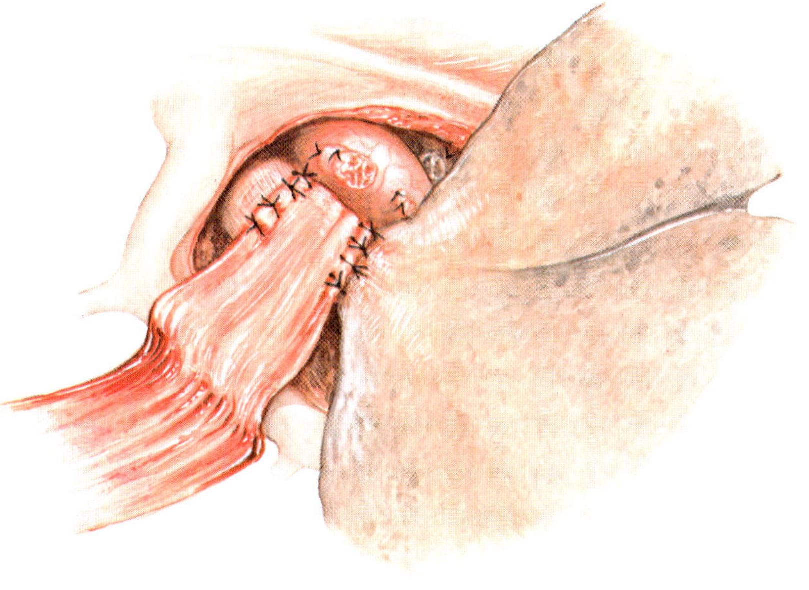

FIG. 4-77.

Right Middle Lobectomy

The middle lobe normally comprises 8% of the total lung mass. The upper surface is usually wholly or partially fused to the upper lobe, and the lower surface may be partially fused to the lower lobe. Because of the close relationship between the middle lobe bronchus and the bronchus to the superior segment of the lower lobe, a centrally occurring carcinoma in either the middle lobe or the superior segment must be removed by a middle–lower bilobectomy rather than by a single lobectomy.

After the exploration of the right thoracic cavity, the depth of the oblique fissure is exposed and dissected between the middle and lower lobe. As the posterior portion of the middle lobe is mobilized, a lymph node is usually encountered and should be carefully removed. Immediately under this node is the interlobar portion of the pulmonary artery. As dissection proceeds superiorly on the lateral surface of this artery, the middle lobe artery or arteries taking origin from the anterior surface and the artery to the superior segment, taking origin from the posterior surface, will be encountered at approximately the same level. Figure 4-78 illustrates the completion of this dissection. The pulmonary artery is shown in the depths of the oblique fissure, which can be seen extending toward the top and the bottom of the figure. The horizontal fissure extends toward the right near the center of the figure. The middle lobe artery is running toward the right, dividing just before it enters the parenchyma of the middle lobe. The artery to the superior segment extends to the left at the same level as the middle lobe artery. The artery to the basilar segments is running down and slightly to the left. The small artery near the top of the dissection is the ascending artery to the upper lobe. The

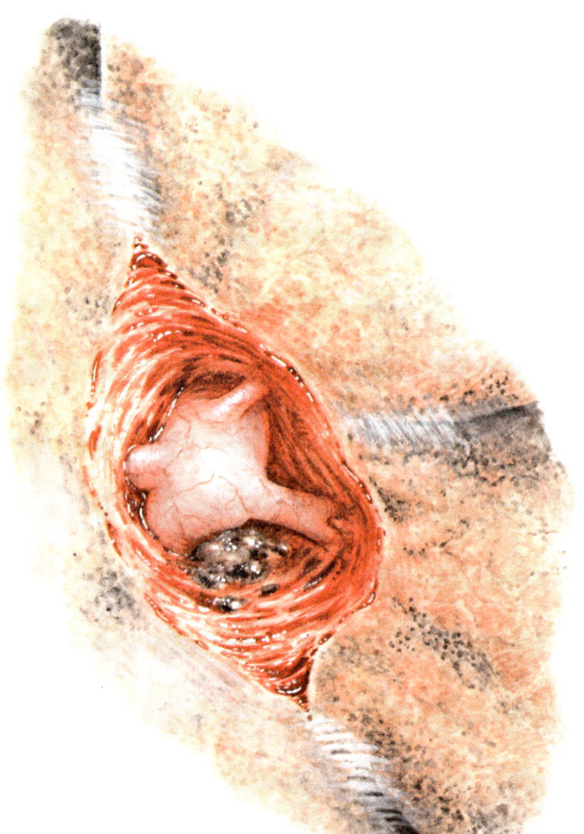

FIG. 4-78.

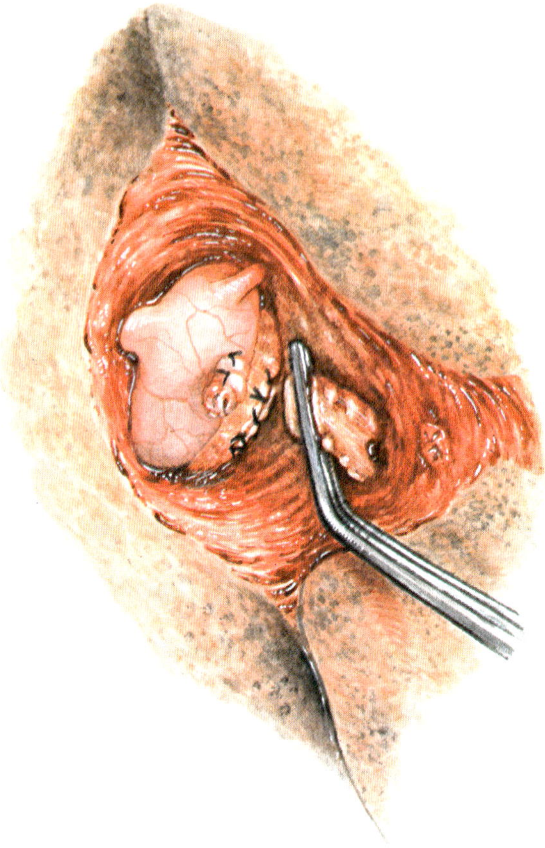

FIG. 4-79.

lymph nodes overlying the artery have been dissected toward the middle lobe and may be seen just under the middle lobe artery. In approximately half of patients, two or three arteries to the middle lobe will be found.

After these arteries are ligated and divided, the bronchus to the middle lobe, which lies just medial to the junction of the middle lobe artery with the basal artery, can be exposed, but often the basal artery must be freed from its attachment to the bronchus intermedius over a short distance to permit good visualization of the origin of the middle lobe bronchus. With traction on the lower lobe, the basilar bronchus and middle lobe bronchus may form a straight continuum and may be misinterpreted as the same bronchus. Such misinterpretation can lead to a division of the wrong bronchus. The bronchus to the middle lobe should be divided close to the lower lobe bronchus and the proximal stump closed with interrupted 4–0 nonabsorbable sutures. In Figure 4-79, the middle lobe bronchus is occluded with a right-angle clamp. The stump of the bronchus, just deep (medial) to the stump of the middle lobe artery, has been closed with five sutures.

The veins from the middle lobe are approached by incising the pleura overlying the anterior portion of the hilus to the level of the inferior pulmonary vein. Both divisions of the superior pulmonary vein should be visualized and the middle lobe veins dissected free for a distance of 15–20 mm. In approximately 50% of patients, a single trunk drains the middle lobe, and in 50%, two or more veins are present. According to Boyden, 14% of those lobes with two or more veins will drain into an upper lobe tributary and in 8% into the inferior pulmonary vein. It is to visualize these anomalies and prevent damage to the upper or lower lobe veins that the more extensive dissection is necessary. Figure 4-80 is a view of the hilus with the lung retracted posteriorly, showing the middle lobe vein ligated prior to its division. The middle

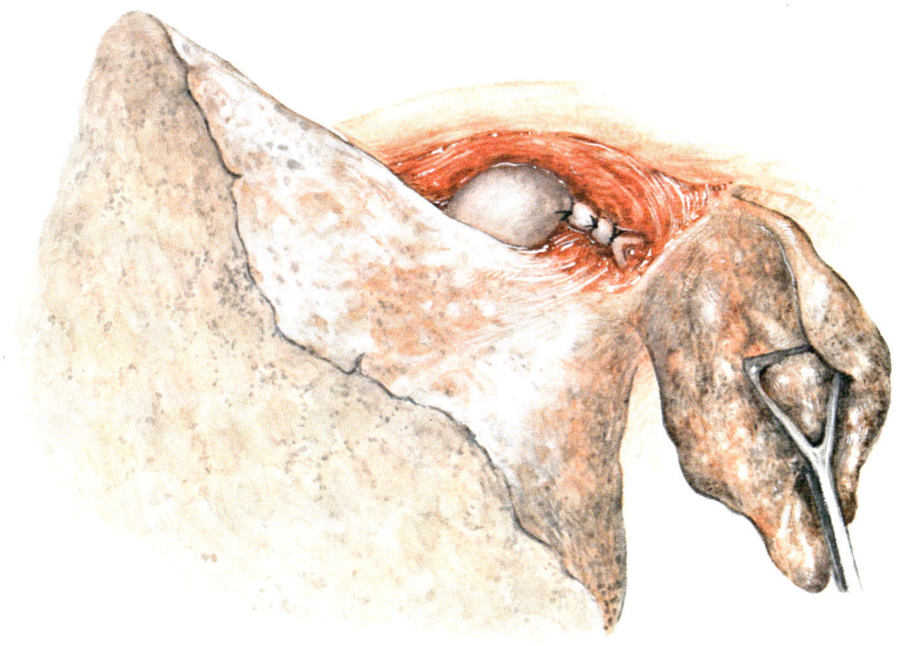

FIG. 4-80.

lobe is held by the lung-grasping clamp, and the upper lobe is on the left. After ligating and dividing the middle lobe veins, the interlobar portion of the pulmonary artery should be visible from the truncus anterior to the arteries of the superior segment so that injury to the upper or lower lobe arteries will not occur when the middle lobe is divided from the upper lobe. Since the fissure between these two lobes is rarely complete, the division is achieved with the GIA (Fig. 4-71) or the TA-90 stapler with 4.8-mm staples.

Right Lower Lobectomy

The normal right lower lobe comprises 25% of the total lung mass. The lobectomy is begun by dividing the pleura at the root of the lung beginning with the pulmonary ligament and extending anteriorly to the level of the superior pulmonary vein and posteriorly to the upper lobe bronchus. The arteries and bronchi of the right lower lobe are best approached through the oblique fissure. The interlobar portion of the right pulmonary artery is found immediately anterior to the junction of the oblique and horizontal fissures. The pleura at the bottom of the oblique fissure should be divided and the posterior portion of the middle lobe reflected superiorly. Often a lymph node lying immediately lateral to the pulmonary artery will be found—it must be carefully removed to expose the artery (refer to Fig. 4-78 and its description). The arterial supply to the superior segment of the lower lobe arises from the posterior portion of the pulmonary artery; in 80% of patients this will be a single artery, but in 20%, two or more arteries to the superior segment are present. These arteries take origin from the interlobar portion of the pulmonary artery either at or only slightly distal to the origin of the middle lobe artery; they must usually be ligated and divided separately from the basal segment artery.

In Figure 4-81, the artery to the superior segment has been doubly ligated and a proximal suture ligature is being placed. In approximately 10% of patients, a branch of a superior segment artery supplies a portion of the posterior segment of the right upper lobe. This branch may not be obvious due to the numerous lymph nodes surrounding the superior segmental artery and bronchus. It should be sought, however, and either spared or ligated as

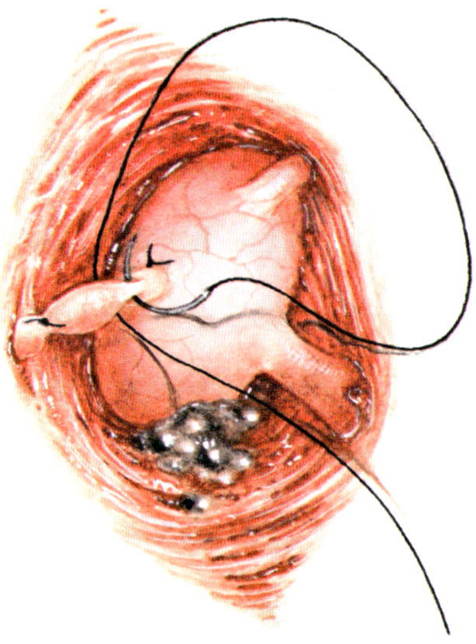

FIG. 4-81.

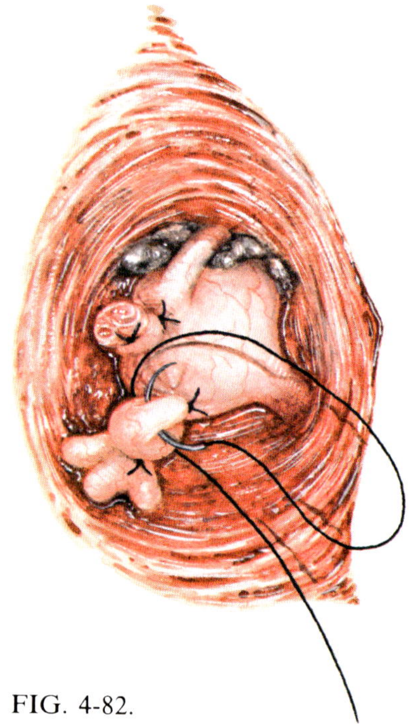

FIG. 4-82.

the clinical situation demands. The basilar portion of the pulmonary artery is then ligated and divided below the middle lobe artery. Figure 4-82 shows the basilar artery doubly ligated and a proximal suture ligature in place. The stump of the divided artery to the superior segment of the lower lobe can be seen at the left. In this patient, one of the ascending arteries to the posterior segment of the upper lobe originated from the pulmonary artery very close to the artery to the superior segment.

The inferior pulmonary vein is found inferior and slightly posterior to the basal bronchus. Unlike its occurrence in the left lung, rarely is there only one pulmonary vein on the right; yet it is well to remember that in one report such a situation existed in 3% of the lungs examined and in 4%, one middle lobe vein drained into the inferior vein. Free the inferior vein for a distance of at least 15 mm; then, using the TA-30 stapler, staple the vein closed with two rows of 30-V staples and divide between them (this is depicted from the anterior aspect of the hilus in Fig. 4-83). The cut edge of the pulmonary ligament extends to the right of the stapler.

The oblique fissure is usually incomplete at its upper end where the superior segment is fused to the posterior segment of the upper lobe, and it is occasionally incomplete at its lower end where the lower lobe may be partially fused to the middle lobe. After the arteries and vein have been divided and the bronchus freed from its surrounding lymph nodes, the areas of fusion in the fissure are divided with the GIA stapler (Fig. 4-84). The divided stumps of the basilar artery and the artery to the superior segment can be seen in the figure. The ascending artery to the upper lobe runs superiorly and to the right; the middle lobe artery is below it.

The bronchus to the lower lobe lies just medial to the pulmonary artery in the oblique fissure and will be apparent after both the basal and the superior segmental arteries are ligated and divided. The bronchus to the superior segment usually arises as a single stem with its orifice nearly opposite that of the middle lobe bronchus. In 5%–6% of patients, two bronchi to the superior segment will be found. Because of its proximity to the middle lobe bronchus,

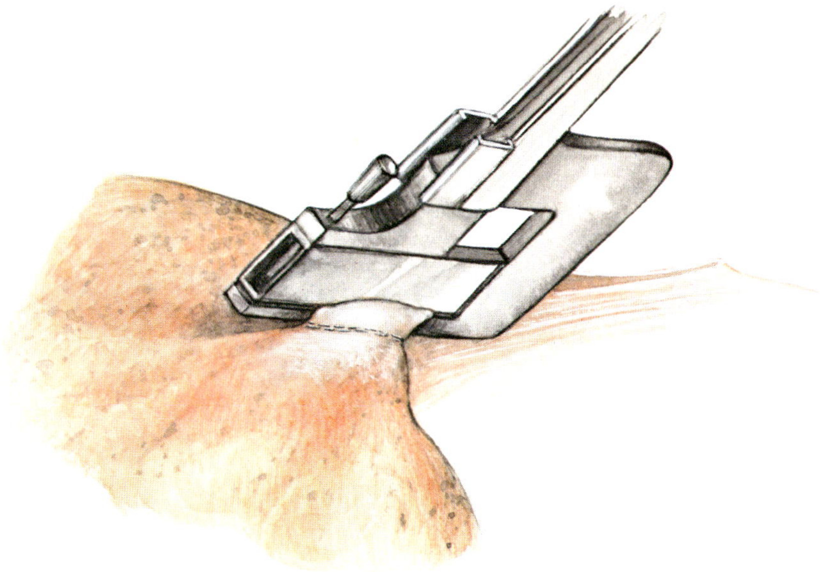

FIG. 4-83.

the superior segment bronchus must be divided separately from the basal bronchus. In Figure 4-85, the superior segmental bronchus has been occluded by the right-angle clamp. The overlying lymph nodes and the interlobar portion of the pulmonary artery have been reflected superiorly; notice the middle lobe bronchus arising immediately opposite the bronchus to the superior segment. The stump of the superior segmental bronchus is closed with four interrupted 4–0 nonabsorbable sutures (Fig. 4-86). The pulmonary artery in this figure is being held away from the bronchus with forceps.

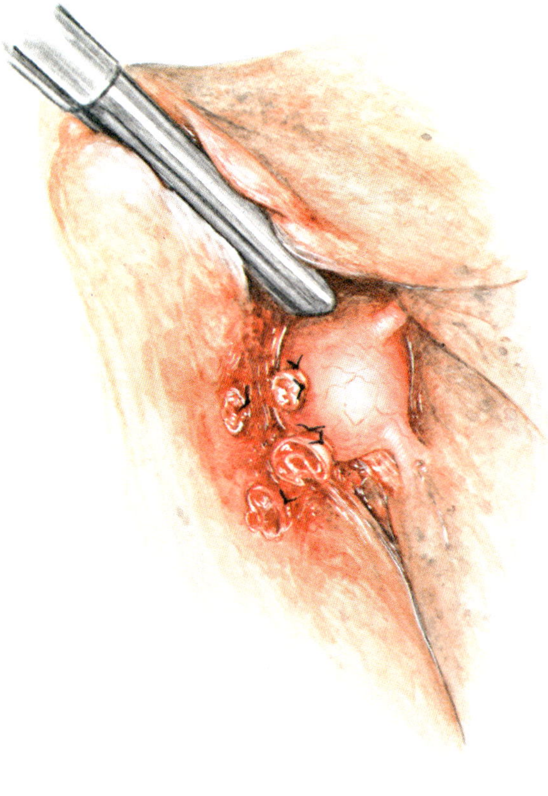

FIG. 4-84.

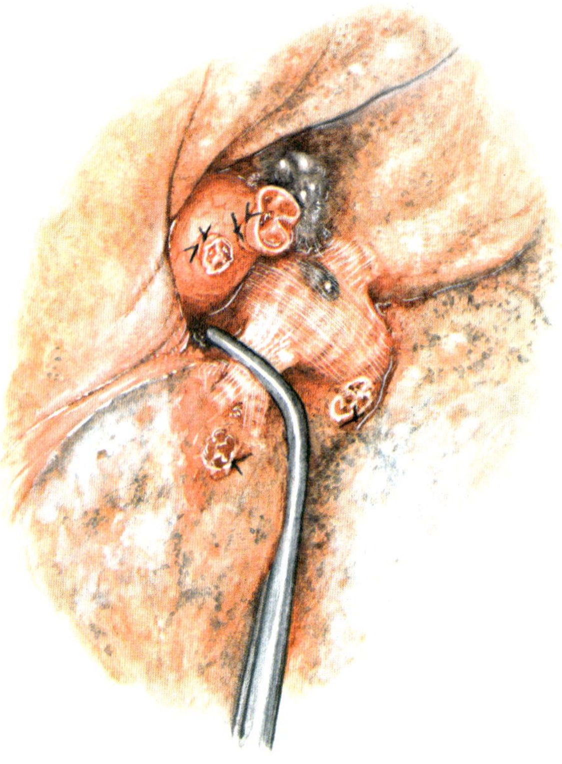

FIG. 4-85.

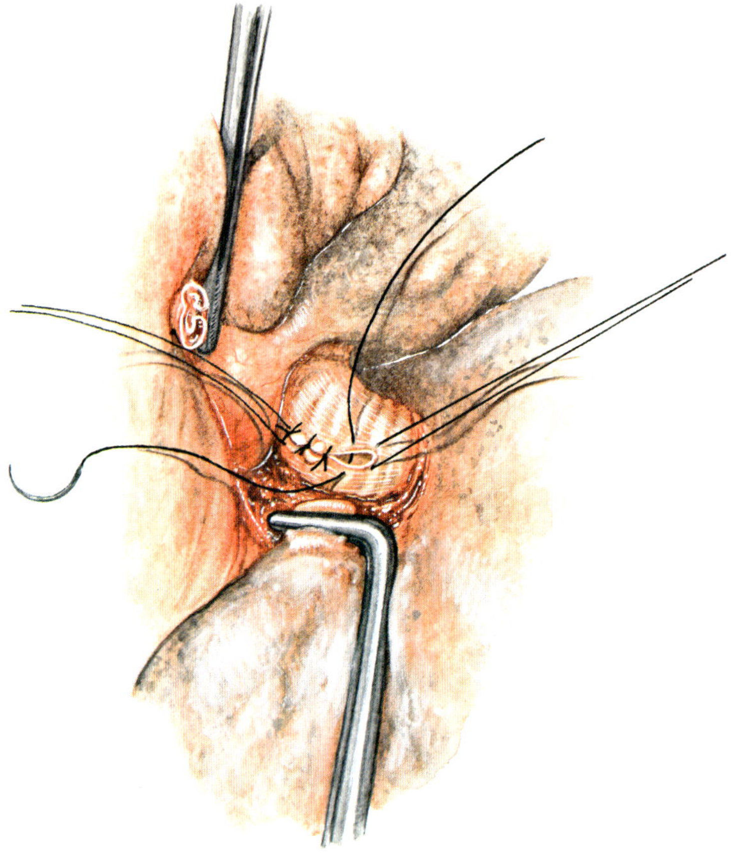

FIG. 4-86.

The basal bronchus is stapled closed distal to the middle lobe bronchus with 3.5-mm staples in the TA-30 stapler and divided distal to the staple line (Fig. 4-87). If the bronchial closure is airtight, a flap of parietal pleura is sutured over the end of the bronchial stump. Figure 4-88 is a view of the hilus after removal of the lower lobe. The upper lobe is at the left of the figure and the middle lobe is being held by the surgeon's hand at the top. The ligated arterial stumps on the interlobar portion of the pulmonary artery are just below the finger; below the artery are the stumps of the superior segmental and basilar bronchi. The stapled end of the inferior pulmonary vein is just to the right of the bronchus. The phrenic nerve can be seen running on the surface of the pericardium.

Left Upper Lobectomy

The left upper lobe comprises about 22% of the total lung mass. The lobectomy is started by dividing the pleura from the level of the pulmonary ligament anteriorly, over the superior part of the hilus, and down the posterior aspect between the vagus nerve and the lung to a level below the interlobar fissure. Figure 4-89 is a view of the anterior superior aspect of the left pulmonary hilus with the main pulmonary artery exposed as it emerges from under the arch of the aorta. The phrenic nerve is anterior, coursing over the pericardium. The vagus nerve is just posterior to the phrenic nerve on the arch of the aorta, but runs posterior to the pulmonary hilus. The lateral surface of the pulmonary artery is exposed from the superior aspect of the hilus, where the artery emerges under the arch of the aorta, to the point where it descends into the interlobar fissure.

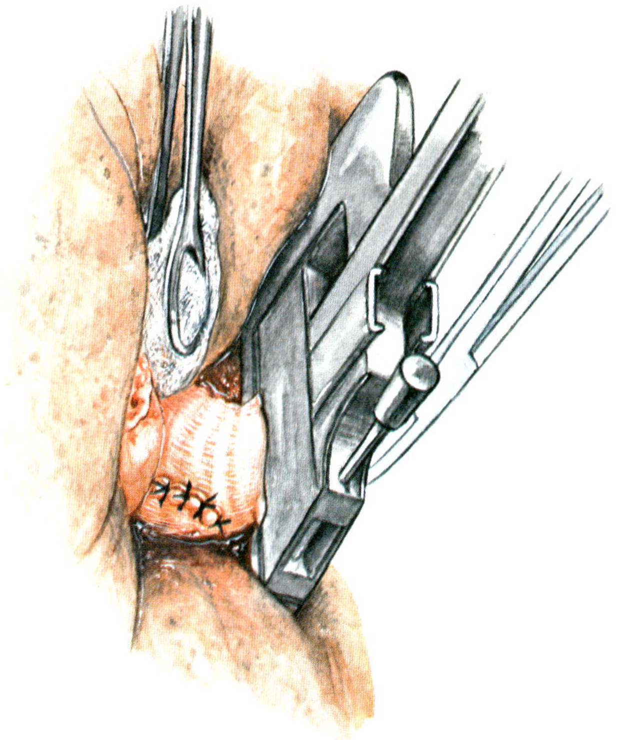

FIG. 4-87.

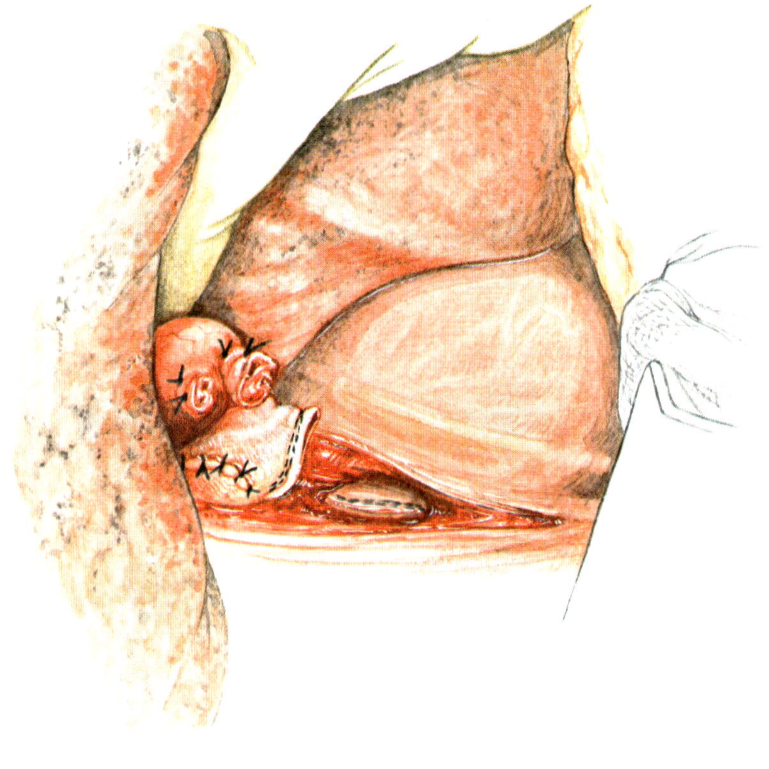

FIG. 4-88.

The left pulmonary artery differs from the right in that it arches over the upper lobe bronchus rather than under it and gives off a greater number, from four to eight, separate arteries to the upper lobe. Care must be taken in exposing the artery because in over one-third of lungs a superior hilar vein arching over the superior aspect of the hilus will be found immediately superficial to the pulmonary artery (Fig. 4-60). This vein, if present, should be ligated and divided before exposing the superior branches of the pulmonary artery. If the lymph nodes under the arch of the aorta are to be removed

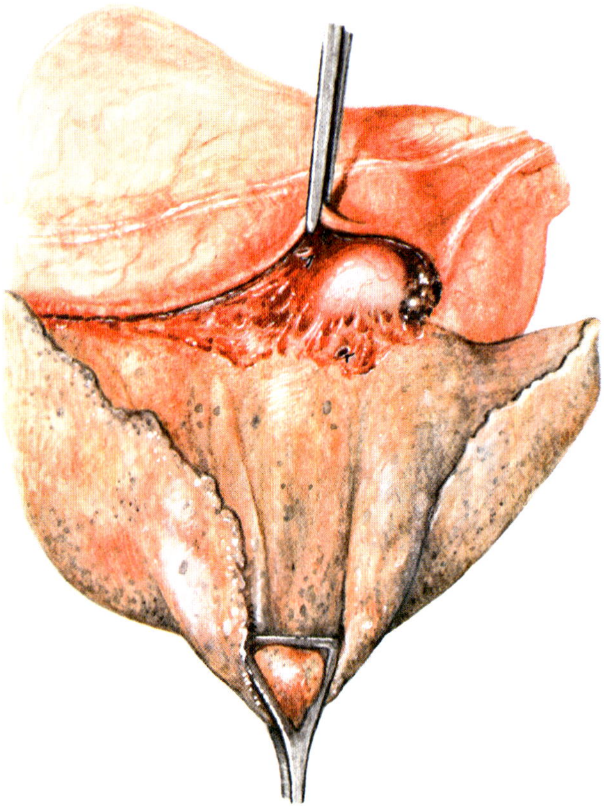

FIG. 4-89.

with the lobe, the left recurrent laryngeal nerve must first be visualized and protected. Figure 4-90 shows the superior pulmonary vein exposed, and the main pulmonary artery with its first branch to the anterior segment dissected out. The vagus nerve can be seen descending over the arch of the aorta and giving off the recurrent laryngeal nerve, which loops around the aorta at the ligamentum arteriosum.

The division of the arterial branches to the upper lobe is begun anteriorly. The first branch usually encountered is either a large short trunk, which immediately divides, or two branches, which arise close together from the pulmonary artery and supply the anterior and apical segments of the upper

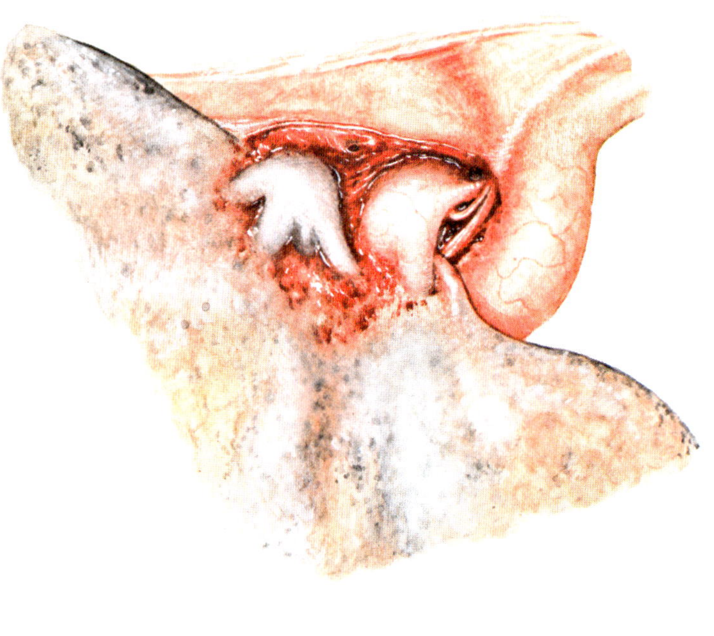

FIG. 4-90.

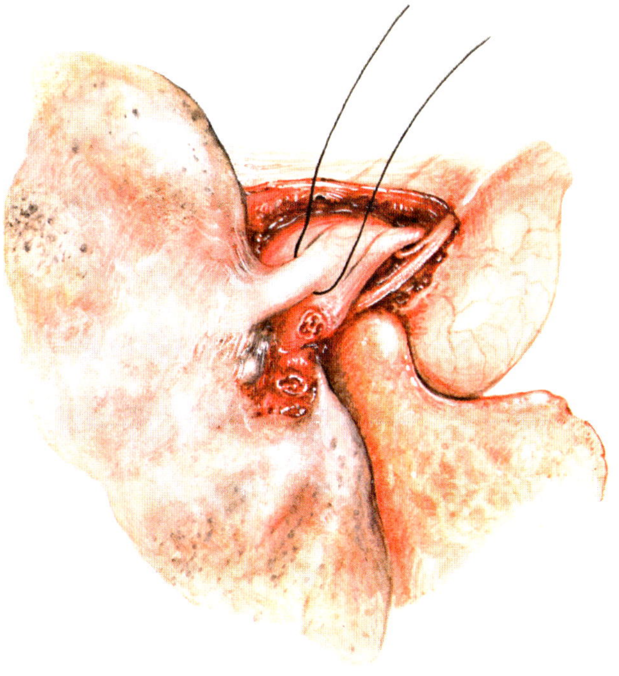

FIG. 4-91.

lobe. This latter situation is shown in Figure 4-91; the apical segmental artery has been divided and the anterior segmental artery is looped with a ligature. A lymph node is routinely found between these branches and the upper lobe bronchus usually adherent to both (Fig. 4-91). This lymph node is often calcified and is commonly the location of a broncholith. If calcified, this node poses a significant risk while freeing and ligating the arterial branches, because the tissue of the artery will tear more readily than will the adhesions to the node; even tightening a ligature around the artery may tear it.

Figure 4-92 depicts a situation found in 20%–30% of patients: a portion or all of the arterial supply to the lingula arises from this proximal portion of the pulmonary artery and passes anterior to the bronchus. These branches are not immediately apparent because they are covered by the apical posterior

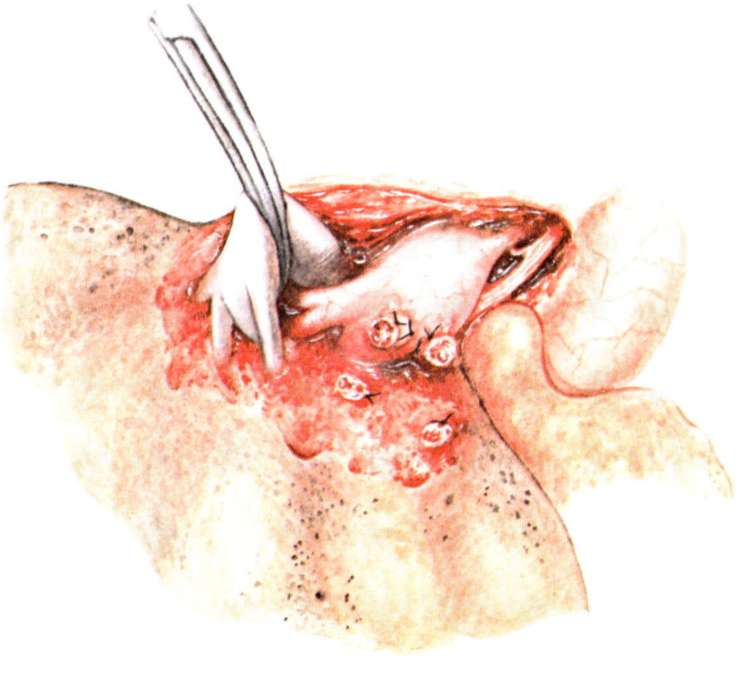

FIG. 4-92.

vein, which is being retracted away. This lingular artery may be damaged if the deep dissection of the anterior and apical branches is made blindly or if the upper lobe bronchus is not freed under direct vision. The two arteries supplying the anterior and the apical segments have been ligated and divided in Figure 4-92. Continuing distally on the pulmonary artery, the various additional branches to the upper lobe, usually to the posterior and to the anterior segments, should be visualized, ligated, and divided. Occasionally one or more arteries to the superior segment of the lower lobe may arise as a branch of one of the arteries to the posterior segment of the upper lobe (Fig. 4-100c).

The arteries to the lingula usually arise from that portion of the pulmonary artery within the interlobar fissure distal to the origin of the artery to the superior segment of the lower lobe. This segment of the pulmonary artery is most easily exposed by placing one finger of the left hand on the pulmonary artery, where it enters the lung substance posteriorly, and dissecting down to the finger through the depths of the fissure. Except for the region of the lingula, the left interlobar fissure is commonly complete. In approximately 50% of patients, the lingular arteries arise from the interlobar portion of the pulmonary artery as a single trunk and in an additional 20%, the two lingular arteries arise separately from this portion. Figure 4-93 illustrates the more common situation in which the two lingular arteries arise as a single trunk. Immediately to the right (posterior) of the lingular artery, a branch to the anterior segment can be seen arising in common with a branch to the posterior segment of the upper lobe. Descending from the portion of the main pulmonary artery just proximal to the lingular artery is the branch to the superior segment of the lower lobe. Two of the basilar segmental arteries are seen at the left. After the artery has been completely exposed, any significant areas of fusion in the fissure are divided with a GIA stapler.

Following ligation and division of all arteries to the upper lobe, the upper lobe is retracted posteriorly and the superior pulmonary vein is isolated (Fig. 4-94 depicts this from the anterior aspect). In 16% of patients there will be a vein crossing the fissure between the lingula and the medial basal segment of the lower lobe, either an inferior lingular vein emptying into the lower lobe vein or a vein from the medial basal segment emptying into a

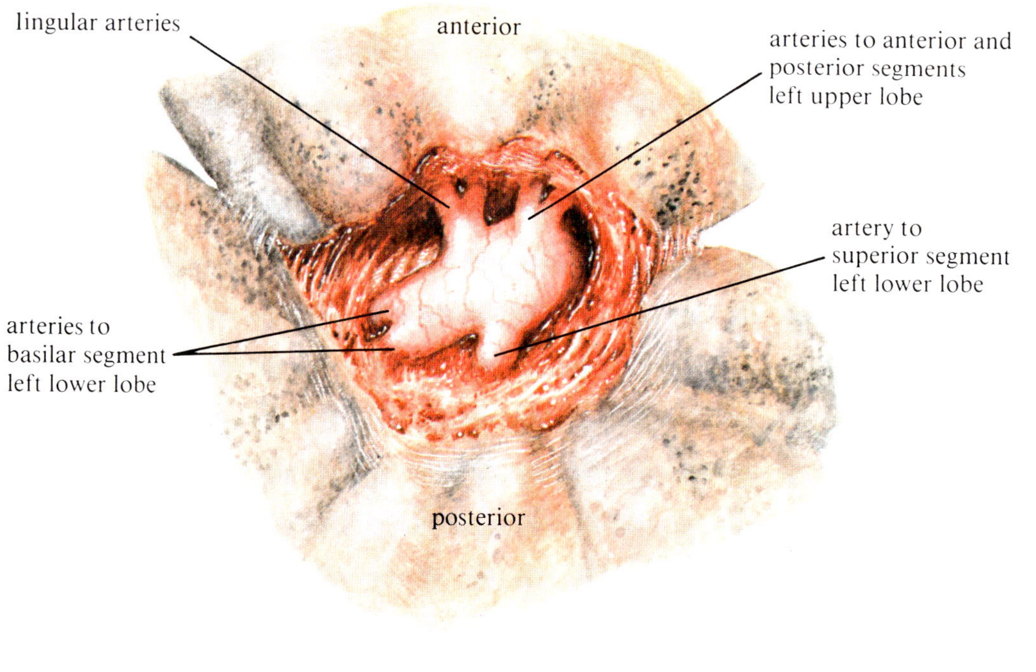

FIG. 4-93.

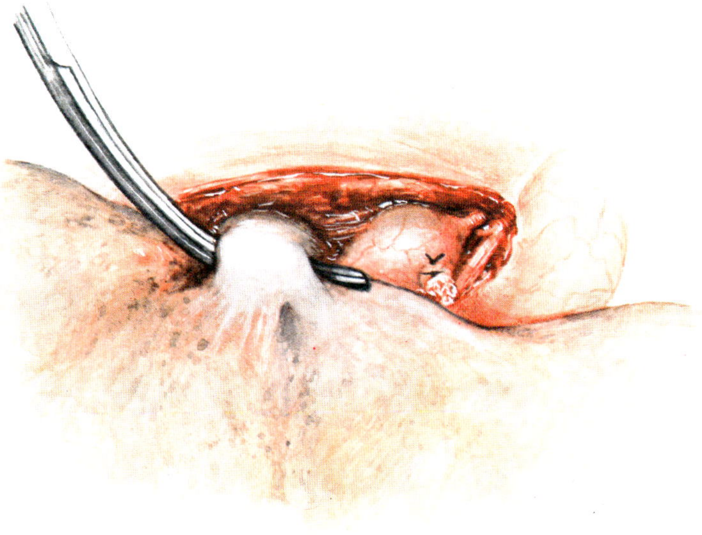

FIG. 4-94.

lingular vein. These veins should be ligated and divided. A dense fascial layer will be encountered posterior to the pulmonary vein connecting it to the bronchus. Because of this layer, forcing an instrument blindly between the vein and the bronchus is hazardous—the dissection should be done under direct vision beginning anteriorly on the vein. During this dissection a small opening may be made into a diverticulum of the pericardium extending out along the vein. This is of no significance. When the superior vein has been freed so that a finger can be placed around it, the vein is closed with two rows of 30-V staples using the TA-30 stapler, then divided between them (Fig. 4-95).

The lymph nodes and fascial strands surrounding the junction of the upper lobe bronchus with the main bronchus should be dissected peripherally so that the junction can be well visualized. Figure 4-96 depicts the upper lobe bronchus and its junction with the main bronchus as seen from the fissure. The four ligated stumps of the pulmonary arterial branches to the

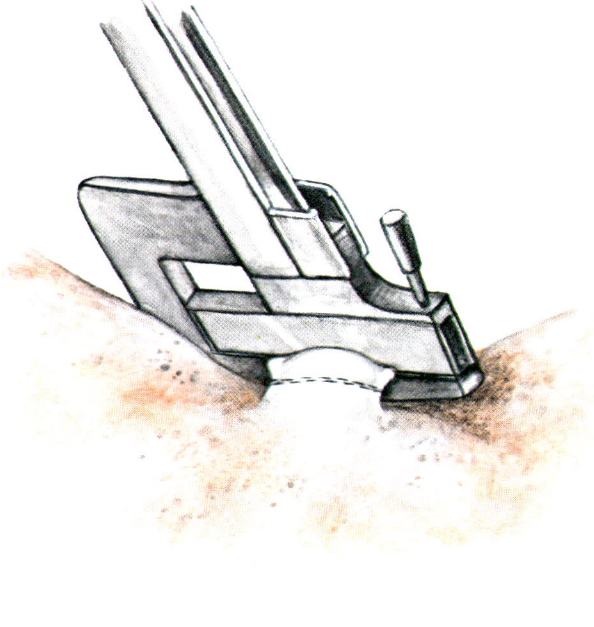

FIG. 4-95.

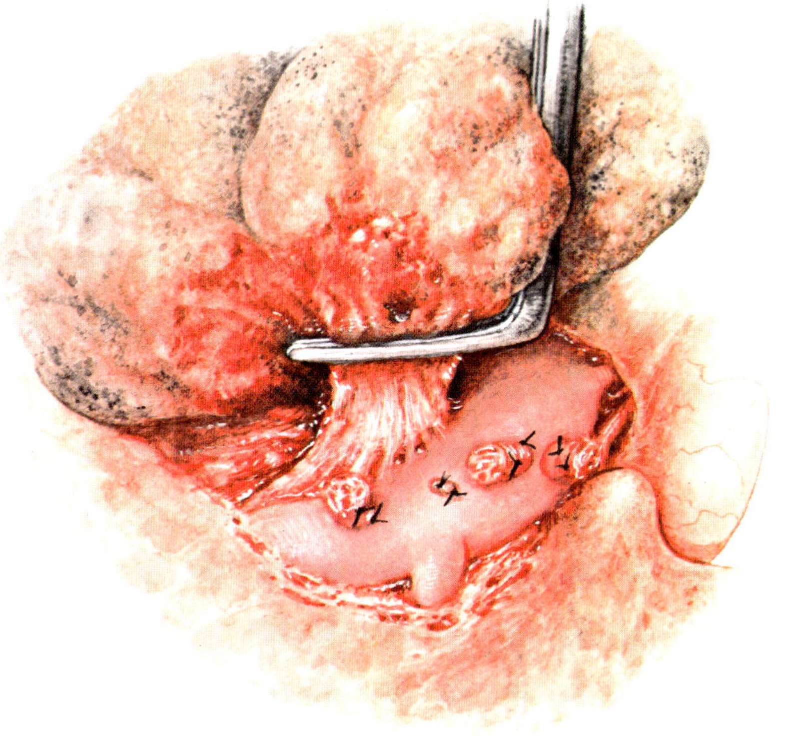

FIG. 4-96.

upper lobe from left to right are lingular, anterior, posterior and apical, and anterior. The intact arterial branch to the superior segment descends into the lower lobe. Using the TA-30 stapler, a row of 3.5-mm staples is placed across the upper lobe bronchus flush with the main bronchus so that a diverticulum where secretions can pool is not created. Care must be taken not to compromise the lumen of the main bronchus, however. A Sarot bronchus

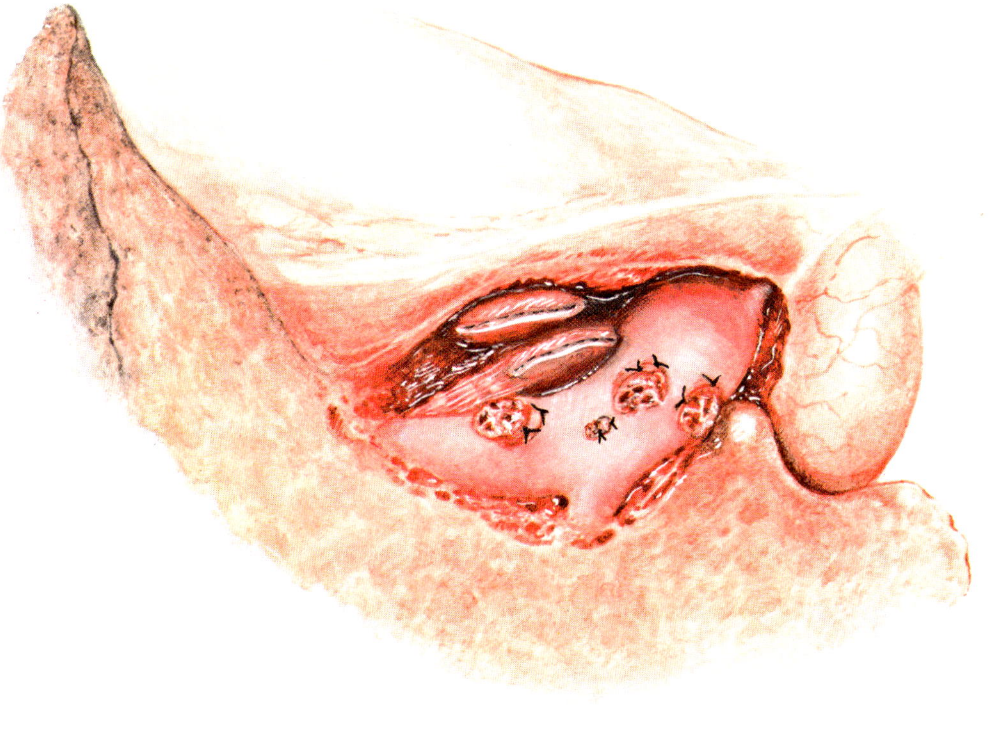

FIG. 4-97.

clamp is placed distally (Fig. 4-96), and the bronchus is divided distal to the staple line. Figure 4-97 is a view of the mediastinum after the upper lobe has been removed. The pericardium, with the phrenic nerve running on it, is anterior. The left lower lobe is posterior. Just posterior to the phrenic nerve is the stump of the superior pulmonary vein, and behind it, the stump of the upper lobe bronchus. The left pulmonary artery, with the stumps of its branches to the upper lobe, is behind the bronchus. After the upper lobe has been removed and the bronchial stump checked for air leaks, the division of the pulmonary ligament is completed in order to permit the lower lobe to ascend in the chest and fill the apical part of the thorax. A flap of pleura, pericardial fat, or pericardium is sutured over the bronchial stump.

Left Lower Lobectomy

The left lower lobe represents 25% of the total lung mass. Initially, the pleura at the hilus of the lung is divided, beginning at the inferior portion of the pulmonary ligament (Fig. 4-98) and extending both anteriorly and posteriorly around the lung. The medial border of the space encompassed by the pulmonary ligament is the esophagus. Often present in this region are blood vessels that can have a troublesome rate of bleeding; they must be coagulated away from the surface of the esophagus, however, to prevent injury to the esophagus. Pulmonary sequestration occurs most commonly in or adjacent to the left lower lobe; if present, there will be systemic arteries of significant size entering the area of sequestration through the diaphragm or directly from the aorta. If these vessels are divided accidentally, an artery traversing the diaphragm may retract and provide the surgeon with some difficult moments. If adhesions are encountered between the lung and the pericardium anterior to the hilus, it is important that the phrenic nerve, as it courses down the pericardium, not be injured by clamping or by coagulating a blood vessel near enough to cause necrosis. The superior border of the pulmonary ligament is the inferior

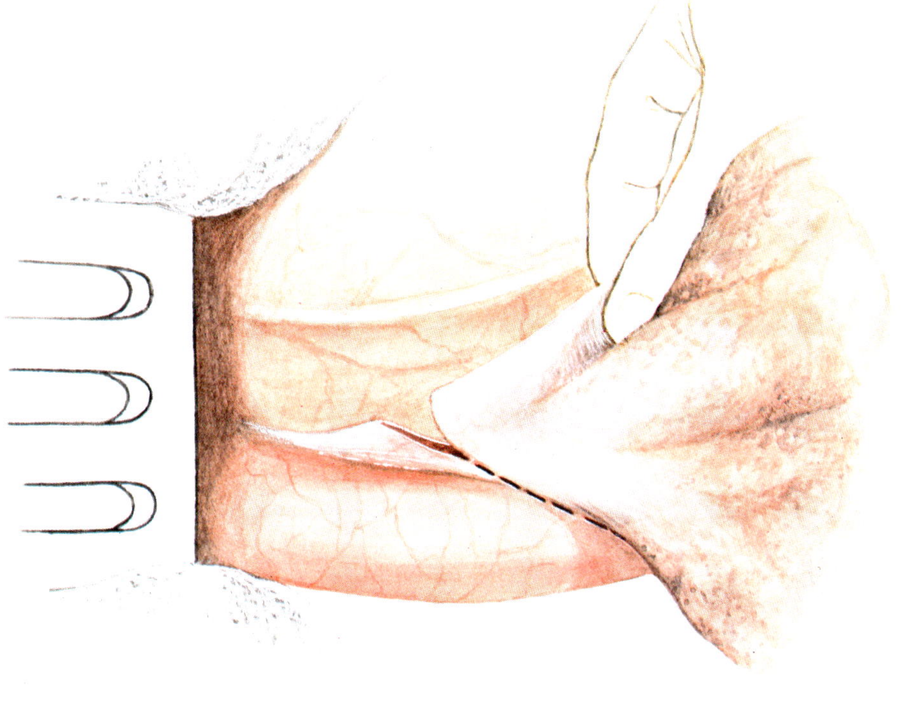

FIG. 4-98.

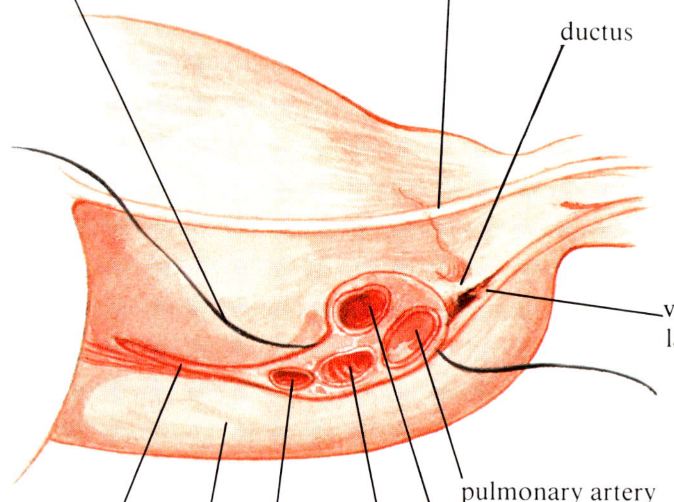

FIG. 4-99.

pulmonary vein. Figure 4-99 is a schematic drawing of the left hilus at the mediastinum with the fissure superimposed. The relationship of the inferior pulmonary vein to the pulmonary ligament can be seen. This vein lies somewhat posterior to the superior pulmonary vein. If the location of this vein is not immediately apparent, a small vein running between the medial and posterior basal segments is present and may be followed down to the pulmonary vein.

This time is often convenient for determining that there is both a superior and inferior pulmonary vein. Although a common pulmonary vein from the right lung is found in only 3% of patients, its occurrence is much higher on the left; Healey and Gibbon (4) give the incidence as 25%. In my experience, the incidence of a common pulmonary vein, external to the pericardium, is closer to 8%. In this 8%, however, if the first pulmonary vein encountered were divided, the blood drainage from the entire left lung would be interrupted.

Following this phase of the dissection, the arterial supply to the left lower lobe should be divided. Division is most readily done by approaching the artery through the fissure, which is complete more commonly than is the similar fissure on the right side. If an area of fusion between the left upper and the left lower lobes is found, it is usually to the lingula rather than between the superior segment and the upper lobe, as is usually the case on the right side. By placing one's third finger underneath the lung posterior to the hilus and one's thumb in the fissure, the pulmonary artery may be easily palpated; it should be exposed first at this point. After the lateral surface of the main pulmonary artery is exposed, the artery to the superior segment of the lower lobe should be isolated. This artery usually arises above the level of the lingular arteries (Fig. 4-93) and must be divided separately. A number of anomalies of this artery exist (see Fig. 4-100A for the usual pattern). The artery to the lingula is on the left and the artery to the superior segment of the lower lobe is on the right. The artery to the posterior segment of the upper lobe runs superiorly. Approximately one-third of patients have two

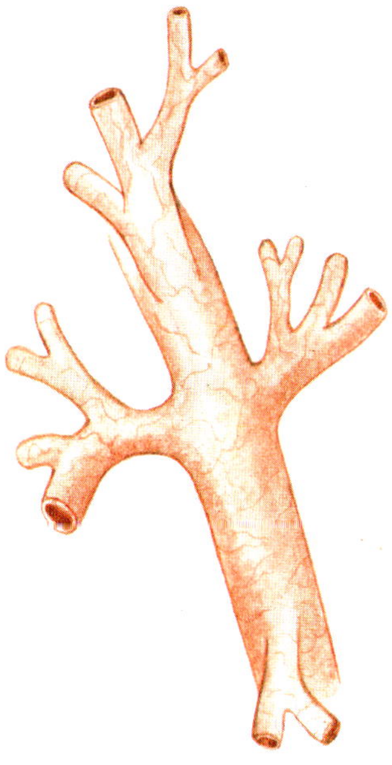

FIG. 4-100A.

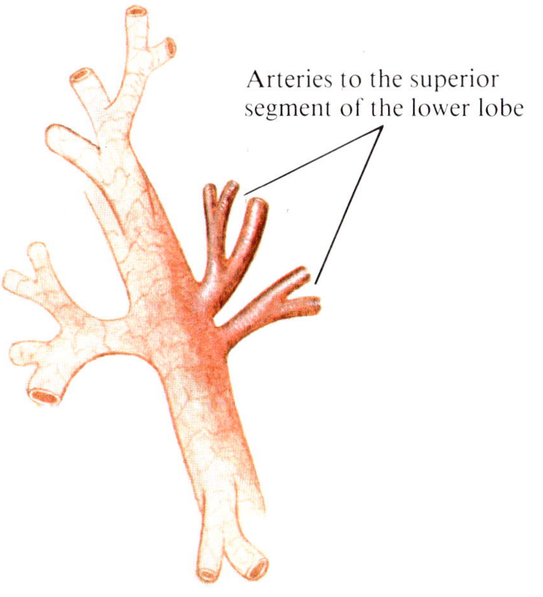

FIG. 4-100B.

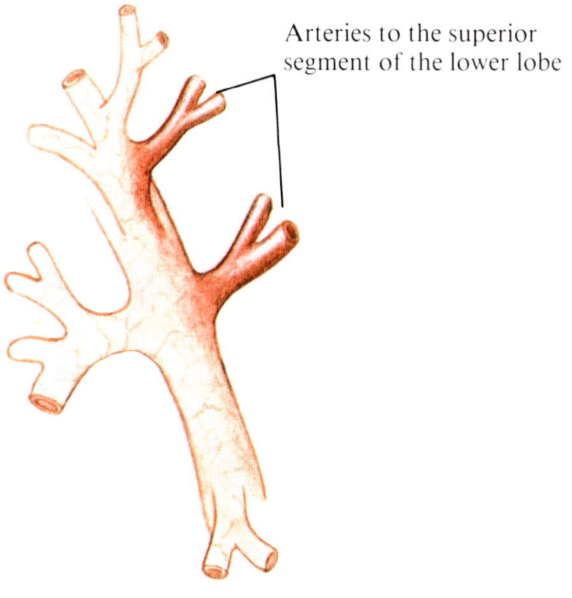

FIG. 4-100C.

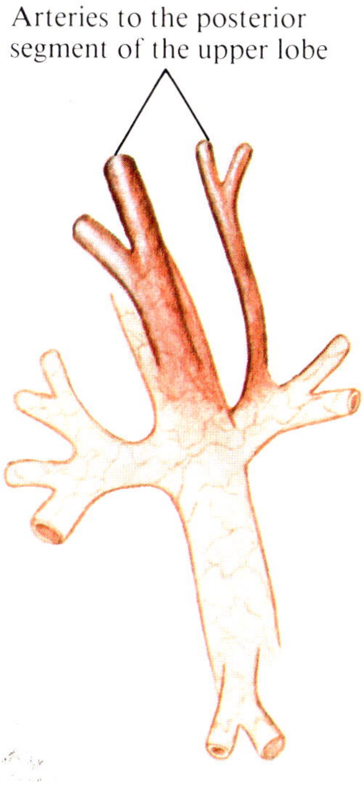

FIG. 4-100D.

arteries to the superior segment (Fig. 4-100B), and about 4% have an aberrant artery to the superior segment arising as a branch of one of the arteries to the posterior segment of the upper lobe (Fig. 4-100C). On the other hand, an artery to the posterior segment of the upper lobe arising from one of the superior segmental arteries may also be found (Fig. 4-100D).

All arteries to the lingular segments must be identified and spared. The artery to the basal segments of the lower lobe is ligated at the level indicated

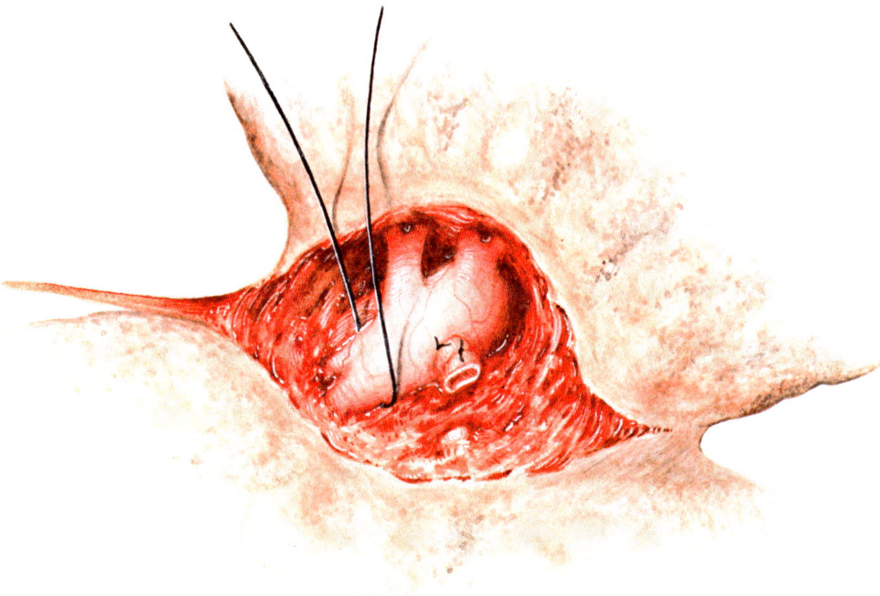

FIG. 4-101.

by the ligature in Figure 4-101 distal to the takeoff of the lingular arteries, then divided.

After dividing these vessels, separation of the fissure between the upper and lower lobes should be completed. If a significant area of fusion is present, this division is done with a GIA stapler; prior to this, however, the area of fusion of the lingula to the lower lobe must be examined, because the inferior lingular vein empties into the inferior pulmonary vein in 10% of patients and in another 6% the inferior lingular vein receives tributaries from the medial basal segment of the lower lobe. Often these tributaries are small and may be divided.

Next, isolate the inferior pulmonary vein. The posterior part of this vein should be freed under direct vision, not by blindly forcing a right-angle forceps around it. If inflammation has occurred in the lobe, the path of least

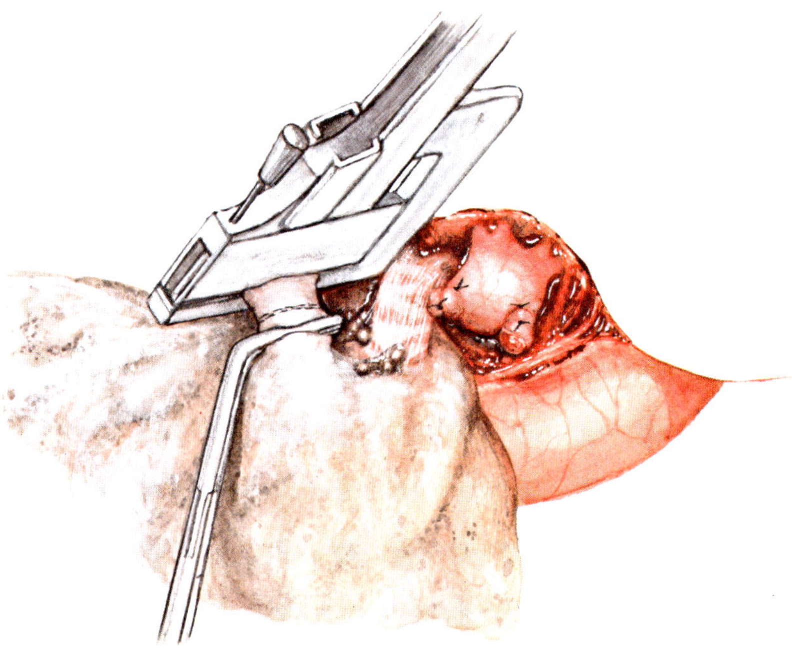

FIG. 4-102.

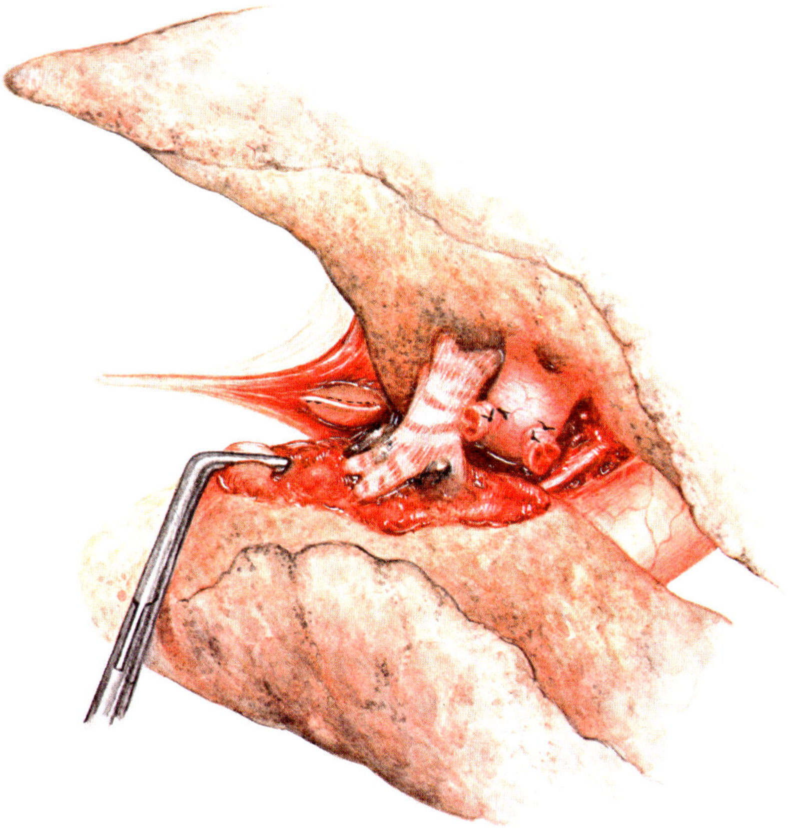

FIG. 4-103.

resistance is often through the vein rather than around it. After this vein has been freed enough to put a finger behind it, the vein is stapled closed with a TA-30 stapler using two rows of 30-V staples (shown from the anterior aspect in Fig. 4-102), then divided between them. If the carcinoma involves the inferior pulmonary vein itself or is very close to its posterior surface, the pericardium should be opened, the vein divided and oversewn at its junction with the left atrium, and a cuff of pericardium removed with the vein.

The lobe is connected now only by the bronchus and the lymph node-bearing connective tissue surrounding it. These lymph nodes medial to the bronchus and anterior to the esophagus should be freed from the mainstem bronchus and removed with the left lower lobe. This dissection serves two purposes: first, it removes more of the lymph drainage area if the lobectomy is for carcinoma, and secondly, it permits a positive identification of the left mainstem bronchus. If traction on the left lower lobe is exerted, the lower lobe bronchus and the upper lobe bronchus will form a straight line, and the upper lobe bronchus may be mistaken for the main bronchus. This situation is illustrated by the linear arrangement of the upper lobe and lower lobe bronchi apparent in Figure 4-103. The left main bronchus in this figure cannot be seen; it is behind the junction of the upper and lower lobe bronchi, perpendicular to the plane of the drawing. Figure 4-104 is a section of the junction of these bronchi with the main bronchus, showing how this relationship occurs with traction on the lower lobe. On the left side the origin of the bronchus to the superior segment of the lower lobe is usually 6–10 mm from the upper lobe bronchus. Consequently, it is seldom necessary to divide the superior segmental bronchus separately. The lower lobe bronchus is closed distal to the upper lobe bronchus with 3.5-mm staples to the TA-30 stapler, then divided distal to the staple line. Figure 4-105 shows the stapler applied to the proximal

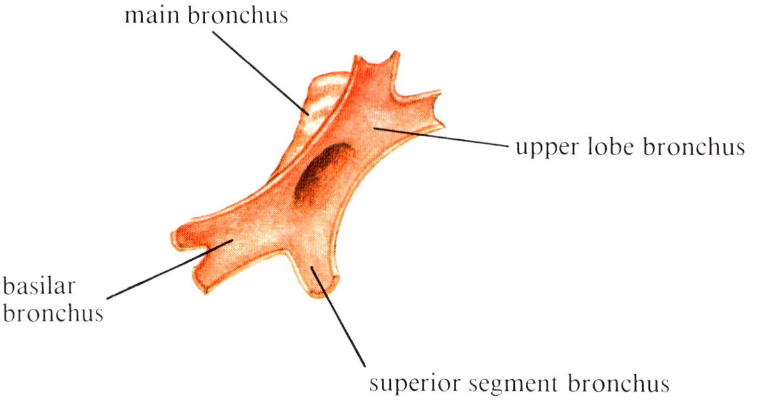

FIG. 4-104.

bronchus and the lower lobe being removed. The relationship of the bronchus to the artery and vein is apparent. The upper lobe, not shown, is to the left and superior.

If the closure of the bronchus is air tight, a small flap of parietal pleura or pericardium is developed, laid over the end of the bronchial stump, and carefully sutured to the bronchus as a cap.

Pneumonectomy

Right Pneumonectomy

Unless the disease process requires a more extensive dissection, an incision is made in the reflection of the mediastinal pleura to the lung, beginning at the inferior edge of the pulmonary ligament, extending superiorly on the anterior surface of the hilus posterior to the phrenic nerve, over the superior surface just below the azygos vein, and down the posterior surface just anterior

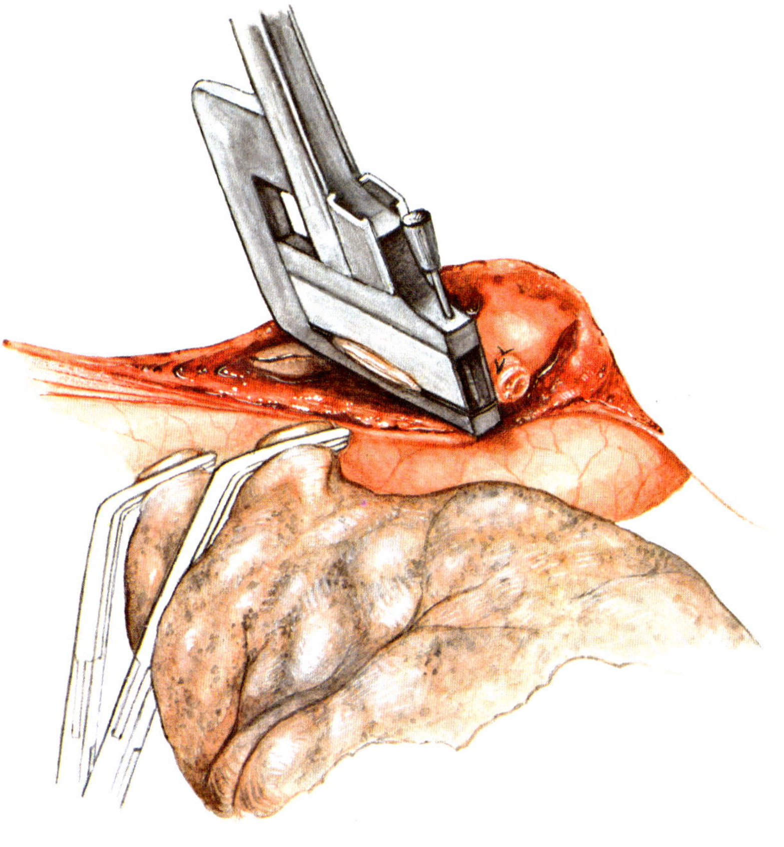

FIG. 4-105.

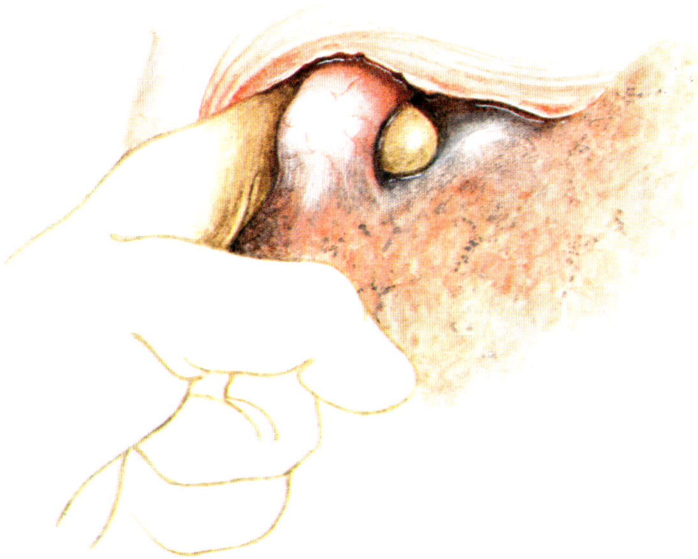

FIG. 4-106.

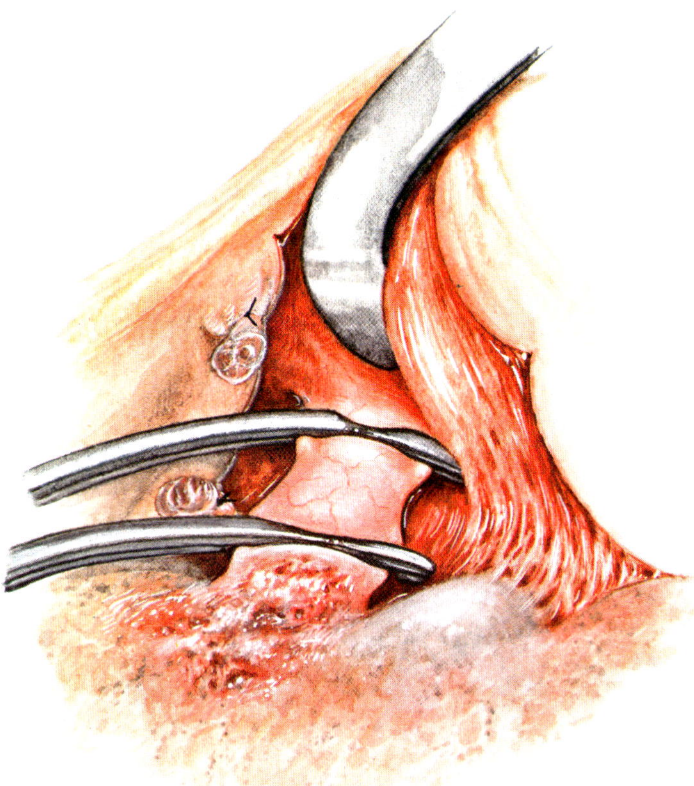

FIG. 4-107.

to the esophagus. At the point that the right main pulmonary artery leaves the pericardium, it is freed of its areolarlike attachments over a length adequate for the surgeon to put one finger around it (Fig. 4-106). The artery is clamped with two curved Glover or similar vascular clamps (Fig. 4-107) and divided between them (Fig. 4-31A). The proximal arterial stump is closed using two continuous 4–0 monofilament sutures (Fig. 4-31B). The distal end is closed with a 2–0 suture ligature. If the carcinoma extends along the pulmonary artery so that an adequate extrapericardial length is not available, the pericardium should be opened, the superior vena cava mobilized, and the portion

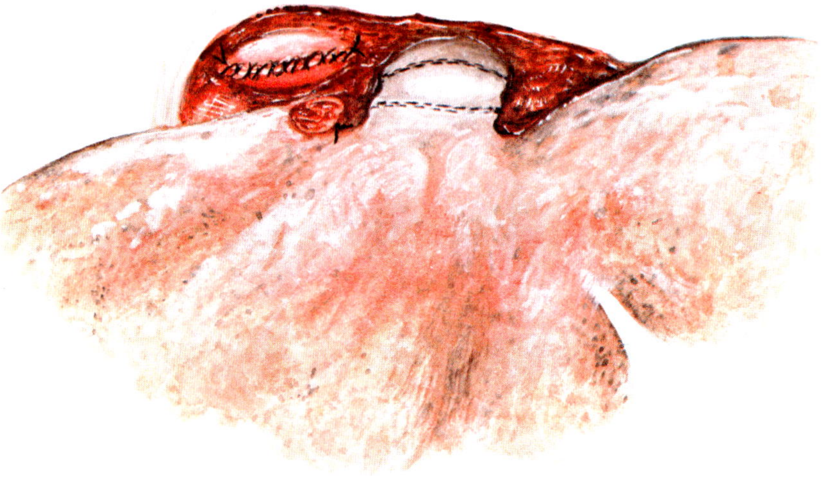

FIG. 4-108.

of the right pulmonary artery that lies lateral to the ascending aorta and behind the superior vena cava freed. If at any time severe hemorrhage from the right pulmonary artery occurs, the artery may be occluded by pressure on that portion posterior to the transverse sinus between the superior vena cava and the ascending aorta.

Following division of the pulmonary artery, the superior pulmonary vein, which is somewhat anterior to the inferior vein, is freed of its attachments; the anterior, superior, and inferior surfaces are attached only to areolar tissue, but posteriorly the vein is attached to a dense fibrous reflection of the pericardium that should be dissected off under direct vision. When the vein has

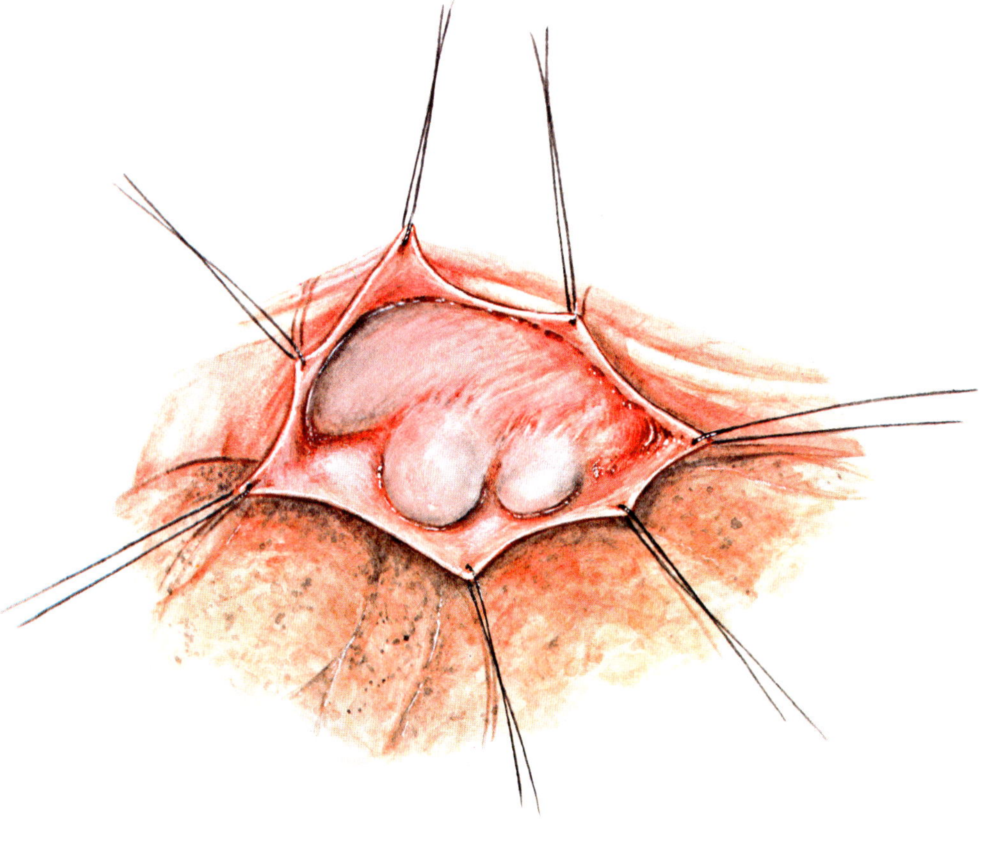

FIG. 4-109.

been freed so that a finger can be placed behind it, the vein is stapled closed using the TA-30 stapler with two rows of 30-V staples and divided between them (see these staple lines in Fig. 4-108). The stump of the transected and oversewn right pulmonary artery can be seen above the vein.

The inferior pulmonary vein, which forms the roof of the pulmonary ligament, is posterior and inferior to the other structures. This vein is likewise freed of its attachments, stapled closed, and divided.

If the tumor margin is too close to permit division of the veins extrapericardially, the pericardium should be opened (Fig. 4-109). The intrapericardial portion of the two pulmonary veins can be seen running toward the lung. Notice the position of the phrenic nerve on the external surface of the pericardium. A small cuff of pericardium is left around the two pulmonary veins, and the veins are stapled closed within the pericardium. Both veins are partially enclosed by a pericardial reflection on the posterior surface, which must be dissected off the vein. Although an intrapericardial length of the superior vein adequate for closure will usually be found, the inferior vein may not have adequate length. If necessary, a portion of the left atrial wall may be removed to gain additional length, but care should be taken not to compromise the orifices of the veins from the opposite lung. If required, the phrenic nerve may be divided with the cuff of pericardium, but the nerve should not be divided electively.

The lymph nodes draining the lung are found principally along the bronchi, with drainage towards the hilus. Those nodes surrounding the lobar bronchi drain to nodes on the anterior–lateral side of the trachea medial to the azygos vein and to lymph nodes medial to the main bronchi and beneath the carina. If the more distal lymphatics are not occluded, the drainage is principally to lymph nodes on the ipsilateral side of the mediastinum, although some crossover from the left lower lobe does exist. Those nodes medial to both main bronchi may be exposed by opening the space between the esophagus and pericardium. In doing a right pneumonectomy, one or two nodes from the left side immediately adjacent to the carina are dissected free of the bronchus. These nodes, together with the subcarinal lymph nodes, are freed and reflected to the right side to expose the carina and at least 1 cm of the right main bronchus. The dissection of these nodes from the left main bronchus and the carina is illustrated from the posterior aspect in Figure 4-110. The

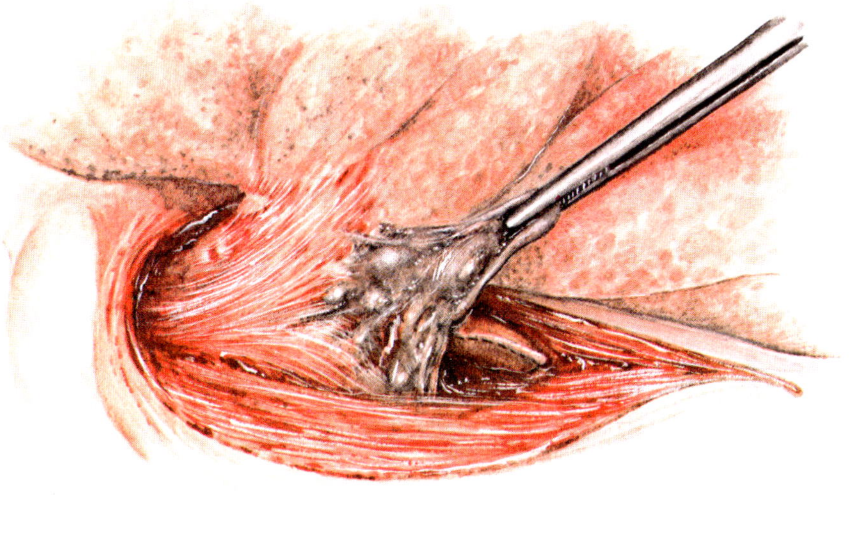

FIG. 4-110.

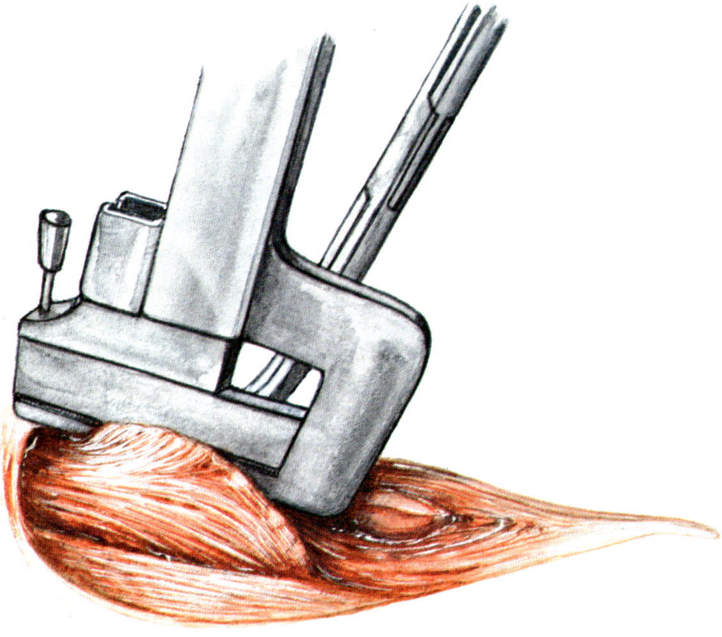

FIG. 4-111.

esophagus is in the foreground, and the left main bronchus is descending behind it. The stump of the inferior pulmonary vein can be seen at the right of the lymph nodes held by the forceps. The right bronchus goes into the visible lung tissue.

The anterior, superior, and posterior surfaces of the bronchus are freed of their fibrous attachments, and the one or two bronchial arteries usually found on the posterior surface of the main bronchus are ligated and divided. The right main bronchus is closed with a row of 4.8-mm staples placed as

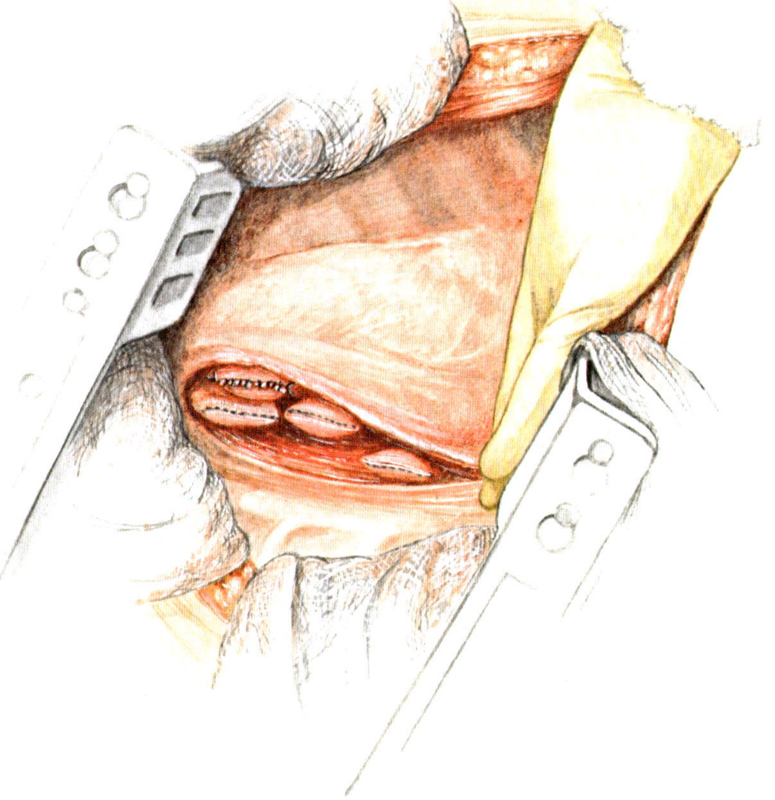

FIG. 4-112.

close to the carina as possible (Fig. 4-111). A Sarot bronchus clamp is placed on the distal portion of the right main bronchus, and the bronchus is divided between the staple row and the clamp. The mediastinal aspect of the right hilus, after the lung has been removed, is shown in Figure 4-112. The stump of the pulmonary artery, closed with sutures instead of staples, is seen in the superior position on the left. The stump of the right main bronchus is just behind it. The other two structures are the stumps of the pulmonary veins.

If the bronchial closure proves to be airtight, a flap of pericardium or pericardial fat is made and carefully sutured over the bronchial stump, in the manner shown for the left lung in Figure 4-119. If the portion of pericardium surrounding the pulmonary artery and veins has been removed, this defect should be loosely laced with a 2–0 absorbable suture to prevent the heart from herniating from the pericardium. It is my practice to leave 1,000,000 units of pencillin in 30 cc saline in the pleural cavity. The chest is closed without drainage tubes, and the intrathoracic pressure adjusted so that no positive pressure phase exists during spontaneous respiration.

Left Pneumonectomy

An incision is made in the mediastinal pleura beginning at the inferior edge of the pulmonary ligament, extending along the anterior aspect posterior to the phrenic nerve, over the superior border below the arch of the aorta, and down the posterior aspect anterior to the descending aorta. The pulmonary artery should be divided first; although its overall length is less than that of the right pulmonary artery, the length available for surgical manipulation is greater. The artery is freed by first clearing the lymph nodes from under the arch of the aorta superior to the pulmonary artery. During the dissection, the left recurrent laryngeal nerve must be identified. This nerve is given off by the vagus on the lateral surface of the aortic arch and swings under the aorta just distal to the ligamentum arteriosum. Often a bronchial artery or other small blood vessels supplying the lymph nodes will be encountered in this area. These blood vessels should not be cauterized near the recurrent nerve, because the cone of heat released may damage the nerve.

In Figure 4-113, the lymph nodes held by the forceps have been dissected from under the arch of the aorta to expose the recurrent laryngeal nerve, which can be seen disappearing under the ligamentum arteriosum. The pulmonary artery is being elevated by the Glover vascular clamp prior to clamping. The vagus nerve distal to the recurrent laryngeal nerve is pictured. The vagus nerve on the left side runs closer to the lung than does that on the right, and it may be near the cancer. If this situation is found, the vagus may be divided distal to the origin of the recurrent nerve with no adverse effects, but division probably should not be done electively.

Figure 4-114 is a posterior view of the superior aspect of the left pulmonary hilus after the pleura has been incised. The vagus nerve descends adjacent to the aorta after it has given off the recurrent laryngeal nerve, seen above the pulmonary artery. The left main bronchus has been exposed and the pulmonary artery penetrates into the posterior surface of the lung at the fissure. The esophagus can be seen below the level of the left bronchus. If required by the position of the tumor, the ligamentum arteriosum may be severed and the left pulmonary artery divided at the bifurcation of the main pulmonary artery, but care must be taken not to compromise the blood flow to the right pulmonary artery. This artery will be directed inferiorly if the patient is in a left straight lateral position. When the pulmonary artery has been freed so that a finger can be placed around it, the pulmonary artery

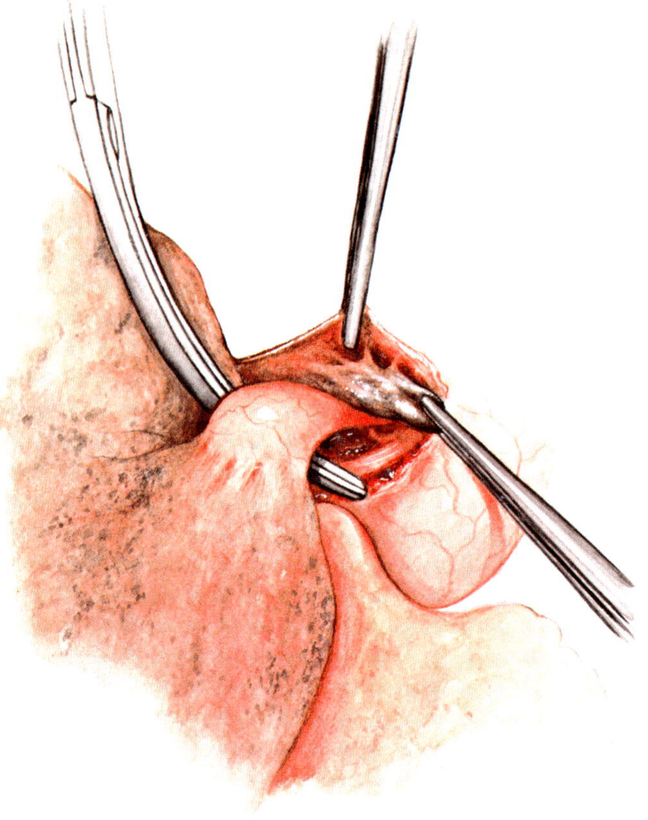

FIG. 4-113.

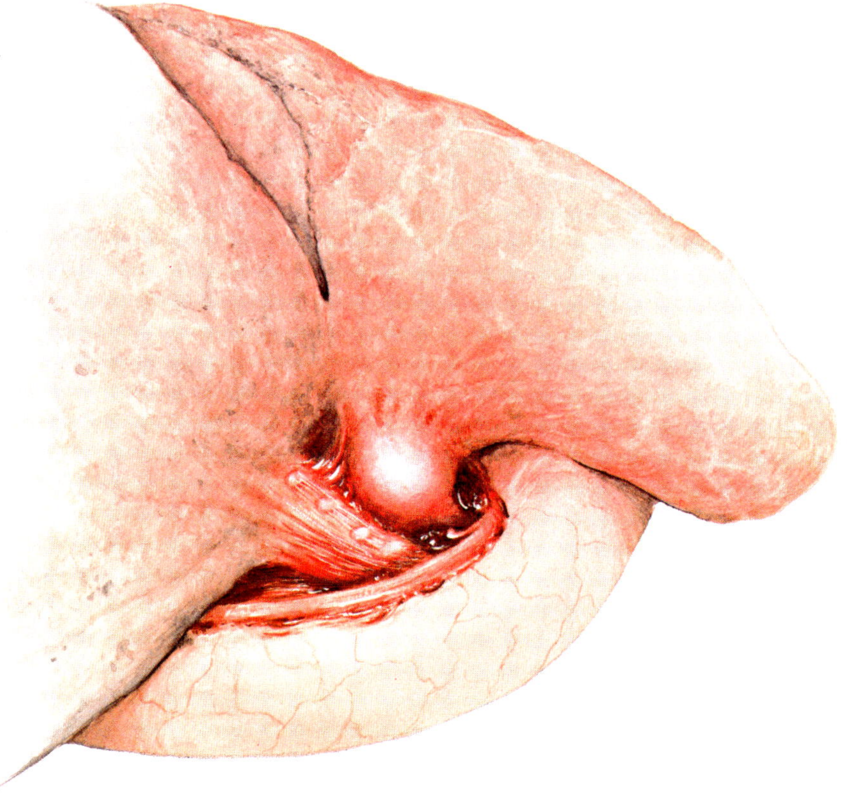

FIG. 4-114.

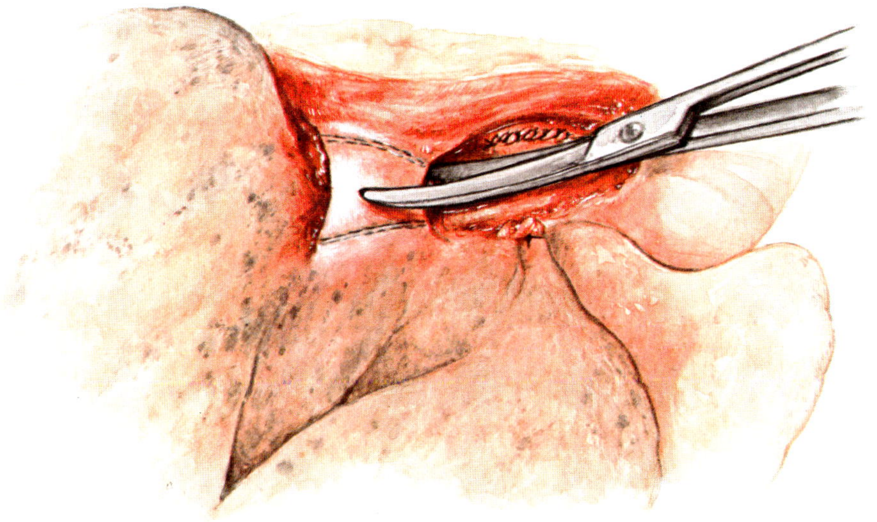

FIG. 4-115.

pressure is measured if it is unknown. Two curved Glover vascular clamps are used to occlude the artery, the vessel is divided between the clamps, and the proximal stump is closed with two superimposed continuous 4–0 nonabsorbable sutures (Fig. 4-31a, b).

Following division of the pulmonary artery, the superior pulmonary vein is freed from its attachments so that a finger may be passed behind it. The vein is closed with two rows of 30-V staples, then divided between them (Fig. 4-115); notice the stump of the pulmonary artery at the right of the

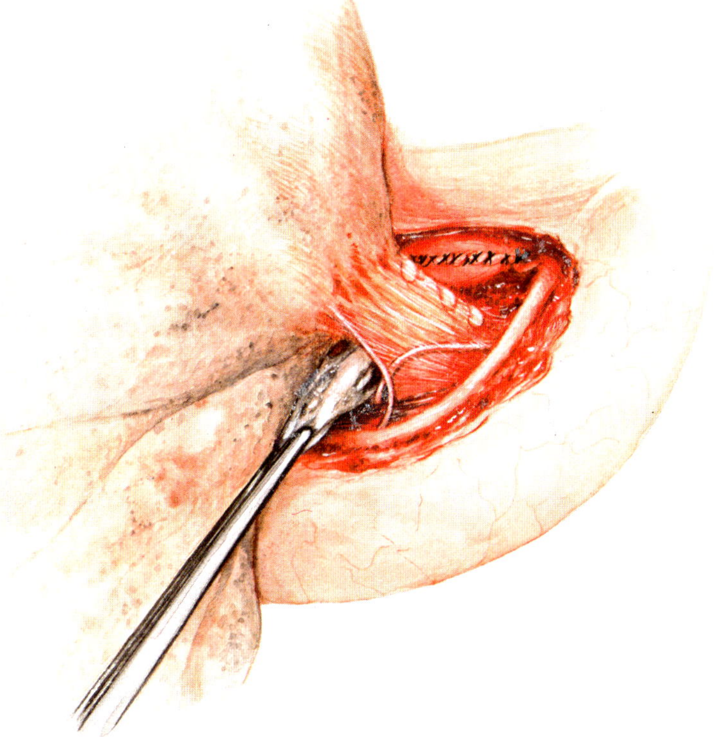

FIG. 4-116.

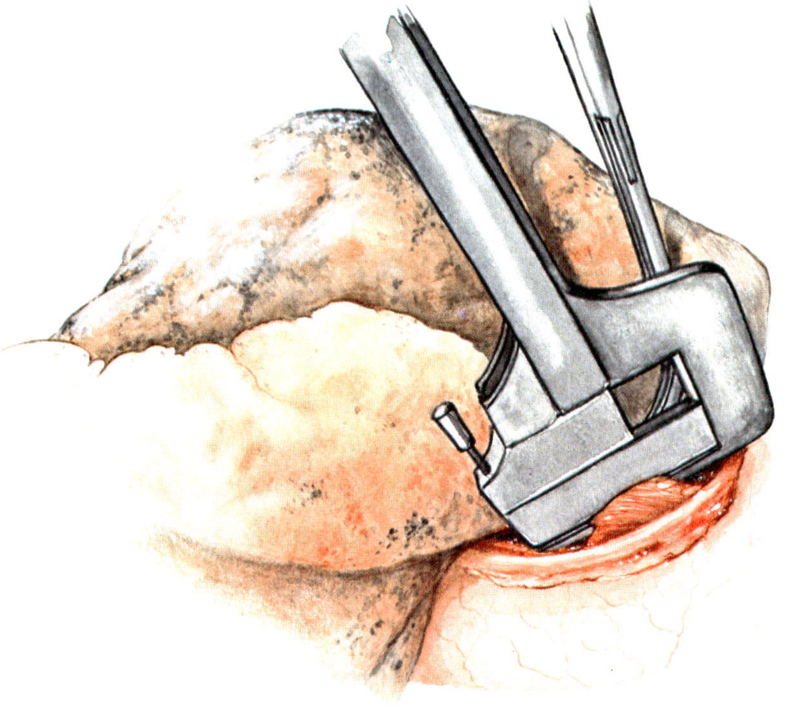

FIG. 4-117.

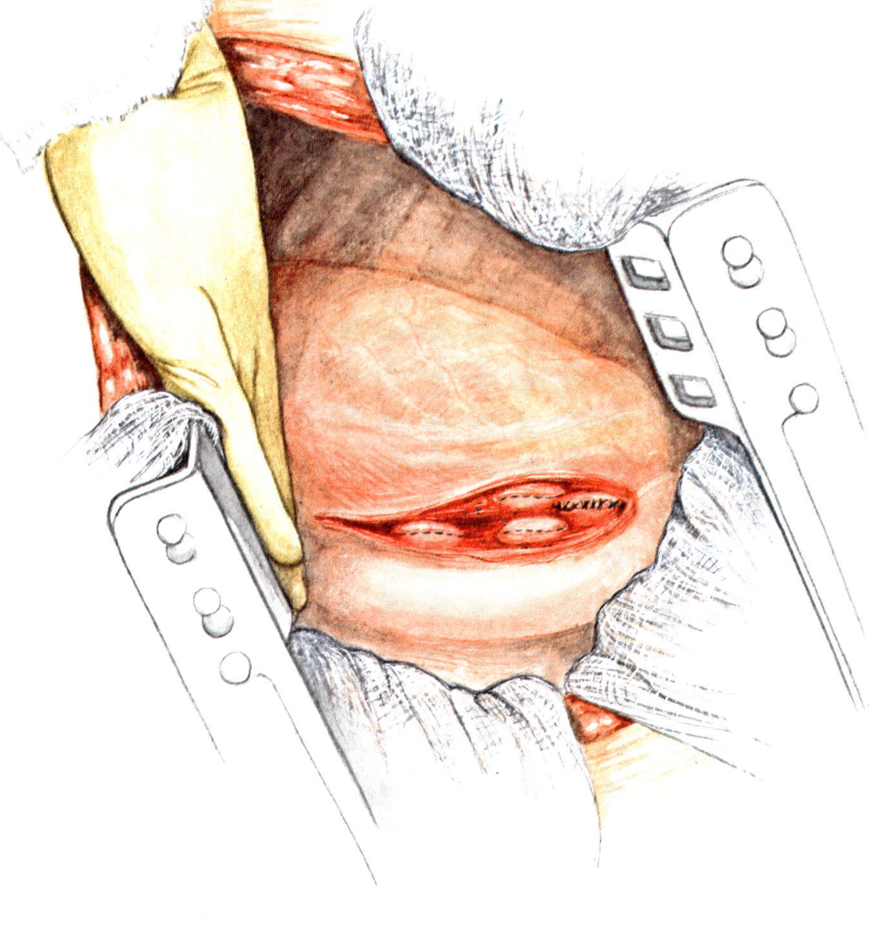

FIG. 4-118.

vein. The inferior pulmonary vein is dissected free, usually most easily accomplished from the posterior aspect of the hilum, closed with staples, and divided in the same manner as was the superior vein.

The removal of the lymph nodes under the carina and along the opposite main bronchus is more difficult from the left side than from the right. Admittedly the role of the lymph node dissection in these patients is unknown; nevertheless this dissection should be done if the operation is for cancer, because occasionally a patient with minimal cancerous involvement of these nodes will have a long survival. In freeing the left main bronchus of the attached lymph nodes and connective tissue, the left bronchial arteries should be ligated and divided. Often one finds on the left two such arteries that arise directly from the aorta; these are shown on the posterior surface of the bronchus in Figure 4-116. The forceps is holding a lymph node dissected from under the carina and from the bronchial arteries. Especially in patients with chronic lung disease, these bronchial arteries may be of significant size.

The origin of the left main bronchus from the carina is immediately under the arch of the aorta. After a 2-cm length of the bronchus has been cleared, the bronchus is closed with a row of 4.8-mm staples placed as close as possible to the carina (Fig. 4-117). A Sarot bronchus clamp is placed distal to the staples, and the bronchus is divided between them. Figure 4-118 depicts the left hilus after the lung has been removed. The stump of the pulmonary artery is at the far right immediately under the arch of the aorta. Left of the pulmonary artery, the stump of the superior pulmonary vein is the anterior structure and the stump of the left main bronchus is the posterior structure. Because of the aorta, the construction of a pleural flap to cover the bronchus is difficult, so instead, a flap of pericardium or pericardial fat is sutured over the end of the bronchial stump (Fig. 4-119).

Extrapleural Pneumonectomy

The usual objective of therapy for chronic empyema thoracis is obliteration of the empyema cavity. This may sometimes be done by a decortication or by a thoracoplasty, but in patients with an almost totally destroyed lung underlying the empyema cavity, especially those with far-advanced tuberculo-

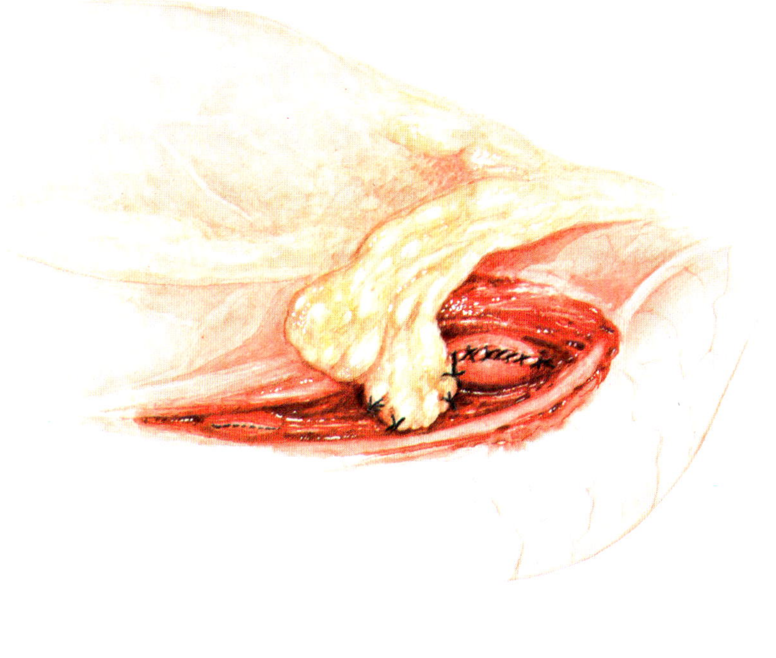

FIG. 4-119

sis, rehabilitation can be accomplished only by removing both the empyema cavity and the underlying lung without infecting the residual thoracic space by entering the empyema cavity.

A double lumen endobronchial tube should be used to prevent aspiration into the dependent lung. With the patient positioned for a lateral thoracotomy, remove the sixth rib and carefully incise the periosteum of the rib bed so that the peel on the parietal pleura is not perforated and the empyema cavity is not entered. To free the wall of the empyema cavity from the chest wall, develop a plane between the periosteum and the parietal peel through the layer of endothoracic fascia. Dissect over the full length of the incision. Working in a limited region invites entry into the empyema cavity; if the dissection becomes difficult in one area, shift to another that is easier, then return to the difficult area after the easier dissection has been completed.

Often an instrument such as a periosteal elevator must be used for this dissection, and occasionally, calcification from the parietal peel will have invaded the chest wall to an extent such that areas of ribs and intercostal muscle must be resected in order to free the wall of the cavity. When the peel has been separated from the chest wall for 4–5 cm above and below the incision, a rib spreader may be inserted to improve the exposure.

As the dissection is continued over the apex of the chest, care must be taken not to avulse the internal mammary vessels or damage the recurrent laryngeal nerve as it passes around the right subclavian artery. The dissection of the empyema wall from the diaphragm is often difficult. The exposure is poor and the planes are obscure, with the result that it is easy to enter the empyema cavity or dissect through the diaphragm at its attachment to the chest wall. It is therefore advisable to delay this dissection until the hilar structures have been divided and the rest of the lung freed. Usually the empyema cavity does not extend onto the mediastinal surface of the lung, so the dissection of the pericardium from the lung and the isolation of the hilar structures is relatively easy. With this accomplished, the pneumonectomy proceeds as described previously.

A similar technique can be used to perform a lobectomy. This is especially applicable for a lobe containing a carcinoma with a distal cavity that has ruptured through the pleura and formed a localized empyema. After the empyema cavity overlying a given lobe has been dissected from the chest wall in the extrapleural plane, the hilus of the lung exposed, and the vessels and bronchus of the involved lobe isolated and divided as previously described, the interlobar fissure is developed, beginning at the hilus. This maneuver is easier than is the attempt to locate the fissure through the thickened lateral peel by guess, and it also permits the dissection of the uninvolved lobes from the peel so that the entire empyema cavity may be resected without entering it.

Wedge Resections and Open Lung Biopsy

Wedge resections of small peripheral pulmonary lesions are done either as excisional biopsies or, in patients with limited pulmonary function, as definitive therapy. To prevent accidental injury to the hilar blood vessels or bronchi, a lesion deep within the lobe should be removed with a formal segmental resection or lobectomy. The same technique of wedge resection is used for an open lung biopsy of generalized pulmonary disease. For this latter use, a wedge of representative lung approximately 3 cm on a side is excised, preferably from some location other than the lingula or the middle lobe, which are often not typical of the lung as a whole.

A wedge resection is usually done through a standard posterior–lateral thoracotomy so that a larger resection, if indicated, can also be performed. In doing an open lung biopsy, a limited interspace incision just large enough to admit a hand and to permit a portion of the lung to herniate out is adequate if the surgeon is confident that no other procedure will be performed. Bilateral wedge resections are commonly performed at one operation through a median sternotomy.

A wedge excision can be done using either the GIA stapler or a clamp and suture technique. To use the stapler, a method considerably faster than suturing, grasp the lobe in the left hand with the lesion to be removed between the thumb and fingers. Apply the GIA stapler to the lung, leaving a 2-cm margin between the lesion and the closest point on the staple line (similar to the method shown in Figs. 4-71 and 4-72). Fire the stapler, then apply it again to construct the second incision of the wedge. To prevent bleeding, the two staple lines should cross at the apex of the wedge; if this is not possible, the wedge may be completed with a third or fourth application of the stapler, or a clamp may be applied across the apex of the wedge and undersewn with a suture ligature. Any air leaks or bleeding from the staple line should be stopped with interrupted figure-of-eight sutures.

The alternative method of using clamps and sutures is by the application of a pair of Buie clamps on each side of the wedge of lung to be excised and cutting between them. The clamp on the specimen side is necessary to prevent the lesion from rupturing through the cut surface of the lung. If the sides of the wedge are longer than the clamps, a second pair of clamps is applied after the incision between the first pair has been completed. With the wedge excised, close the cut edge of the lung by undersewing the clamps with a continuous horizontal-loop (Heidenhain) suture to hold the two pleural surfaces together. Remove the clamp and place a second continuous suture in an over-and-over manner distal to the first line of sutures. The suture line should be examined for bleeding and air leaks prior to closing the chest. As a rule, one intercostal catheter is adequate for drainage following this procedure.

References

1. Boyden EA: Segmental Anatomy Of The Lungs. New York, McGraw-Hill, 1955.
2. Churchill ED, and Belsey A: Segmental pneumonectomy in bronchiectasis. Ann Surg 109:481–499, 1939.
3. Harlan BJ, Starr A, Harwin F: Manual of Cardiac Surgery, Vol II. New York, Springer-Verlag, 1981.
4. Healey JE Jr, Gibbon JM: Intrapericardial anatomy in relation to pneumonectomy for pulmonary carcinoma. J Thorac Surg 19:864–874, 1950.
5. Merendino KA, Johnson RJ, Skinner HH, Maguire RX: The intradiaphragmatic distribution of the phrenic nerve with particular reference to the placement of diaphragmatic incisions and controlled segmental paralysis. Surgery 39:189–198, 1956.
6. Overholt RH, Woods FM, Ramsay BH: Segmental pulmonary resection. J Thorac Surg 19:207–220, 1950.

Resection of the Trachea and Bronchi 5

Indications for Tracheal Resection

Primary Tumors of the Trachea

Primary tumors of the trachea are rare. This, plus the nonspecificity of their early symptoms (cough, dyspnea, and hemoptysis), usually results in a significant delay in diagnosis. The number of patients seen at any one institution has been too small to develop a general characterization of the disease or the results of its treatment. The frequency of the several histologic types from three of the larger series in the recent English literature are summarized in Table 5-1.

Anterior–posterior and lateral tomograms of the trachea are helpful in the detection of these lesions and should be done to locate the tumor precisely within the trachea, but the final diagnosis is made by bronchoscopy and biopsy.

Squamous cell carcinoma is the most common malignant tumor of the trachea and also the most common tumor of the trachea in adults. It is frequently part of the syndrome of multiple squamous cell carcinomas of the airways and oral cavity that occurs in cigarette smokers. These carcinomas are usually polypoid and will invade the tracheal wall and surrounding mediastinal structures. They metastasize to regional lymph nodes, but uncommonly develop distant metastasis; most patients die with the disease confined to the chest and obstructing the airway. Reports of long-term survival following treatment of this tumor are only anecdotal. Houston et al. (8) found one patient alive and free of tumor 5 years after radiotherapy. Hadju and coworkers (7) reported on five patients that survived at least 5 years free of disease; two of his patients had undergone surgical removal of their lesion and three had radiation therapy only. In Grillo's series (4), two patients had survived free of disease more than 5 years after primary resection and anastomosis of the trachea.

Adenoid cystic carcinoma, the second most common tracheal tumor in adults, is histologically identical to the adenoid cystic carcinoma of the salivary glands. The tumors are polypoid and often extensively infiltrate the tracheal wall and surrounding mediastinal structures. This tumor is characterized particularly by its tendency to extend in the submucosa for long distances from the gross tumor. In contrast to squamous cell carcinoma, it may metastasize widely to distant organs. Survival for 5 years following therapy is not uncom-

TABLE 5-1 Primary Tumors of the Trachea.

	Houston (8)	Hajdu (7)	Grillo (4)
Squamous cell carcinoma	24 (45%)	30 (73%)	42 (52%)
Adenoid–cystic carcinoma	19 (36%)	7 (17%)	29 (36%)
Adenocarcinoma	1	4	
Small cell undifferentiated carcinoma	2		
Mucoepidermoid carcinoma	1		
Leiomyosarcoma	3		
Other malignant tumors	3		10
Total malignant tumors	53	41	81
Total benign tumors	37		9

The number of reported cases is given. The figures in parentheses are the percent of the total malignant tumors in the series. Other malignant tumors that have been reported to be primary in the trachea are carcinoid, plasma cell myeloma, carcinosarcoma, chondrosarcoma, fibrosarcoma, and angiosarcoma.

mon, but unfortunately, death from a recurrence of this tumor more than 10 years following therapy is also not uncommon. Of Hadju's seven patients, two developed recurrent disease more than 5 years and two more than 10 years after resection and radiation therapy, while one patient was alive and free of disease 18 years after a resection. In Houston's series, 13 patients survived 5 years, and eight of these survived 10 years. Grillo reported three patients alive, free of disease, and one patient alive with a recurrence more than 5 years following a tracheal resection. Pearson et al. (12) had five patients alive and free of disease more than 5 years after resection.

At the present, tracheal resection seems to offer the greatest opportunity for long-term survival from these malignant tumors. Grillo has recommended that 5000 rads of postoperative irradiation be used if the resectional margins are short or if the regional lymph nodes are involved by tumor. Although Pearson has utilized 3500–4000 rads preoperatively and has performed the tracheal resection safely one month later, it seems to me unwise to attempt a tracheal resection and anastomosis after previous high-dose radiotherapy. In several instances, however, a resection of the larynx and cervical trachea with the construction of a low tracheostomy has been successful months or years after high-dose radiotherapy if the cervical skin is replaced by a thoraco-acromial flap.

Benign tumors of the trachea are less frequent overall than are malignant tumors, but they are relatively more common in children. A full circumferential resection of the trachea is rarely required for their treatment; many can be removed through an endoscope. Some lesions, such as squamous papilloma in children, may regress spontaneously. Benign mixed tumors of the trachea, however, should be removed by a tracheal resection. Other reported benign tumors of the trachea are hemangioma, lipoma, fibroma, hamartoma, neurilemmoma, chondroma, chondroblastoma, and granular cell myoblastoma.

Secondary Tumors in the Trachea

Exclusive of metastasis to the trachea, which is extremely rare, secondary involvement of the trachea is commonly from carcinoma that is primary in the larynx, thyroid, esophagus, or lung. I have considered any extension of carcinoma of the esophagus to the trachea to contraindicate resection. This is in contrast to involvement of the esophagus by a carcinoma of the trachea. The course of carcinoma of the esophagus is more aggressive either because it is discovered at a more advanced stage, because the structure of the esophagus allows earlier and wider spread, or because of the intrinsic nature of the tumor itself. Any involvement of the trachea or carina by an extension of a carcinoma of the lung other than a carcinoid or adenoid cystic carcinoma also contraindicates a resection if more than a limited lateral excision would be required to remove it. On the other hand, some patients may survive long term following a resection of the trachea that has been secondarily invaded by a carcinoma of the thyroid or larynx; such resections should be performed more commonly when no other location of tumor spread is apparent.

Postintubation Stenosis of the Trachea

If the defect in the anterior tracheal wall after a tracheostomy is excessively large either from removing too much of the tracheal wall during the tracheostomy or, as Andrews and Pearson have observed (1), from force applied to the anterior tracheal wall from cumbersome connecting systems, the stoma will heal by scarring and contraction to form a stricture. However, a more common cause of the tracheal strictures I have seen has been erosion from the pressure of a tube cuff. The pathology and etiology of postintubation tracheal stenosis and malacia have been described extensively by Grillo (3). With his introduction of soft, high volume cuffs that provide a tracheal seal with low inflation pressures (5), the incidence of such abnormalities has been significantly reduced.

Patients with this lesion usually present with severe dyspnea, cough, and stridor that appear within days to weeks after extubation following either a tracheostomy or the use of an endotracheal tube. Commonly one finds a 1–3 cm length of stenosis in which the normal tracheal wall has been replaced with fibrous tissue plus varying amounts of granulation tissue and inflammation. This inflammation extends transmurally and may involve the innominate artery or the esophagus. The area of stenosis is usually associated with an adjacent area of tracheal malacia, which must also be resected to restore a functional airway.

The diagnosis of benign tracheal stenosis must be confirmed by bronchoscopy, but the length of the abnormality, particularly distal to the superior portion of the stricture, is determined best by the use of tomograms and fluoroscopy. Although tracheal obstructions due to granulation tissue may be treated by endoscopic removal, and occasional minor areas of stenosis will respond to progressive dilitation, most significant postintubation strictures should be treated by tracheal resection and reanastomosis. Since these patients can be satisfactorily managed for prolonged periods by a Montgomery T tube, the resection can be postponed until all sources of infection, such as esophageal fistula, are healed and the patient's nutritional status is optimal.

Operative Procedures for Tracheal Resection

Major resections of the trachea have been a relatively recent addition to the armamentaria of the thoracic surgeon. The delay in the development of this procedure was due to the belief that two to four tracheal rings comprised the maximum resection possible with a primary anastomosis and to the knowledge that no prosthesis exists which can be used successfully to replace circumferential defects of the trachea. The present ability to resect increased lengths of the trachea with restoration of continuity is due principally to the work of Grillo.

The adult human trachea is supported by 17 or 18 cartilaginous rings, and it averages 11 cm in length; the lower 6 cm are intrathoracic and the upper 5 cm are within the neck when the neck is in a neutral position. In a detailed study of the human trachea, Salassa and co-workers (13) concluded that the blood supply of the cervical trachea is usually from two to three tracheoesophageal branches of the inferior thyroid artery, the most superior branch of which courses through the substance of the thyroid gland. They found the carina to be supplied by the superior and middle bronchial arteries. The branch of the superior bronchial artery that runs anterior to the carina also supplies the carinal lymph nodes and is immediately adjacent to them. In addition to the above, the blood supply of the thoracic trachea is from segmental tracheoesophageal arteries coursing in the lateral tracheal pedicles and arising from the supreme intercostal, the subclavian, the internal mammary, or the innominate arteries [Fig. 5-1, from the work of Salassa and colleagues (13)]. These segmental arteries anastomose with one another as well as with the inferior thyroid and bronchial arteries by a small longitudinal vessel on each lateral surface of the trachea.

Although the amount of trachea that may be resected with restoration of continuity is still limited, the limits are not as confining as previously believed. From cadaver studies, Grillo and co-workers (6,11) have reported that 5–6 cm of thoracic trachea can be resected and reanastomosed with a tension of 1000–1200 g after division of the right pulmonary ligament, hilar mobilization, pericardial dissection, and flexion of the neck from 15° to 35°. Using the same anastomotic tension, he found the length of cervical trachea that could be resected and primarily reanastomosed, with the neck flexed, averaged 5.8 cm. Intrathoracic and intrapericardial dissection of the hilus of the right lung increased this length by an average of 1.4 cm. He warned, however, that total mobilization of a long length of distal trachea, including the carina and including division of the lateral tracheal pedicles, may result in necrosis of the upper portion of this lower segment.

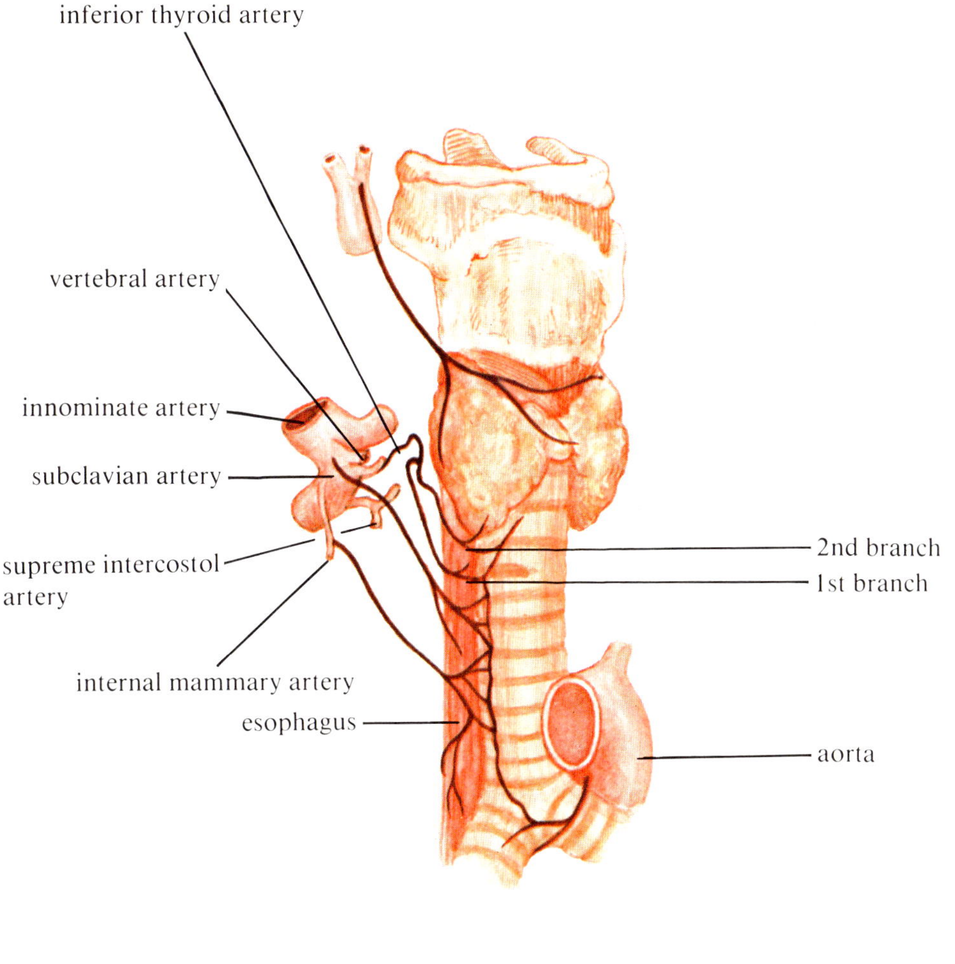

FIG. 5-1. From Salassa JR, Pearson B, Payne WS. Growth and microscopic blood supply of the trachea. Ann Thorac Surg 24:100–107, 1977. Courtesy of Little, Brown.

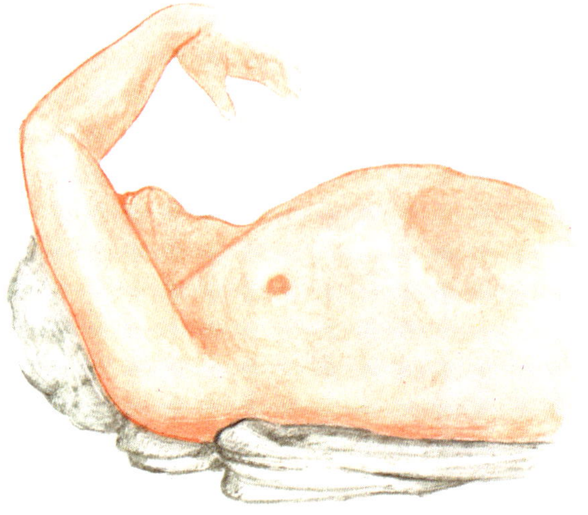

FIG. 5-2.

Resections of the Upper Trachea

The patient should be placed supine with the right arm abducted and the elbow flexed (Fig. 5-2). Provision must be made first to extend the neck and later to flex it slightly. In addition, provision should be made for elevating the right side of the chest so that an incision can be made from the sternum to the posterior axillary line, if necessary. These two maneuvers are achieved most easily by the use of two inflatable bags, one placed high between the shoulders and the other under the right chest near the spine; however, the same position may be attained by the use of sand bags and a tilting operating table. In addition to the usual anesthesia apparatus, a set of sterile corrugated gas tubes must be available to connect the ventilator to a sterile auxiliary endotracheal tube across the operative field.

The incisions for resections of the upper trachea should be performed in the sequence indicated in Figure 5-3, as the need for additional exposure develops. Most such operations can be performed solely through a cervical collar incision, thus this incision is made first. If the patient has had a previous tracheostomy, the tracheal stoma is included within the incision. If no tracheostomy is present, the incision should be placed somewhat lower than usual so if a tracheostomy becomes necessary, the stoma can be made through the superior skin flap rather than through the operative wound.

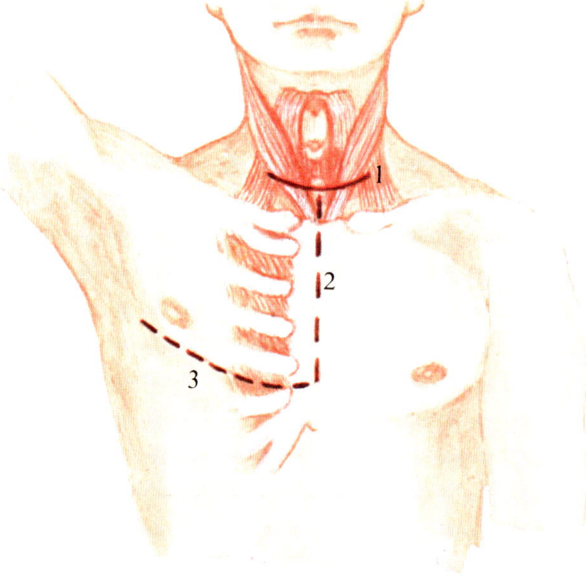

FIG. 5-3.

Although the trachea can usually be dissected to the carina through a cervical incision if the neck is extended, the placement and tying of sutures in the distal trachea is difficult when the end is more than a centimeter below the manubrium, and it is occasionally difficult to dissect the inominate artery from the trachea when both are enveloped by scar tissue. In such instances, the sternum should be split from the manubrium to the fourth intercostal space. Then, if the right lung must be released to permit the distal tracheal segment to ascend further, the sternal incision can be extended into the right fourth interspace as far as the posterior axillary line.

The skin and platysma in the superior flap of the cervical incision should be dissected to the margin of the thyroid cartilage, the strap muscles freed, and the thyroid isthmus divided to expose the anterior surface of the cervical trachea (Fig. 5-4). The extent of the resection and the consequent dissection varies with the nature of the lesion and its location. Occasionally in resections for carcinoma, the strap muscles, one or both lobes of the thyroid, and even a portion of the esophagus will require resection with the trachea. Conversely, if the resection is for treatment of a stricture, the dissection should be as close to the trachea as is possible. All care must be taken to preserve as much of the tracheal blood supply as is possible; the trachea should be freed circumferentially only over the segment to be resected. Especial care must be given to the preservation of the tracheal branches of the inferior thyroid arteries, which pass behind the common carotid arteries, descend posterior to the thyroid gland (Fig. 5-1), and enter the trachea through its lateral pedicles.

In the presence of a tracheal stricture, dense scar tissue often involves both the trachea and the esophagus near the stricture. When this occurs, the separation of the trachea from the esophagus is facilitated by putting a #40 Hurst or Maloney dilator in the esophagus. With the patient's neck extended, the anterior surface of the trachea should be freed to the carina. Below the diseased segment, this dissection can usually be done with a finger, but if difficulty is encountered, a mediastinoscope and a suction tip can be used to complete it. If the distal segment is not mobile enough, after the

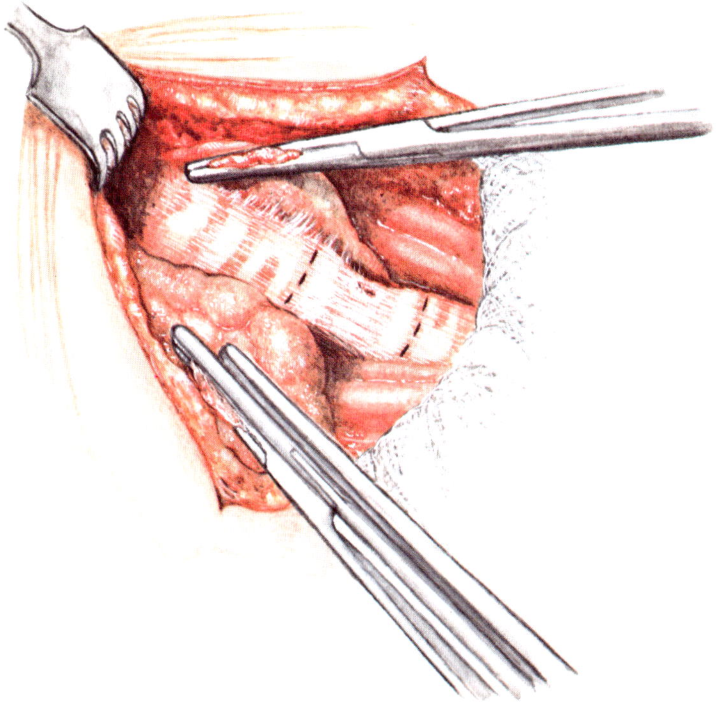

FIG. 5-4.

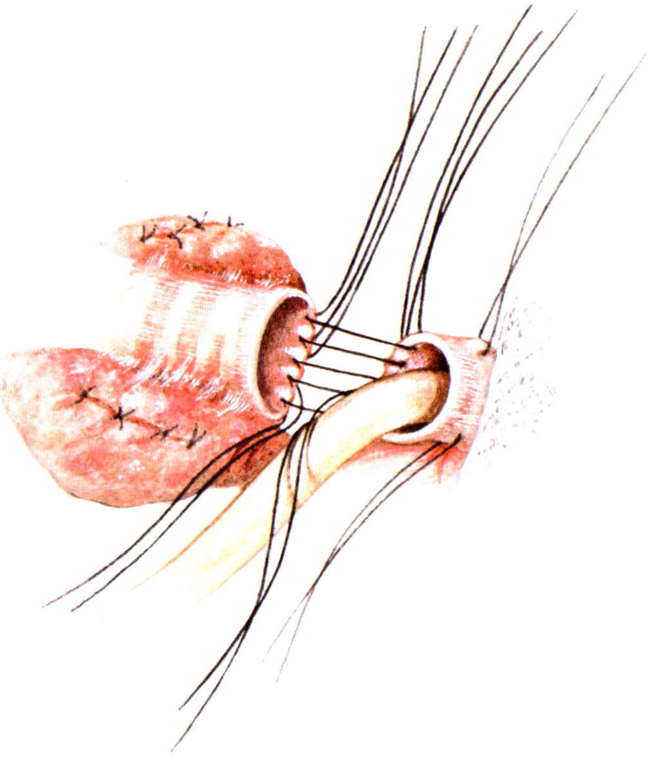

FIG. 5-5.

trachea has been divided the posterior wall of the trachea may be freed from the esophagus, leaving the lateral tracheal attachments intact. If the length is still inadequate, free the carina and the hilus of the right lung, as described for a resection of the lower half of the trachea. To control the position of the distal segment after tracheal section, place two 2–0 stay sutures in the trachea, 1.5–2 cm below the proposed level of distal division (these sutures are shown in Fig. 5-5 just above the gauze wound protector). The division of the trachea below the lesion should be done first so the distal trachea

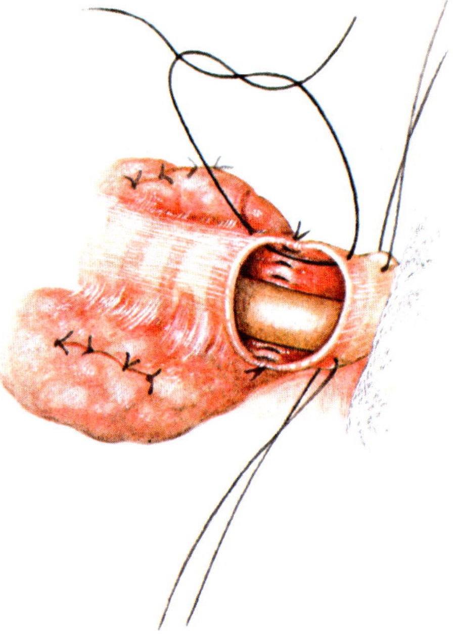

FIG. 5-6.

can be intubated and ventilation resumed immediately. If the resection is to remove a benign stricture, make the initial division through the lower part of the diseased segment; then, with the trachea open, trim off the rest of the diseased tissue under direct vision, so that no normal trachea is removed. If the resection is to remove a carcinoma, open the trachea on the side away from the tumor first so that if necessary, the level of division may be corrected without cutting into the tumor.

The distal tracheal segment is intubated with a sterile auxiliary endotracheal tube across the operative field (Fig. 5-5), and ventilation is resumed. This distal segment is short, so when positioning the endotracheal tube, take care not to obstruct the left main bronchus with the cuff of the tube. A suture from the anterior wall of the trachea tied around the tube helps to prevent this complication. Pull the peroral endotracheal tube back above the site for proximal division of the trachea, and perform this division also under direct vision of the tracheal interior. If, after flexion of the neck and mobilization of the carina and the right lung, the tension on the suture line still seems too great to permit a primary tracheal anastomosis, an additional 1.5 cm length may be obtained by a suprahyoid release using the technique described by Montgomery (10).

The anastomosis in the neck is performed with 4–0 Ethabond™ sutures with Tapercut needles. The sutures are placed 3 mm apart and about 3 mm deep; all knots are tied on the outside of the trachea (Fig. 5-5). This results in a minimum of granulation tissue and postoperative hemoptysis. To prevent an excess of tension developing on a few sutures, as they are tied the two ends of the trachea should be approximated by the assistant using the previously placed stay sutures. After the posterior row of sutures has been placed and tied, the auxiliary endotracheal tube is removed and the peroral tube advanced into the distal trachea to continue ventilation while the anterior suture line is completed (Fig. 5-6). The adequacy of the tracheal closure should be tested by positioning the cuff of the endotracheal tube proximal to the anastomosis and ventilating the patient while dropping saline on the suture line to detect air leaks. Any leak at all should be closed.

If the tracheal anastomosis is immediately adjacent to the innominate artery, other tissue should be interposed between these two structures. A flap of pericardium has proven adequate and convenient to construct. Others have recommended the use of sternocleidomastoid muscle or one of the strap muscles.

It is my practice to use for 24 hours only a Hemovac drain under the skin flap, placed well away from the anastomosis. The routine use of a tracheostomy is not necessary and risks infecting the region of the anastomosis and the mediastinum. If assisted ventilation is necessary in the postoperative period, the endotracheal tube may be left in place for 4 or 5 days, but the cuff must not be against the anastomosis. Bronchial secretions the patient is unable to cough up are best removed by use of the flexible bronchoscope. In accordance with Grillo's recommendation, the patient's neck should be kept flexed for the first 8–10 days (2).

Because of the multifocal nature of squamous cell carcinoma of the airway, it is sometimes necessary to do a tracheal resection in a patient who has had a previous laryngectomy. In such a patient, the maximal length of trachea that may be resected is less than the length which may be resected in a patient with a previously intact larynx and trachea. If the length of trachea available to make a tracheostomy above the manubrium is inadequate, the disparity in reach may be decreased somewhat by resecting the manubrium below the first ribs and removing the medial third of the clavicles and the

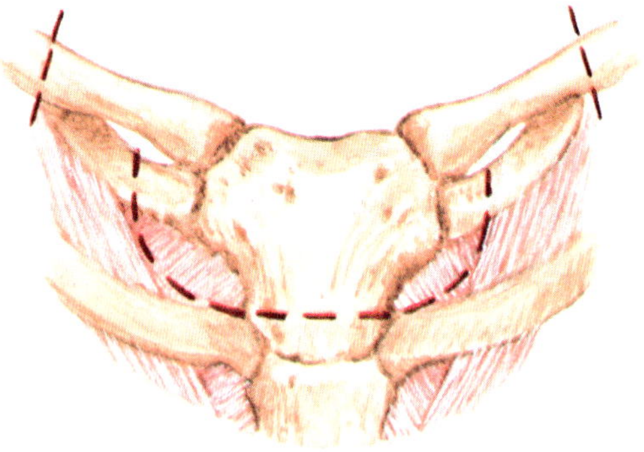

FIG. 5-7.

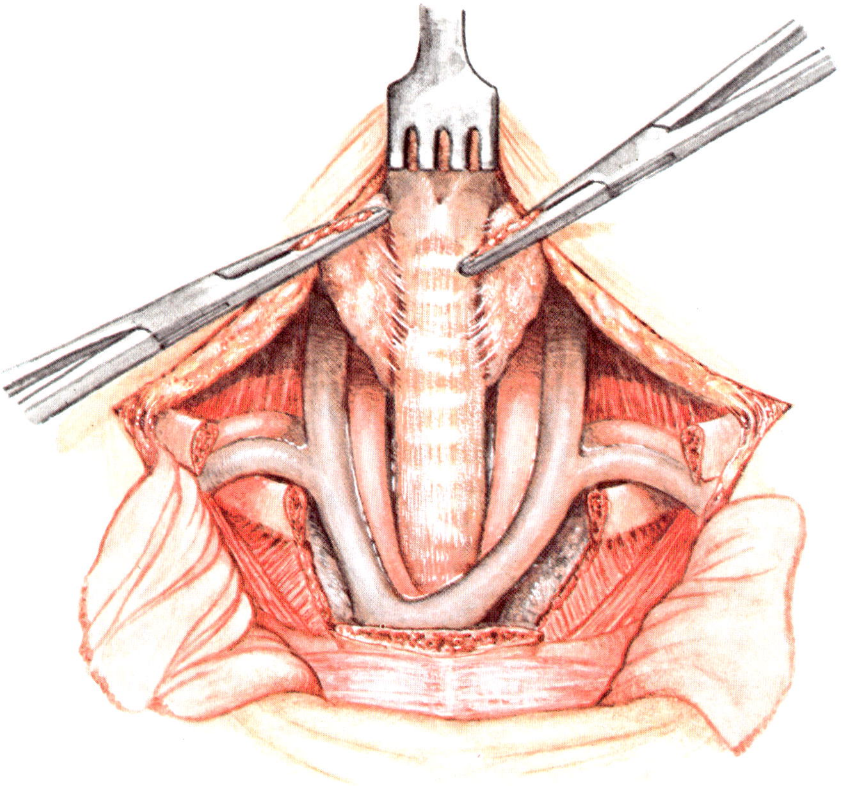

FIG. 5-8.

first costal cartilages (Fig. 5-7). A sternal resection greater than this results in little improvement, because the increase in length of trachea available as the tracheostomy site is moved inferiorly is matched by the increase in distance between the trachea and the sternum; as the trachea descends into the chest, it moves posteriorly, parallel to the spine, while the sternum tends to angle anteriorly. The major anatomic structures of this operative field are depicted in Figure 5-8. In addition, as described by Terz et al. (14), the risk of herniations of the lung through the anterior chest wall defect increases as more of the sternum and upper ribs are removed. Every effort should be made to preserve as much of the posterior tracheal wall as is consistent with complete removal of the cancer, since a greater length of posterior than of anterior tracheal wall is required to reach the skin.

When a tracheal resection is performed for a recurrence of tumor at a prior tracheostomy site, the combination of carcinoma and skin necrosis from previous irradiation will usually require a wide resection of skin over the anterior aspect of the neck. A full-thickness thoracoacromial flap (Fig. 5-9A and B), a bipedicled upper thoracic flap (Fig. 5-10), or a myocutaneous flap of the pectoralis major (described in Ch. 6) may be used to cover such a defect. The tracheostomy stoma is made through the flap. If a bipedicled flap is used, the lower incision should be extended down the anterior axillary fold so enough length is available to permit moving the flap to the neck.

When complete removal of the cancer requires resection of a portion of the cervical esophagus, the esophagus should be closed distal to the tumor with a TA-30 stapler. Divide the esophagus above the staple line and let the thoracic end retract into the mediastinum. Divide the esophagus above the tumor and make a pharyngostomy or esophagostomy from the remaining

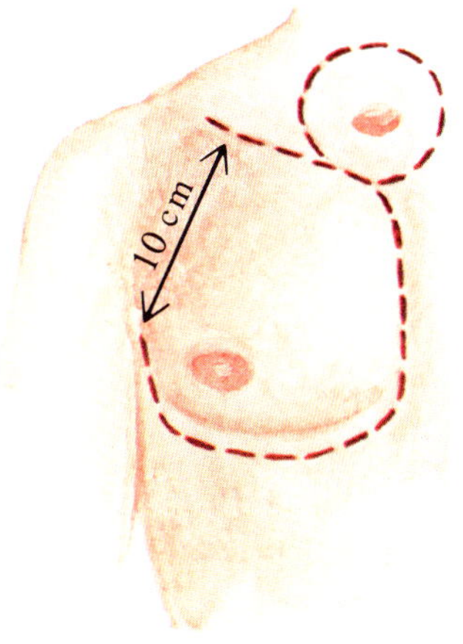

FIG. 5-9A.

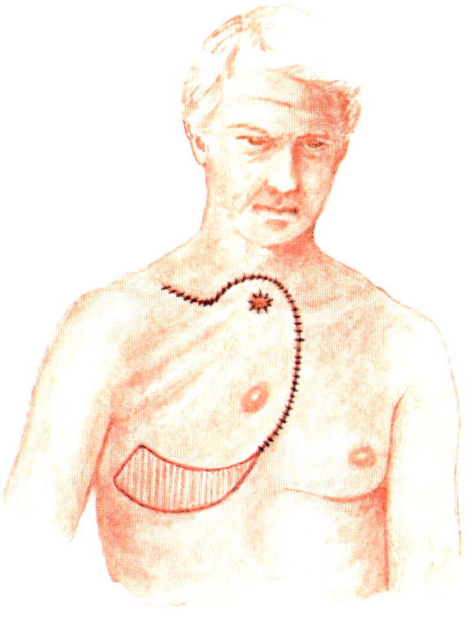

FIG. 5-9B.

cervical esophagus. Complete the tracheal anastomosis or the construction of a tracheostomy, close the cervical wound, and construct a Stamm gastrostomy. After a 3-week interval to permit the patient to return to a positive nitrogen balance, allow the mediastinum to seal and any cervical flaps to heal, I use either the right colon and terminal ileum pedicled on the middle colic vessels (Fig. 5-11) or the transverse colon pedicled on the left colic artery to restore deglutition. I have never had any problem with insufficient length using either of these two methods. In patients with a permanent tracheostomy or a tracheal anastomosis, the colon is placed in a subcutaneous position over the anterior chest and the anastomosis to the esophagus is placed

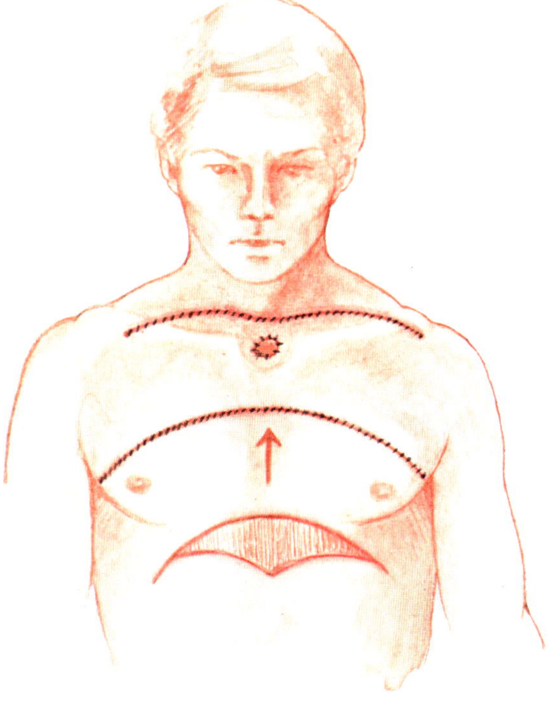

FIG. 5-10.

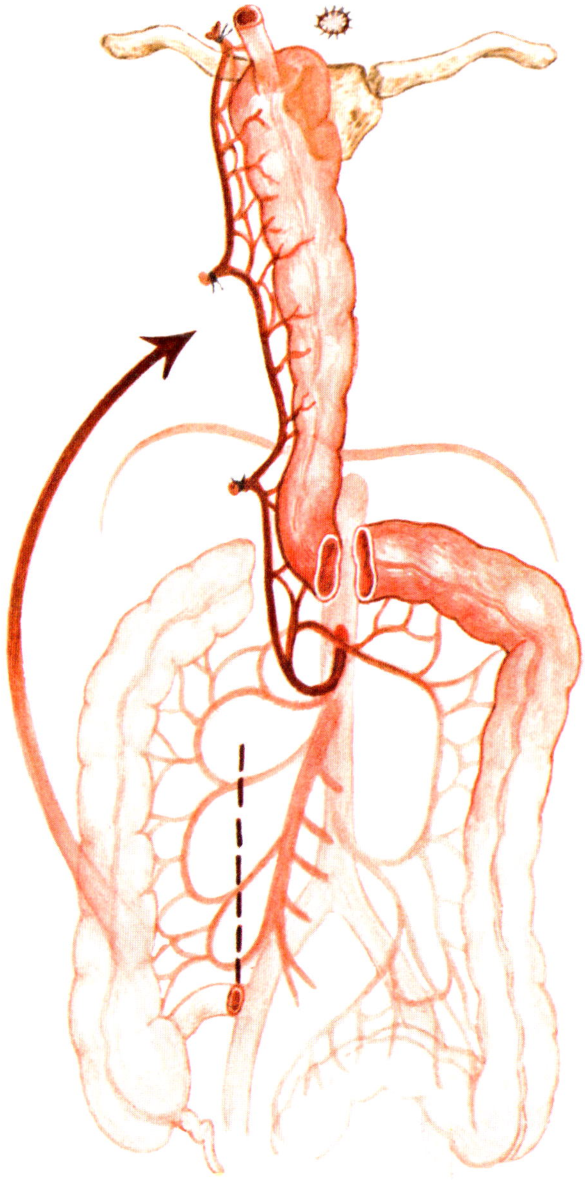

FIG. 5-11.

laterally so the tracheal anastomosis will not be exposed to the risk of contamination from a leak at the esophageal anastomosis, if such should occur. The anastomosis of the bowel to the esophagus is performed using two layers of interrupted 5–0 Ethabond™, and the cologastrostomy is done with a typical two-layered open technique.

Resections of the Lower Trachea

The patient's trachea should be intubated transorally with an endotracheal tube 35–36 cm in length to permit passing the tube into the left main bronchus after the auxiliary transthoracic endobronchial tube is removed. The patient is placed in a straight lateral position for a standard right posterior–lateral incision through either the fourth interspace or the bed of the fifth rib. The head must be free enough to permit flexing the neck 30°.

It is advisable to complete all of the necessary mobilization prior to resecting the lesion. Begin by dividing the pleura between the esophagus and trachea from the level of the innominate artery to the azygos vein. In Figure

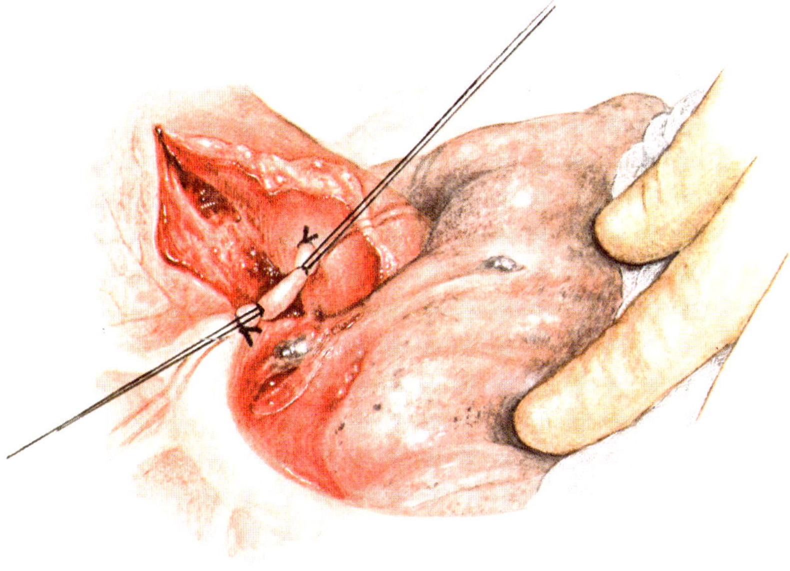

FIG. 5-12.

5-12, the patient's head is on the left; as this figure depicts, isolate the azygos vein, ligate it anterior and posterior with 2–0 ligatures plus 3–0 suture ligatures, and divide the vein between them. Separate the trachea from the esophagus over the length of the tumor and for approximately 2 cm above it, but do not divide the lateral tracheal pedicles above this point. Separate the superior vena cava from the lesion and from the lymph nodes and connective tissue that lie between the trachea and the vena cava; dissect the anterior surface of the trachea free to the thoracic outlet, leaving the lymph nodes attached to the area of the tumor. Figure 5-13 shows the azygos vein divided and the trachea separated from the superior vena cava above and the esophagus below. If the tumor is resectable, incise the pleura that reflects onto the posterior aspect of the lung from the azygos vein down to the diaphragm, and divide the pulmonary ligament. Free the carina and both the right and left main bronchi from the esophagus, but unless the carina is to be resected, leave the lymph nodes under the carina intact in order to preserve the bronchial artery on the surface of the carina. (These lymph nodes with the bronchial artery can be seen in Fig. 5-13.)

Separate the right main bronchus anteriorly from the vena cava and the pericardium to the level of the right pulmonary artery, and separate

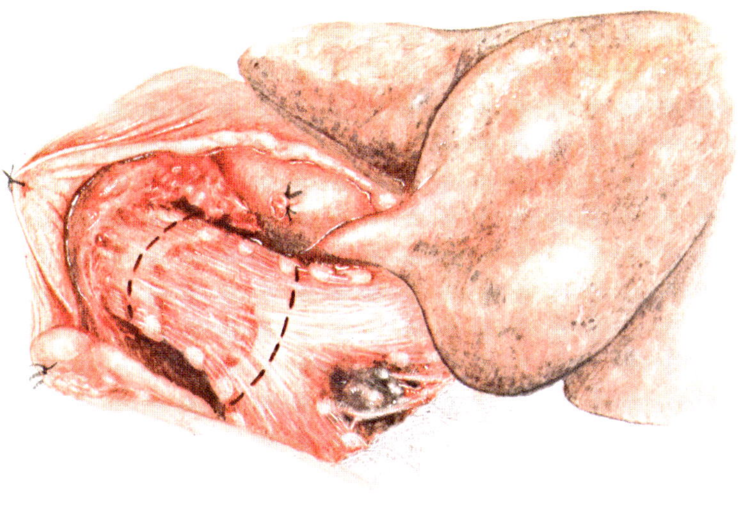

FIG. 5-13.

2–3 cm of the left main bronchus from the aorta. Dissect the left side of the trachea and its adjacent lymph nodes free of the ascending aorta down to the left main bronchus, but do not clean off either the trachea or bronchi, for the longitudinal anastomotic vessels may be damaged. Test the mobility of the right hilus and the carina; if additional mobility seems to be required, open the pericardium between the phrenic nerve and the right superior pulmonary vein. Extend this incision from the pulmonary artery to the inferior vein and then superiorly on the posterior side of the hilus, freeing both the anterior and posterior aspect of the pulmonary veins from the pericardium. Some additional mobility may be obtained by freeing the right pulmonary artery from the pericardium behind the superior vena cava.

The trachea should be divided first below the tumor so the left main bronchus can be intubated immediately. The site for this initial incision into the trachea is difficult to determine, because the internal extent of the tumor cannot be palpated and it frequently does not correspond to the external abnormality. (The tumor has been ghosted in for Fig. 5-13 and the extent of the resection noted by the dashed lines.) Because of the difficulty in determining the extent of the tumor, it is important to measure the distance from the inferior limit of the tumor to the carina on both posterior–anterior and lateral tomograms and during bronchoscopy. These measurements are used to determine the site of the incision which should be at least one full ring and preferably two rings below the lowest mucosal abnormality. If possible, the incision should be started on the side opposite the principal mass of the tumor so that, if the choice of site was incorrect, the incision may be altered without cutting into the tumor.

Prior to dividing the trachea, a sterile endotracheal tube of the proper size should be connected to the gas tubes already in the operative field (Fig. 5-14). As soon as the trachea has been divided, the left main bronchus is intubated, taking care not to obstruct the left upper lobe, the tube cuff is inflated, and ventilation of the left lung through this transthoracic system is started. (This intubation of the left main bronchus is shown in Fig. 5-15.) It should be an assistant's responsibility to continually aspirate blood from the distal end of the trachea, for if blood is allowed to remain in either main bronchus, the patient's postoperative course may be significantly complicated.

Withdraw the oral endotracheal tube to a position above the proposed proximal site of tracheal division, but leave it within the trachea so that it may be advanced easily after the posterior–medial sutures on the left side are placed. Place two nonabsorbable 2–0 stay sutures in the trachea 1.5–2 cm above the site of division to control the position of the proximal tracheal segment (Fig. 5-15). Divide the trachea above the tumor and remove the diseased segment. In doing this it may be necessary to resect a segment of the right vagus nerve because its proximity to the trachea in this region makes it liable to involvement with the disease process. I have not found any disability from dividing the vagus at this level.

Prior to making the anastomosis, the anesthesiologist should flex the patient's neck by about 30°. The anastomosis is performed using 4–0 Ethabond™ sutures in the manner described previously for an upper tracheal anastomosis (depicted here in Fig. 5-15). The endobronchial tube in the distal tracheal segment is retracted out of the way and the sutures in the left half of the anastomosis are placed first. If there is a discrepancy in size between the upper and lower segments, this discrepancy is most easily corrected on the membranous portion of the trachea. After all the sutures on the left side have been placed, they are tied while the assistant approximates the two ends of the trachea so that the tension on any single suture is not enough

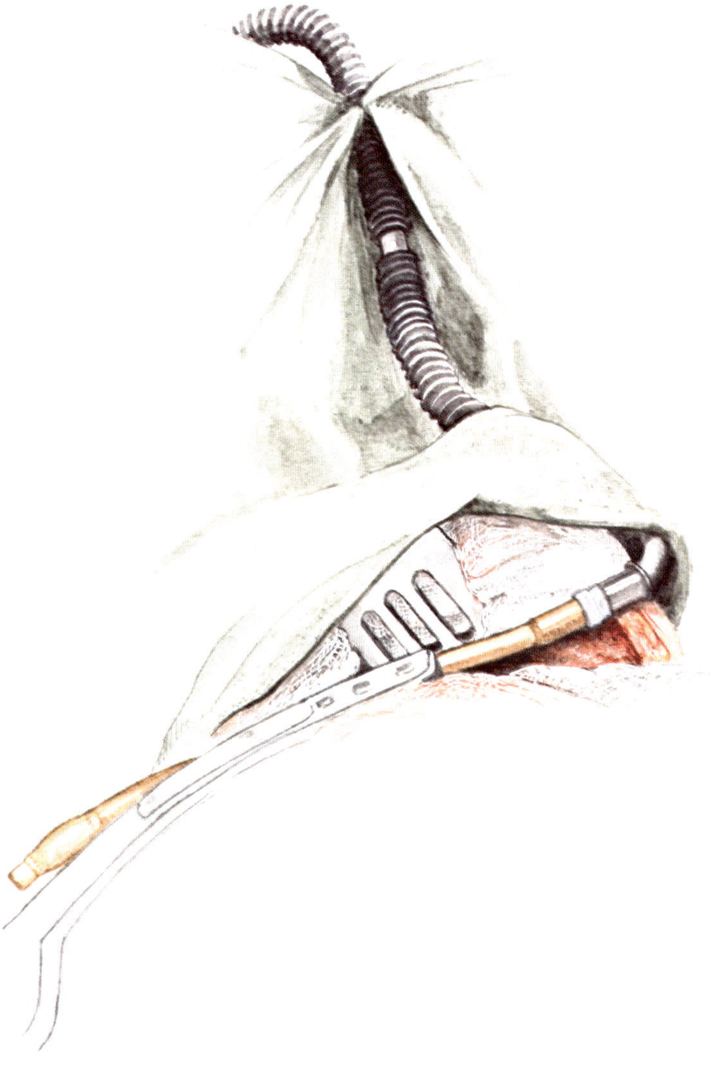

FIG. 5-14.

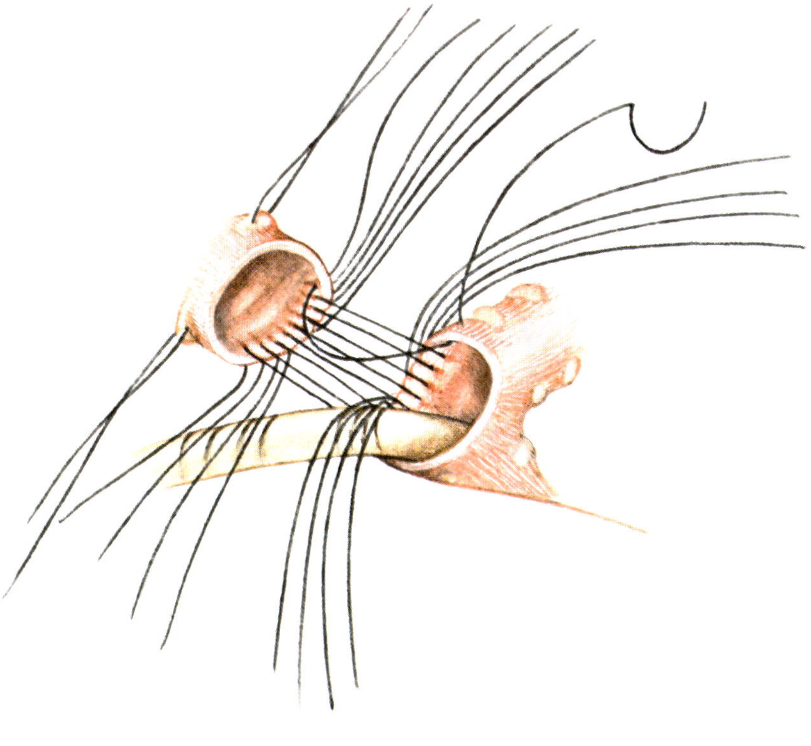

FIG. 5-15.

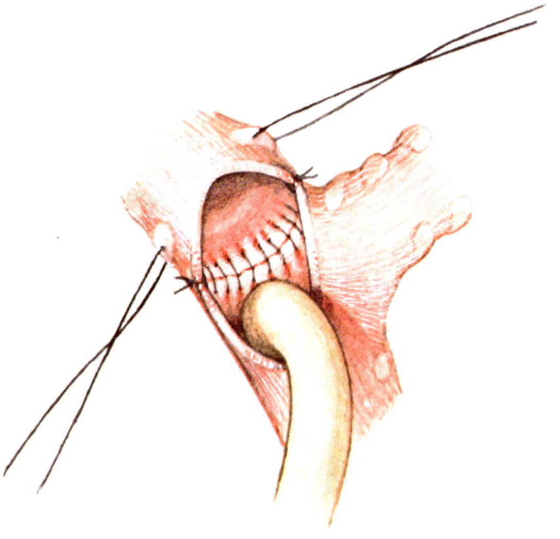

FIG. 5-16.

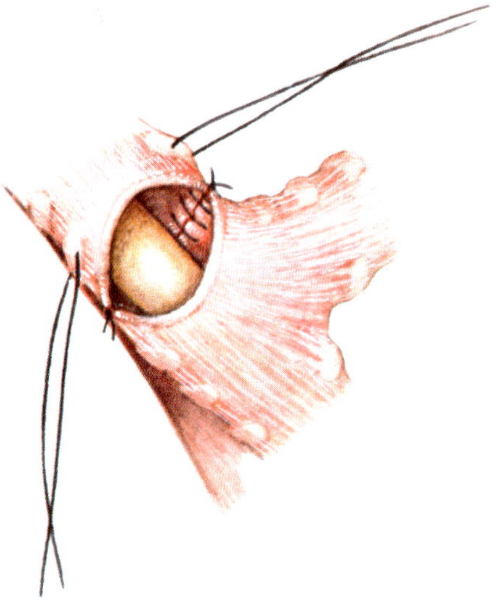

FIG. 5-17.

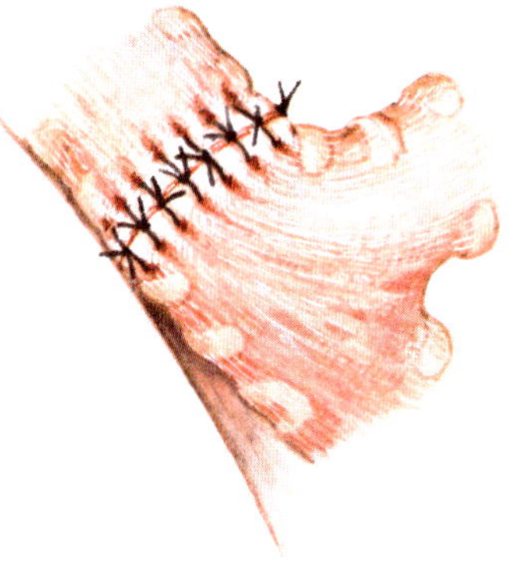

FIG. 5-18.

to cut through the tracheal wall. In Figure 5-16, the left half of the anastomosis has been completed with all knots on the outside.

When all sutures on the left half of the anastomosis have been tied, the transthoracic endobronchial tube is removed, the trachea suctioned well, and the oral entotracheal tube advanced past the anastomosis into the left main bronchus (Fig. 5-17); the cuff is inflated and ventilation of the left lung is resumed by this route. The sutures on the right side of the anastomosis are placed and tied as on the left side. After the anastomosis has been completed, it should appear similar to that in Figure 5-18. The cuff on the endotracheal tube is then deflated, the tube pulled back proximal to the anastomosis, and the cuff again inflated. Test the anastomosis for air leaks by covering it with saline and increasing the airway pressure to 20 cm H_2O. If no air leaks are found, construct a broad-based flap of parietal pleura and suture this carefully over the anastomosis to buttress the seal (Fig. 5.19). The completed covering can be seen in Figure 5.28. A tracheostomy should not be done because the space has been developed from the site of a potential tracheostomy to that of the anastomosis, and the possibility of an infection in this space would exist if a tracheostomy communicated with it.

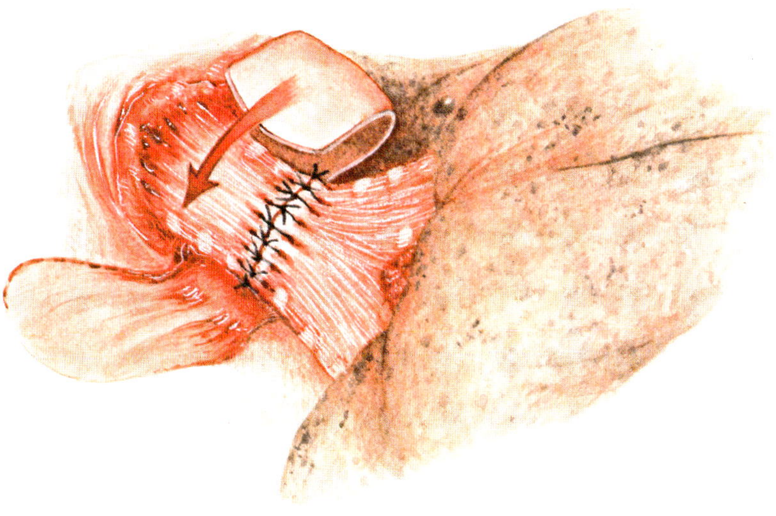

FIG. 5-19.

In the postoperative period the patient's neck should be kept flexed for the first 8–10 days. Instruct the personnel to insert suction catheters only to the length of the endotracheal tube; any deeper suctioning ought to be done with a flexible bronchoscope.

Resections of the Carina

The procedure for a carinal resection is usually similar to the one described for a resection of the lower half of the trachea, except that a carinal resection must be tailored to the location of the lesion, which may involve primarily the trachea, the right main bronchus, the left main bronchus, or any combination of these three structures. Although a tumor of the carina will usually require a circumferential resection of either the right or the left main bronchus, it does not always require a completely circumferential resection of the trachea and of both bronchi. Because of the various possible resections, it is difficult to plan the reconstruction before the necessary excision has been completed. This is particularly true of resections done for adenoid cystic carcinoma that may have submucosal extensions for a considerable distance beyond the gross tumor margin.

In situations for which a left pneumonectomy, in addition to a carinal resection, is necessary (Fig. 5-20A,B), the approach should be through a left thoracotomy utilizing the bed of the fifth rib and mobilization of the arch of the aorta to expose the lower trachea. This operation requires ventilation of the right lung by transthoracic intubation of the right main bronchus, a procedure which is hazardous because the orifice of the right upper lobe bronchus begins only 1–2 cm from the carina. All other types of carinal resections are performed preferably through a right thoracotomy.

The right hilus, the right main bronchus, the carina, the left main bronchus, and the trachea should be mobilized, preserving the lateral blood supply of the trachea (as previously depicted in Fig. 5-13). If the right main bronchus is primarily involved and a right upper lobectomy is required without a circumferential resection of the trachea or left main bronchus, the right bronchus intermedius should be sutured to the lower portion of the defect in the left main bronchus and the trachea (Fig. 5-21A and B). This anastomosis should be done even if the patient could tolerate a right pneumonectomy, for it not only preserves a significant volume of functioning lung, but permits the closure of the defect in the trachea and left bronchus without narrowing the airway. The residual defect in the trachea may be closed in an anterior–posterior

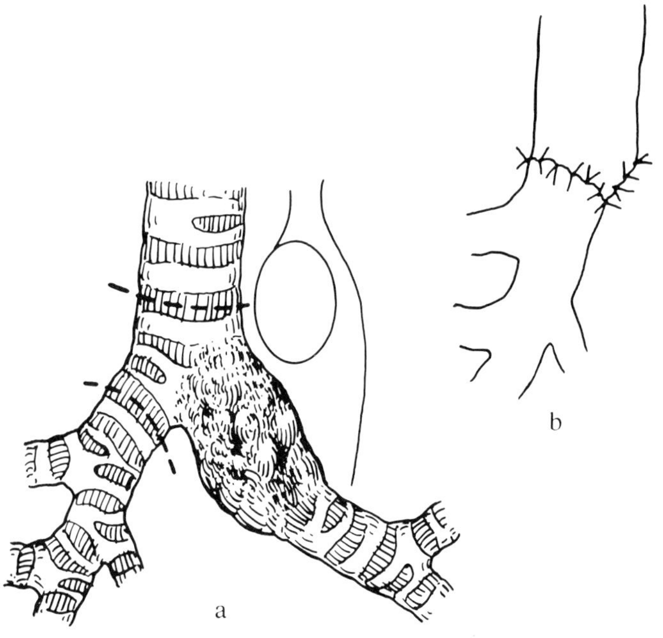

FIG. 5-20A,B.

direction (as the suture line in the trachea above the anastomosis of the right bronchus to the trachea in Fig. 5-21B depicts). If such a closure causes significant narrowing of the trachea, the trachea must be shaped and anastomosed to the bronchus as described by Grillo (4) and illustrated in Figure 5-22A and B. Because the left main bronchus is relatively fixed, in patients for whom complete circumferential resections of the trachea and both main bronchi must be done, it is usually easiest to anastomose the left main bronchus end to end to the proximal trachea, and anastomose the right main bronchus to the side of the trachea (Fig. 5-23A and B).

If the length of lower trachea that must be removed is too great to permit an anastomosis of the trachea to the left main bronchus, the right main bronchus can be anastomosed to the residual trachea and the left main

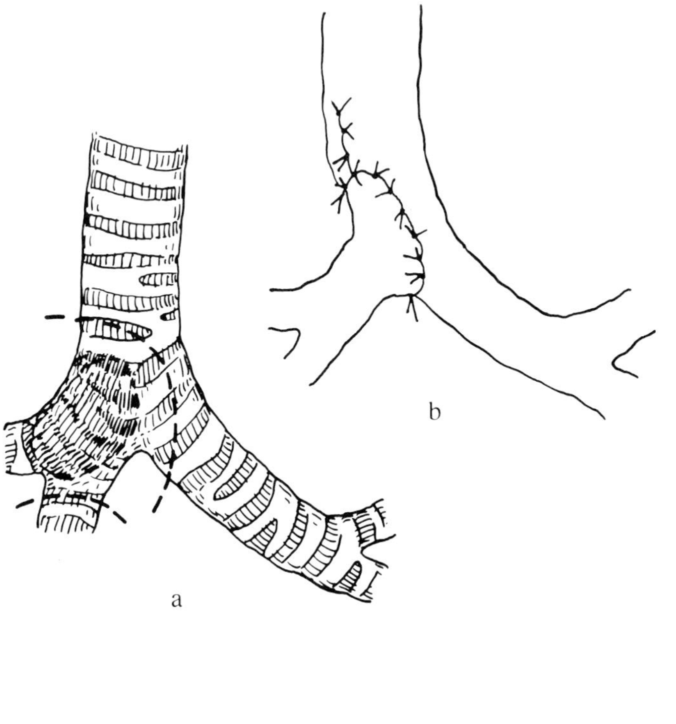

FIG. 5-21A,B.

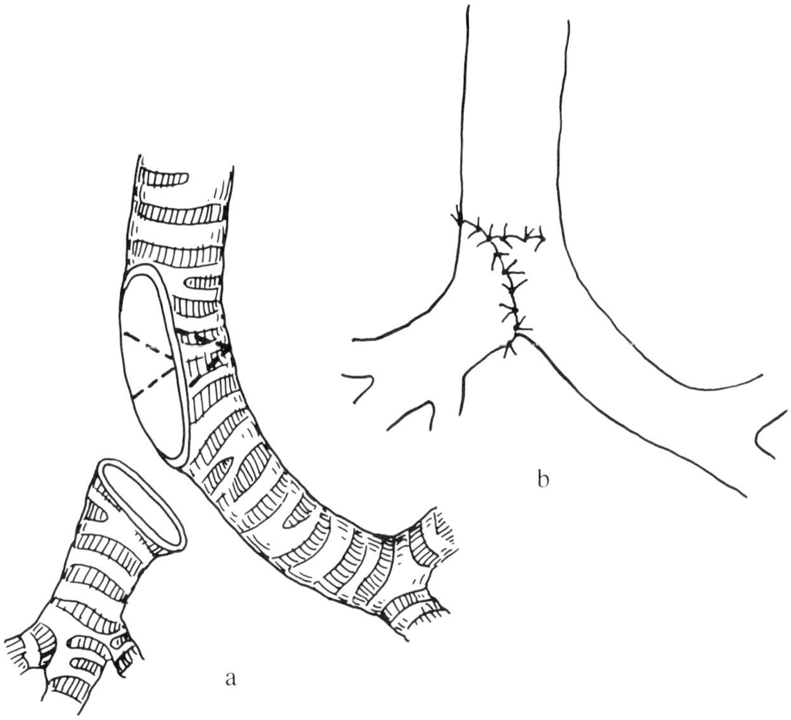

FIG. 5-22A,B.

bronchus anastomosed end to side to the bronchus intermedius (Fig. 5-24A and B). This operation should not be attempted for a lesion much above the carina if a significant length of distal trachea must be used for the anastomosis. In one such patient with a midtracheal carcinoma, after completely mobilizing the carina and transecting the left bronchus, a 3.5-cm length of trachea above the carina was anastomosed to the proximal trachea high in the chest. This anastomosis did not heal and the patient ultimately died from an erosion of the innominate artery 6 weeks after surgery.

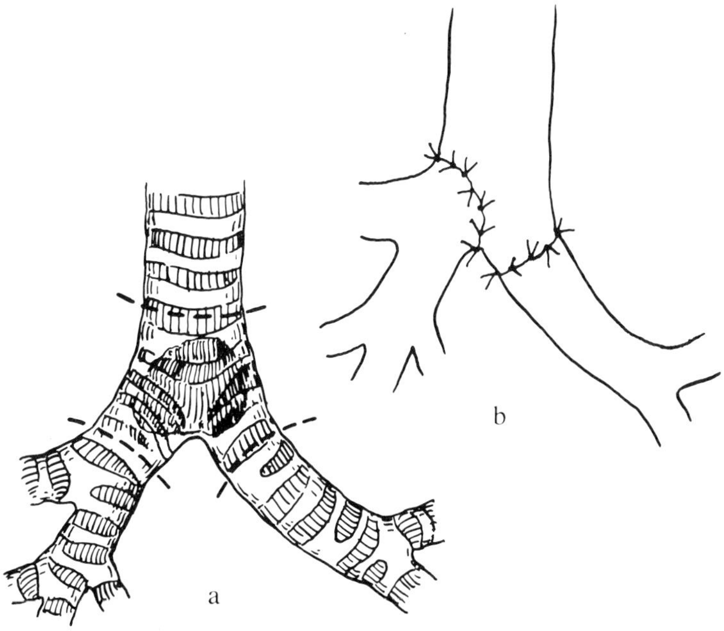

FIG. 5-23A,B.

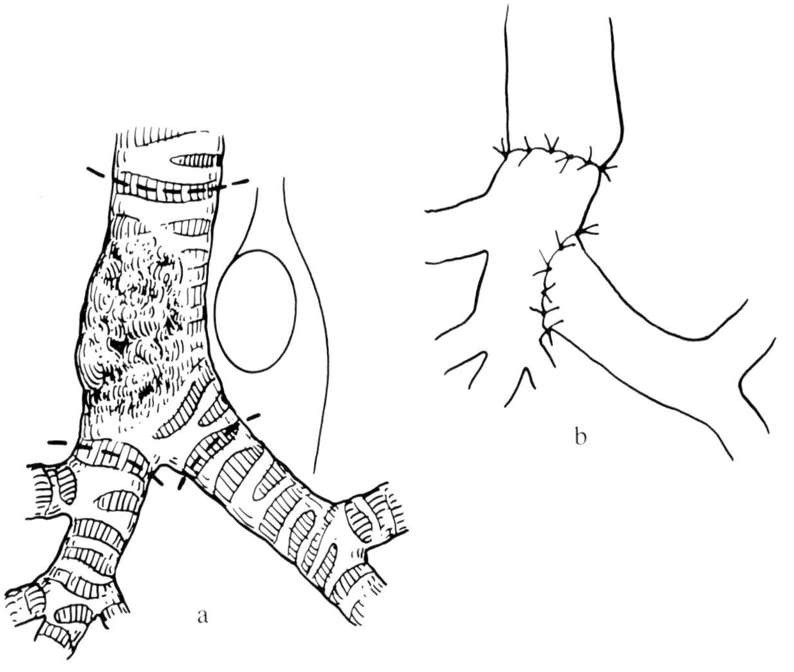

FIG. 5-24A,B.

Bronchoplastic Procedures

Over the past 20 years, it has become evident that patients with a carcinoma of the lung completely removable by a lobectomy have as good a long-term survival if treated by a lobectomy as when treated by a pneumonectomy. It has also become evident that patients treated by a pneumonectomy will develop, in time, an increasing respiratory and cardiac disability. These conclusions have motivated surgeons to extend the indications for lobectomy, by the use of bronchoplastic procedures on the main bronchus, to patients that would otherwise have required a pneumonectomy. The operation of lobectomy with a bronchoplasty, termed a sleeve resection of the main bronchus, permits the complete removal of some carcinomas involving the main bronchus in patients who could not tolerate a pneumonectomy. Bronchoplasty without lobectomy is indicated to repair a traumatic transection or tear of a main bronchus either early after the trauma or late after a bronchial stricture has formed.

In most published series of lobectomy with a bronchoplasty performed for a carcinoma of the lung, the patients are highly selected, but in these series, the results have been superior. Jensik et al. (9) reported a projected 10-year survival of 30.3% with an operative mortality of 1.8% in 57 patients having a sleeve lobectomy for carcinoma of the lung. Weisel et al. (15) performed the same operation on 27 patients having compromised pulmonary function and on 43 having uncompromised function, with an overall 11% postoperative mortality. Of those patients with complete resection of the tumor and uncompromised pulmonary function, 36% survived for 5 years. At the Minneapolis Veterans Administration Medical Center and the University of Minnesota, 25 patients with compromised pulmonary function underwent a lobectomy and a sleeve resection of the main bronchus with an 8% postoperative mortality. Fifty percent of the patients who had resection for a squamous cell carcinoma of the lung survived 5 or more years.

The various combinations of lobectomy and bronchial resection that have been done are depicted in Figures 5-25A (right upper lobectomy), 5-25B (left upper lobectomy), and 5-25C (left lower lobectomy). A right upper lobectomy

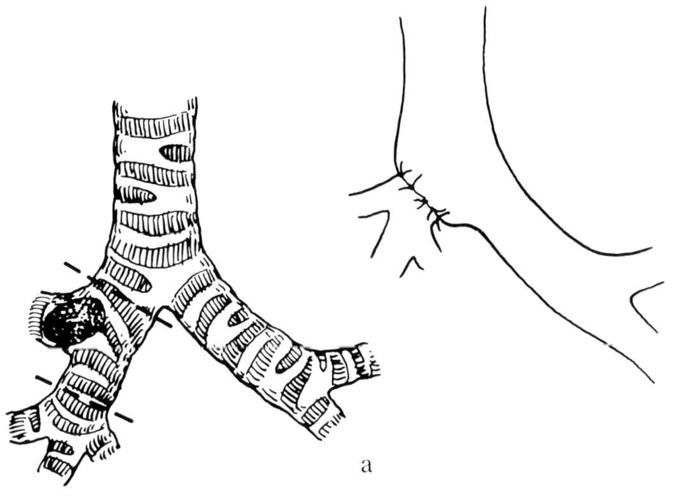

FIG. 5-25A.

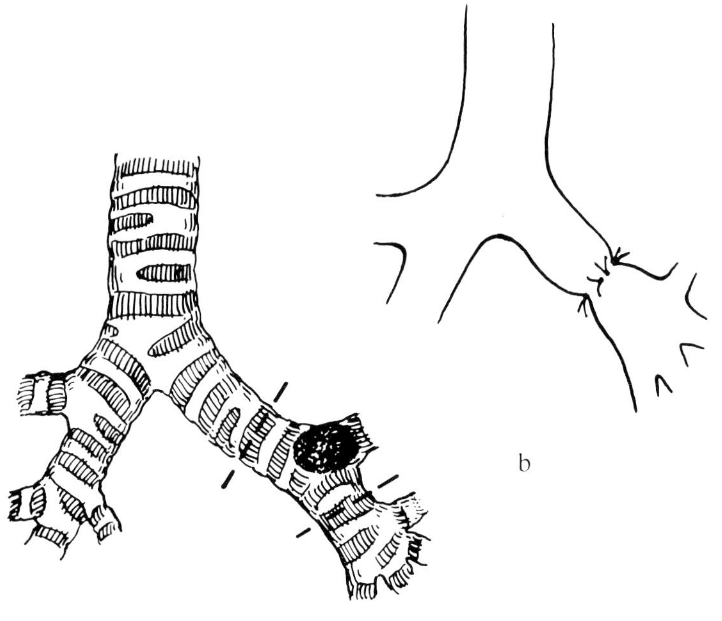

FIG. 5-25B.

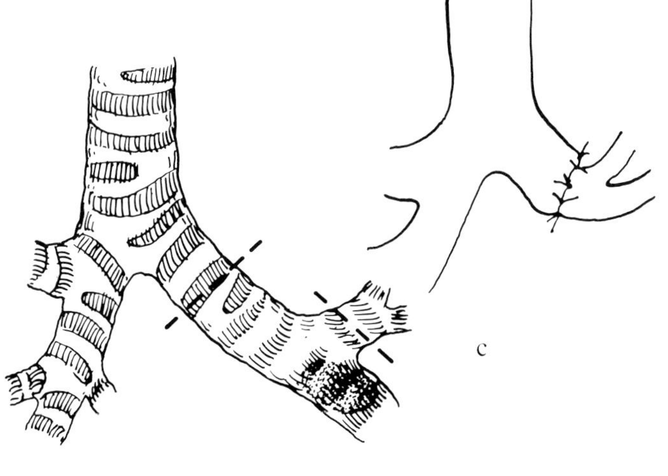

FIG. 5-25C.

with a resection of the right main bronchus and an anastomosis of the bronchus intermedius to the carina is the most commonly performed operation because the main pulmonary artery and the artery to the superior segment of the lower lobe are not as close to the upper lobe bronchus on the right as they are on the left, so they are less apt to be involved with an upper lobe cancer. Resections of the lower lobes plus the main bronchi, with an anastomosis of the upper lobe bronchus to the carina, may be useful for extensive submucosal extension of carcinoma, but this requires biopsy evidence that the upper lobe bronchus has not also been invaded.

In addition to the usual operative findings contraindicating a resection, the specific adverse findings for a sleeve lobectomy are three: 1) invasion of the trachea or carina above the proposed level of resection or extension of the carcinoma to the segmental bronchi or arteries of the remaining lobe, 2) invasion of the parenchyma of the remaining lobe by cancer, and 3) extension of carcinoma to the main pulmonary artery or to the pulmonary vein from the remaining lobe. On occasion, it has been possible to resect a segment of the left main pulmonary artery and reanastomose it, but the situation in which such a procedure will remove all obvious disease is rare.

Only the technique of right upper lobectomy with a bronchoplasty of the main bronchus will be described here since the principles are similar for all bronchoplastic operations. The patient should be intubated with a double-lumen endobronchial tube such as the Robertshaw tube. This permits making the anastomosis without applying clamps to the bronchus, thus avoiding the risk of damage to the bronchial blood supply or mucosa. If an intraoperative situation arises in which a bronchoplasty is indicated but the patient has not been intubated with a double-lumen tube, the proximal bronchus may be occluded with a vascular clamp, but this is an inferior method. A Robertshaw tube is preferred to a Carlens tube because the former has no spur crossing over the carina to interfere with the bronchial anastomosis.

The dissection of the right upper lobe should progress (as described in Ch. 4) until the arterial supply and the venous drainage have been divided and the parenchyma of the upper lobe has been separated from that of the middle lobe and the lower lobe. Next, ligate the azygos vein near its junction with the superior vena cava using two 2–0 nonabsorbable ligatures and two 3–0 suture ligatures. Divide the vein between the ligatures. Dissect the divided vein from the lateral surface of the trachea and expose both the anterior and posterior aspects of the carina, together with 1–2 cm of the trachea and left main bronchus, but do not clean them off or free them more extensively because such dissection may impair the blood supply to the anastomosis. Free the right pulmonary artery from its attachments to the bronchus so it can be retracted anteriorly if necessary. Expose the bronchus intermedius and the origins of the superior segmental bronchus and the middle lobe bronchus by dissecting the hilar lymph nodes overlying the bronchus toward the upper lobe. To prepare the carina for anastomosis, dissect the subcarinal lymph nodes toward the right side, but leave them attached to the segment of the right main bronchus that will be resected (Fig. 5-26 depicts the dissection completed to this point). Mobilize the lower and middle lobes by dividing the pulmonary ligament and the pleural reflections from the mediastinum to these lobes. It is advisable to complete all of the dissection and mobilization prior to dividing the bronchus so that the time available for entry of blood into the bronchus or for contamination of the pleural cavity with endobronchial organisms will be as short as possible.

With all preparation for the anastomosis complete, inflate the tube cuff in the left main bronchus and discontinue the ventilation of the right lung

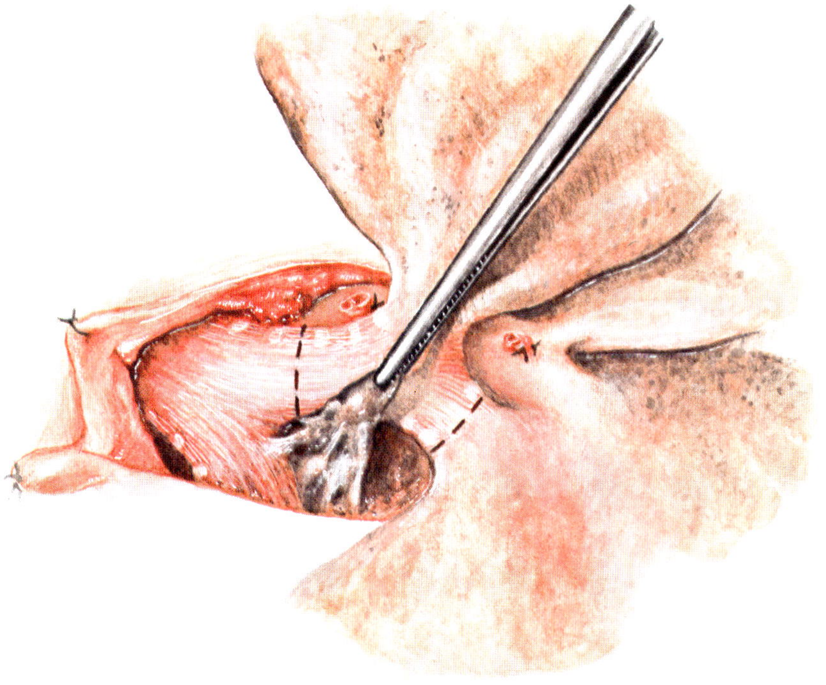

FIG. 5-26.

while continuing it to the left lung. Divide the bronchus intermedius distal to the tumor first at the level indicated by the dashed line in Figure 5-26. This division should be between the cartilaginous rings so that no fragmentation of the cartilage will interfere with the anastomosis. Divide the right main bronchus at the carina and remove the upper lobe with the resected segment of the right main bronchus and the attached lymph nodes. During the period the bronchus is open, keep all blood sucked out of the bronchi, for intrabronchial blood can be the cause of a severe postoperative pneumonia.

The anastomosis is performed using interrupted sutures of 4–0 Ethabond™ with tapercut needles; the sutures are placed so all knots are tied on the outside. Commonly, the stump of the right main bronchus will be larger than is the bronchus intermedius. This discrepancy should be eliminated by closing the lateral portion of the right main bronchus with a few interrupted 4–0 Ethabond™ sutures to the degree necessary to make the size of this opening equal to that of the bronchus intermedius. (This is illustrated in Fig. 5-27A by the three sutures in the trachea above the opening in the right main bronchus.) Place the sutures for the anastomosis of the cartilaginous portion of the bronchi first, beginning in the middle of the medial wall and tagging and arranging the sutures (Fig. 5-27A). The sutures should be placed 3 mm apart and about 3 mm deep. Prior to tying these sutures, the bronchus intermedius should be approximated to the carina by pushing up on the remaining lobes so the tension developing on any one suture from pulling the bronchical ends together will not be great enough to cut the bronchial wall. The sutures must be tied only tightly enough to approximate the ends of the bronchus; greater tension than this may cause the suture to cut through the wall. When the sutures in the cartilaginous portion of the bronchial wall have been tied, the sutures in the membranous portion are placed (Fig. 5-27B) and tied in a similar manner. Ventilation of the right lung can then be resumed. The completed anastomosis of the bronchus intermedius to the stump of the right main bronchus is illustrated in Figure 5-27C.

To inspect the anastomosis for air leaks, cover the bronchus with saline and ask the anesthesiologist to maintain an airway pressure of 20 cm H_2O

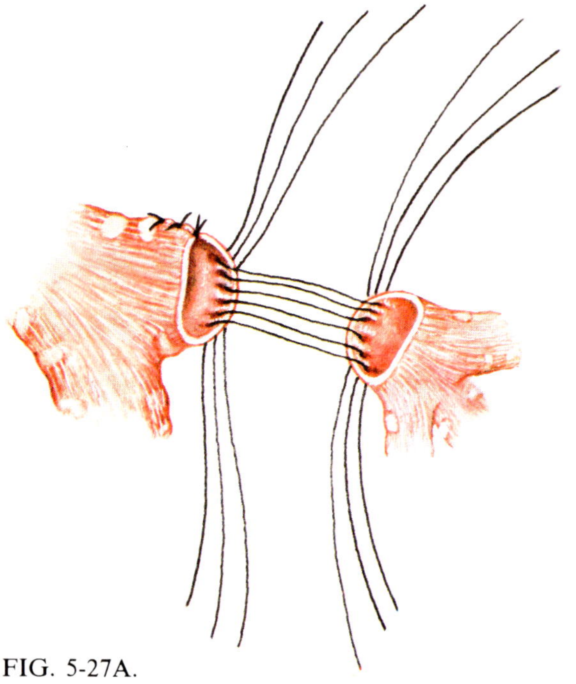

FIG. 5-27A.

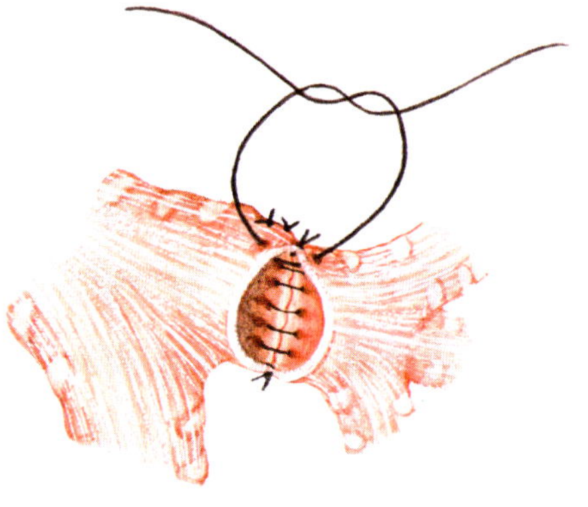

FIG. 5-27B.

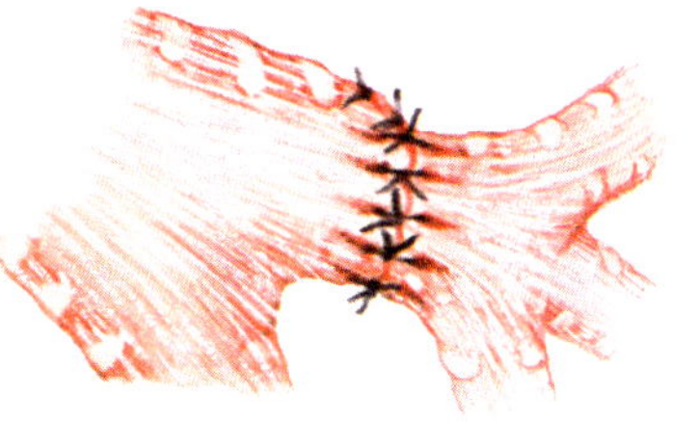

FIG. 5-27C.

for a few seconds. If any bubbles are seen coming from the anastomosis, the leak should be stopped with additional sutures, placed as horizontal mattress sutures if the leaks are from tears by previous sutures. When the suture line is air tight, it should be further buttressed by covering it with a pleural flap carefully sutured to the bronchus (Figure 5-28). The stump of the transected azygos vein often serves admirably for this purpose.

It has been my practice to examine the inside of the bronchial anastomosis with a flexible bronchoscope and to thoroughly clean out the bronchi prior to extubating the patient. For the first few postoperative days there may be enough swelling around the anastomosis to impair the patient's ability to clear bronchial secretions. If this occurs, the bronchoscopic removal of mucous should be repeated as often as necessary to prevent atelectasis or pneumonia. A tracheostomy is not necessary. If a problem with inadequate ventilation is encountered, the double-lumen endobronchial tube should be replaced with a single lumen endotracheal tube. Such a tube may be left in place for 5 or 6 days if necessary while the patient's respiration is assisted by mechanical ventilation.

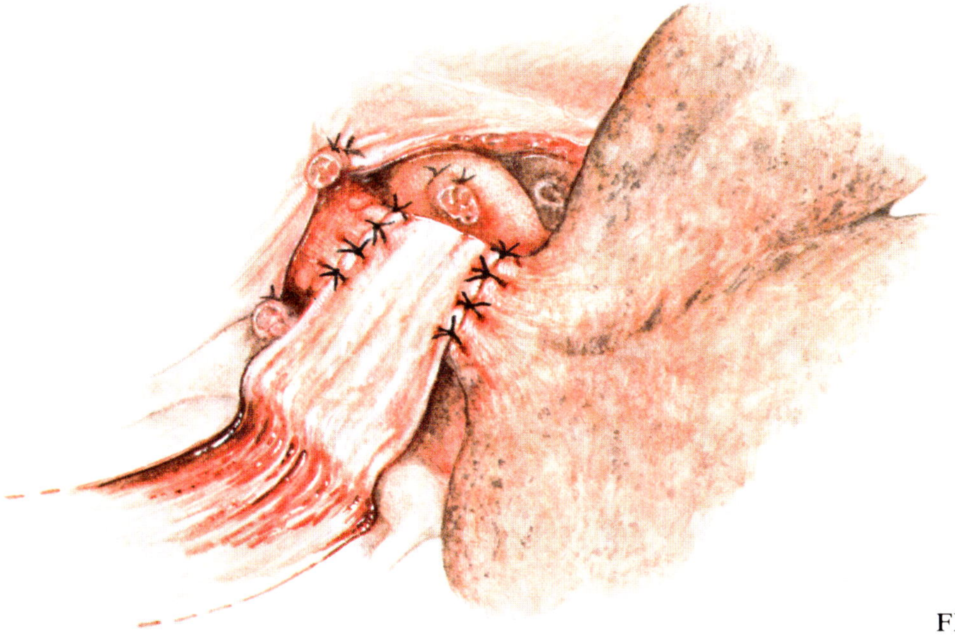

FIG. 5-28.

References

1. Andrews MH, Pearson FG: Incidence and pathogenesis of tracheal injury following cuffed tube tracheostomy with assisted ventilation. Ann Surg 173:249–263, 1971.
2. Grillo HC: The management of tracheal stenosis following assisted respiration. J Thorac Cardiovasc Surg 57:52–68, 1969.
3. Grillo HC: Surgery of the trachea. Curr Prob Surg July 1970.
4. Grillo HC: Tracheal tumors: Surgical management. Ann Thorac Surg 26:112–125, 1978.
5. Grillo HC, Cooper JD, Geffin B, Pontoppidan H: A low-pressure cuff for tracheostomy tubes to minimize tracheal injury. J Thorac Cardiovasc Surg 62:898–907, 1971.
6. Grillo HC, Dignan EF, Miura T: Extensive resection and reconstruction of mediastinal trachea without prosthesis or graft: An anatomical study in man. J Thorac Cardiovasc Surg 48:741–749, 1964.
7. Hajdu SI, Huvos AG, Goodner JT, Foote FW, Beattie EJ: Carcinoma of the trachea. Cancer 25:1448–1456, 1970.
8. Houston HE, Payne WS, Harrison EG, Olsen AM: Primary cancers of the trachea. Arch Surg 99:132–140, 1969.
9. Jensik RJ, Faber LP, Milloy FJ, Amato JJ: Sleeve lobectomy for carcinoma. J Thorac Cardiovasc Surg 64:400–412, 1972.
10. Montgomery WW: Suprahyoid release for tracheal anastomosis. Arch Otolaryngol 99:255–260, 1974.
11. Mulliken JB, Grillo HC: The limits of tracheal resection with primary anastomosis: Further anatomical studies in man. J Thorac Cardiovasc Surg 55:418–421, 1968.
12. Pearson FG, Thompson DW, Weissberg D, Simpson WJK, Kergin FG: Adenoid cystic carcinoma of the trachea. Ann Thorac Surg 18:16–29, 1974.
13. Salassa JR, Pearson B, Payne WS: Growth and microscopic blood supply of the trachea. Ann Thorac Surg 24:100–107, 1977.
14. Terz JJ, Wagman LD, King RE, Brown P, Neifeld JP, Lawrence W: Results of extended resection of tumors involving the cervical part of the trachea. Surg Gynecol Obstet 151:491–496, 1980.
15. Weisel RD, Cooper JD, Delarue NC, Theman TE, Todd TRJ, Pearson FG: Sleeve lobectomy for carcinoma of the lung. J Thorac Cardiovasc Surg 78:839–849, 1979.

The Chest Wall and Diaphragm

6

Primary Chest Wall Tumors

Tabulations of primary benign and malignant tumors of the chest wall are commonly presented in a form such as Table 6-1, but the exact diagnosis of a chest wall tumor is often not evident before surgery. Consequently, based on the history and the radiologic findings, the surgeon must make two decisions: (1) Should the initial approach to the lesion be a biopsy, a total excision, or neither? (2) If the lesion is to be excised with or without a preliminary biopsy, how extensive should the resection be? Most published series of primary rib tumors have reported 50%–60% malignancy. Overall, the most frequent tumors of the bony thorax are metastatic deposits from other primary malignancies. Such lesions need biopsy only if the histology is in serious doubt. The most common lesion confused with a neoplasm is a fractured rib with nonunion.

Almost 50% of all chest wall tumors originate from cartilage. Because the radiologic and histologic appearance of chondrosarcomas and benign chondromas are often indistinguishable (1) in or near the costochondral junction, any tumor that expands and replaces normal bone, particularly with a characteristic mottled calcification of the matrix, must be assumed to be a chondrosarcoma and removed by a wide resection without a preliminary biopsy. These tumors may also occur in other regions of the chest wall; if such a diagnosis is suspected, and the lesion is growing or is over 4 cm in diameter, it should also be resected without a preliminary biopsy.

A bony excresence on a stalk with a cartilaginous cap having a distinct outer margin and containing a mottled calcification is characteristic of an osteochondroma. Although fewer than 1% of solitary osteochondromas are malignant, pain or growth of such a lesion after puberty suggest a sarcomatous change and are indications for resection. This principle also implies that any osteochondroma arising after puberty should be resected. In an adult an osteochondroma that is not on a stalk cannot be reliably distinguished from a chondroma. If such a tumor is over 4 cm, it should be resected.

Fibrous dysplasia is a slowly growing, solitary, expansile lesion with a central trabecular pattern. It occurs most commonly in the posterior aspect of the ribs. Although the diagnosis is often suggested radiologically, it may

TABLE 6-1 Primary Chest Wall Tumors (Excluding Skin Tumors).

Ribs	Sternum	Soft Tissues
	Benign	
Chondroma	Chondroma	Desmoid
Osteochondroma	Aneurysmal bone cyst	Lipoma
Fibrous dysplasia	Giant cell tumor	Hemangioma
Eosinophilic granuloma	Hemangioma	Neurilemmoma
Giant cell tumor		
Aneurysmal bone cyst		
Osteoblastoma		
Hemangioma		
	Malignant	
Chondrosarcoma	Chondrosarcoma	Fibrosarcoma
Plasmacytoma	Plasmacytoma	Liposarcoma
Ewing's sarcoma	Malignant lymphoma	Rhabdomyosarcoma
Malignant lymphoma	Osteosarcoma	Malignant Schwannoma
Osteosarcoma	Ewing's sarcoma	
Fibrosarcoma	Fibrosarcoma	
	Angiosarcoma	

be difficult to distinguish from the sarcomas that arise in the same region. If fibrous dysplasia is the most likely preoperative diagnosis, it is my practice to plan the surgery so that a preexcisional biopsy may be done. If the preoperative diagnosis was correct, a conservative resection of the lesion is performed, but if the diagnosis was incorrect and the tumor is a chondrosarcoma, osteosarcoma, or fibrosarcoma, a radical resection with total excision of the biopsy tract is required. If the preoperative evaluation suggests one of the latter three sarcomas, a radical resection without a preliminary biopsy is used. A lesion thought to be a Ewing's sarcoma, a plasmacytoma, or a malignant lymphoma is biopsied, then treated with irradiation. Desmoids are aggressive nonmalignant lesions with a proclivity for recurrence. Although they develop most commonly in the anterior abdominal wall, they may also occur in the muscles or fascia of the chest. They should be treated by a wide resection of the full thickness of the thoracic wall with 4 cm lateral margins, if possible.

The sternum is a frequent site of metastasis from distant malignant tumors, and in addition, 80%–85% of all primary sternal tumors are malignant, commonly chondrosarcomas or osteosarcomas. The most common benign tumor of the sternum is a chondroma, which cannot with certainty be differentiated histologically from a chondrosarcoma. These data have led to the conclusion that all primary tumors of the sternum should be considered malignant and treated by a wide resection without preliminary biopsy unless evidence of multiple myeloma, malignant lymphoma, or some other disseminated malignancy is found.

Wide Resection of the Chest Wall

The best opportunity to cure a patient of a chest wall malignancy belongs to the surgeon performing the first excision; therefore, he should make every effort, within reason, not to err by resecting too conservatively. The reconstruction of the chest wall should be planned prior to the resection, for it may influence the placement of the incision. When possible, the skin incision should not immediately overlie the closure of the skeletal portion of the chest wall. However, if the tumor is large enough to put the skin in jeopardy of invasion, or if a previous biopsy has been done, the overlying skin and the entire thickness of the chest wall, with a 4–5 cm margin, should be resected. If the resulting defect is large enough to require the use of sizable rotational flaps, preliminary

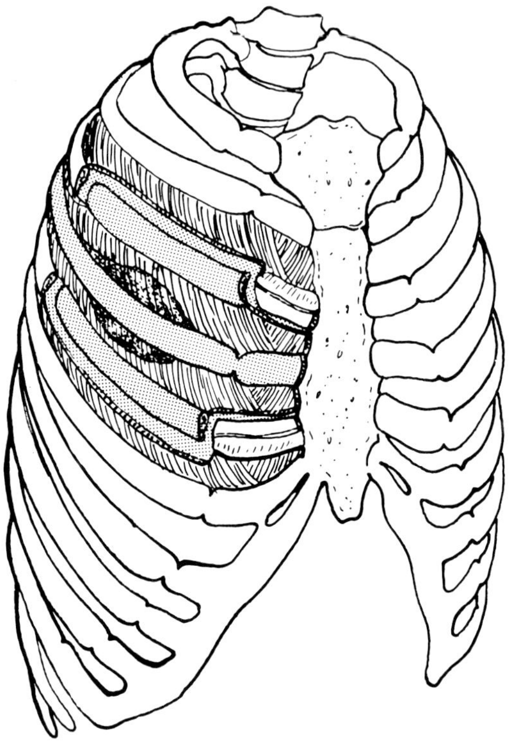

FIG. 6-1.

obliteration of the pleural cavity by a pleural abrasion performed 2–3 weeks prior to the resection may be advisable. This procedure will prevent collapse of the lung and possible pulmonary insufficiency if necrosis of the flaps should occur. The wide resection of a malignant chest wall tumor often necessitates the removal of a portion of those muscles, such as the serratus anterior and the pectoralis major, which insert directly on the involved ribs. However, the more superficial layer of muscles can often be spared. Due to the utility of a latissimus dorsi myocutaneous flap in the reconstruction of the chest wall, a particular attempt should be made to spare this muscle if it can be done without compromising the resection.

Because of the risk of spread within the marrow cavity, the resection of a malignant primary rib tumor should include the entire rib of origin. In addition, lengths of all grossly involved ribs plus one uninvolved rib above and below the tumor should be resected with 5-cm margins anterior and posterior to the tumor. (Such a resection is shown in Fig. 6-1 for a tumor of the right fourth rib that extends anteriorly to about the midclavicular line. The darkened, stippled segments of ribs are to be removed.) To perform an adequate resection, it may be necessary to resect some or all of the sternum or the transverse processes and up to 20% of the bodies of adjacent vertebra. The resection for tumors arising from the lower ribs may include a portion of the abdominal wall, the diaphragm, or the pericardium. If the lung is adherent to the tumor, the adherent portion should be resected in continuity with the chest wall.

Make an incision large enough to insert a finger in the interspace beyond the first uninvolved rib above or below the tumor and palpate the pleural surface to determine if tumor extension beyond that visible on the chest radiogram has occurred. If the chosen rib and interspace are indeed free of tumor, extend the interspace incision from a point 5 cm posterior to the tumor to one 5 cm anterior to the tumor. Reflect the periosteum from a 2-cm segment of this rib at both ends of the interspace incision and divide the rib at both places. Doubly ligate the intercostal vessels under the rib and divide them between the ligatures. If the lung is adherent to the tumor (as illustrated in Fig. 6-2), no attempt should be made to dissect it free. Instead, place an adequate sized stapler, usually the TA-55 with 3.5-mm staples, around the adherent slip of lung, staple across the involved portion of lung, as shown in the figure, and divide the lung distal to the staple line, leaving the amputated portion of lung attached to the tumor.

Continue to divide the ribs and interspaces to be resected above and below the rib of origin until only that rib remains attached. Divide the pleura and intercostal muscles in the center of the interspace above and below the rib of origin from the site of the posterior division of the other ribs to the transverse process of the vertebra and from the position of anterior division to the sternum. Doubly ligate and divide the internal mammary vessels at the anterior end of these two interspaces; with a scalpel divide the costal cartilage at the site of its attachment to the sternum. If this site of division would not provide an adequate tumor-free margin, the next step in extending the resection is to remove an adjacent segment of sternum to its midline; if this is also inadequate, the entire width of the sternum should be removed. Insert a finger under the sternum and sweep the pericardium away from the posterior surface of the bone over the area to be resected. Using an air driven sternal saw with a pleura-guard attachment, cut a section out of the sternum (as shown in Fig. 6-3 for a tumor located in the region indicated by the dashed circle). With the anterior end of the chest wall section free, loosen the posterior end of the remaining rib by inserting an osteotome between the rib and the transverse process as an assistant puts inward pressure on the anterior end of the rib (similar to the maneuver illustrated in Fig. 6-11, but without resecting the transverse process). Ligate the intercostal vessels at the posterior end of the interspace and complete the separation of the rib from the vertebral body with the osteotome.

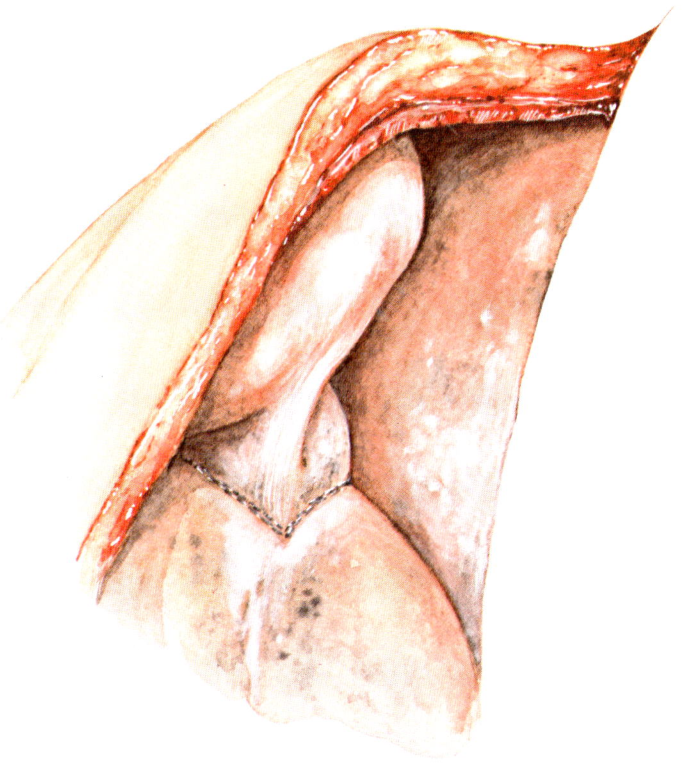

FIG. 6-2.

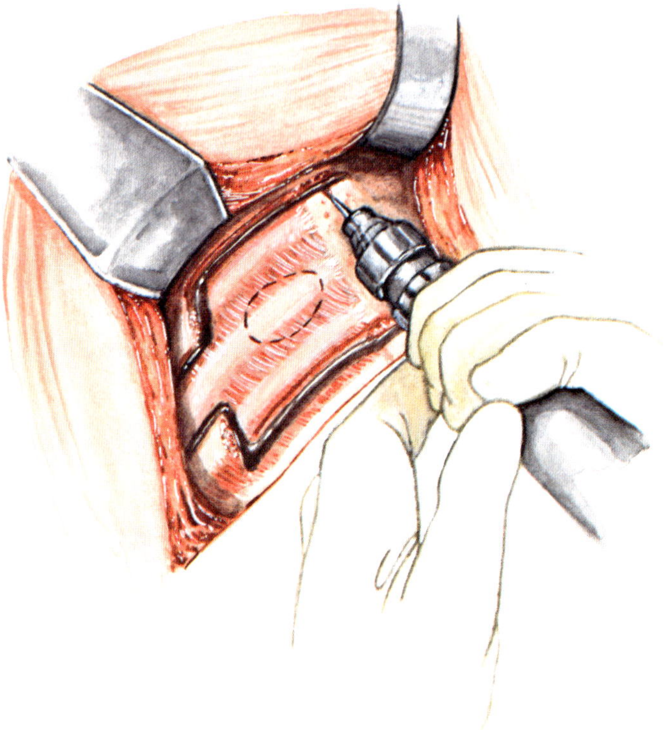

FIG. 6-3.

The resection of a sternal tumor should be planned so that at least a 5-cm margin of uninvolved sternum and chest wall around the tumor is removed. Figure 6-4 shows the defect created by the resection of a tumor in the lower sternum at the level of articulation with the fifth rib; the entire lower sternum, with a portion of both cartilaginous webs, has been resected. A resection of such a large tumor arising in the lower sternum will often result in the development of a significant ventral hernia from denervation of the anterior abdominal musculature. Usually a portion of the sternum can be spared, but occasionally an adequate resection will require the removal of the entire sternum, the costal cartilages, and segments of ribs bilaterally or of portions of the pericardium, diaphragm, or anterior abdominal wall.

For small or moderate-sized sternal tumors, make a transverse incision that curves under the tumor from one anterior axillary line to the other. Large tumors often require a vertical midline incision, and because of the lack of tissue between the sternum and the skin, an elliptical piece of skin overlying the tumor must often be excised. To determine the deep extent of a tumor in the lower portion of the sternum, extend the incision through the linea alba, and palpate the posterior surface of the sternum through a defect made in the diaphragm at its insertion onto the xiphoid process. If the tumor is in the upper sternum, divide the external cervical fascia and palpate the deep surface through the suprasternal space. In the manner previously described, resect a 2-cm segment of a rib, 5 cm lateral to the tumor, and insert a finger into the right pleural cavity to determine if tumor has invaded the pericardium or other adjacent mediastinal or chest wall structures.

Continue to divide the ribs on both sides of the tumor, ligating the intercostal bundles with 2–0 suture ligatures and incising the pleura over the full extent of both lateral incisions. If the incisions cross the cartilages of ribs 5 through 9 (as would be required for the resection shown in Fig.

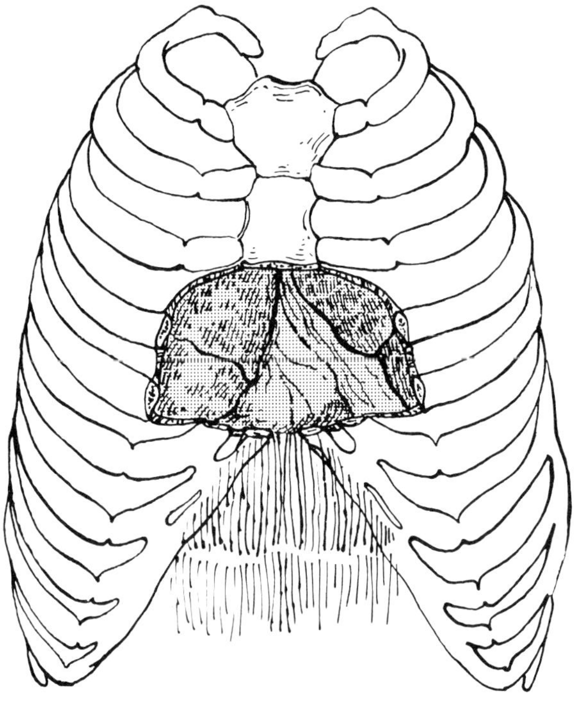

FIG. 6-4.

6-4), care must be taken not to leave devitalized or denuded cartilage in the wound. The sternum should be divided at least 5 cm from the gross margin of the tumor. Because most tumors tend to occur toward the ends of the bone, the sternum is usually divided at just one point and the upper or lower portion containing the tumor removed. However, if a tumor does occur toward the middle, less postoperative disability will occur if the two ends of the sternum with attached ribs are left intact.

The interspaces at the level of sternal division should be incised from the lateral incisions that divide the ribs to the sternum. Doubly ligate and divide the internal mammary vessels on both sides; then insert a finger under the sternum to create a retrosternal space. Divide the sternum at this point with the air-driven sternal saw. If the pericardium or other mediastinal structures have been invaded by tumor, the area of involvement can now be excised under direct vision. Resection of the lower sternum will often require resection of portions of the diaphragm, the rectus abdominis, and other anterior abdominal muscles after the sternum and attached tissue has been separated from the mediastinum. During this dissection, the superior epigastric vessels should be isolated, ligated, and divided below the costal margin and anterior to the transversus abdominis muscle; the bleeding points on the cut edge of the diaphragm are ligated with figure-of-eight suture ligatures.

A resection of the manubrium is illustrated in Figure 6-5. As shown on the left side of the figure, separate the sternocleidomastoid and the pectoralis major muscles from their origins on the clavicle and the anterior surface of the manubrium. Divide the sternohyoid and sternothyroid muscles and identify the subclavian veins as they descend under the clavicles. Both clavicles should be divided at approximately their midpoints with an air-driven saw. After the subclavian and innominate veins have been visualized and protected, divide the first ribs. Under direct vision, the internal mammary vessels are ligated and divided near their origins, and the separation of the upper portion of the sternum from the underlying mediastinal structures is completed.

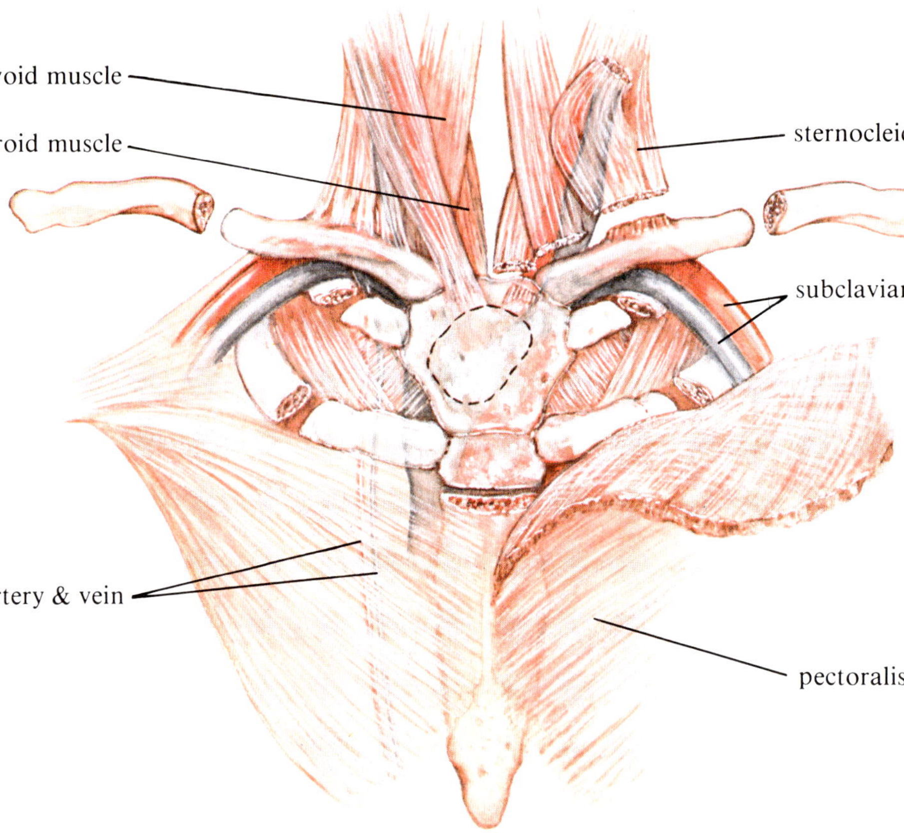

FIG. 6-5.

Pulmonary Resection with Resection of the Chest Wall

If the chest wall is invaded posteriorly by direct extension of a carcinoma of the lung above the level of the fifth rib, the patient is placed in a straight lateral position with the arm internally rotated, the elbow flexed, and the hand fixed at the hip (Fig. 6-6). This position causes the weight of the arm to pull the scapula forward and expose the upper chest wall. Make a high parascapular incision from the level of the scapular spine to the anterior axillary line (shown by the line in Fig. 6-7). Divide the latissimus dorsi, the rhomboideus major, and the portion of the trapezius below the spine of the scapula. Before entering the chest, insert a hand under the scapula and palpate the area of the brachial plexus above and posterior to the middle of the first rib. If the tumor is palpable along the vertebral column at this level, I consider the patient unresectable and discontinue the operation since the actual extent is always greater than that palpable. When the region of invasion is anterior or low in the chest, a standard posterior–lateral incision is used.

The chest should be entered some distance from the tumor. For example, if the chest x-ray shows the tumor overlying the posterior portion of ribs 3 and 4, the chest should be entered by resecting the anterior portion of rib 5. Before removing the posterior portion of rib 5, palpate the pleural surface underlying it to prevent accidentally cutting through the cancer, which may extend on the pleural surface or in the plane of the endothoracic fascia for 3–4 cm from the location visible on the chest radiogram. Examine the chest for evidence of unresectability; in addition to the usual reasons, a cancer invading the chest wall may be unresectable because of spread to the vertebral bodies. Although 20% of a vertebral body may be resected, a useful action

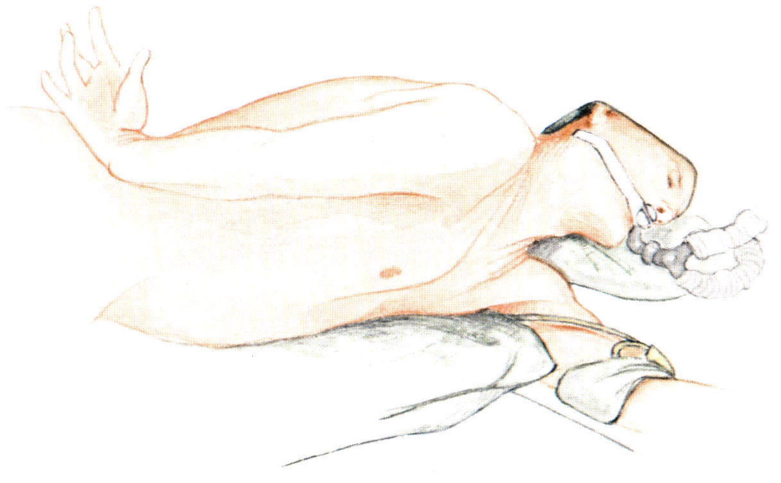

FIG. 6-6.

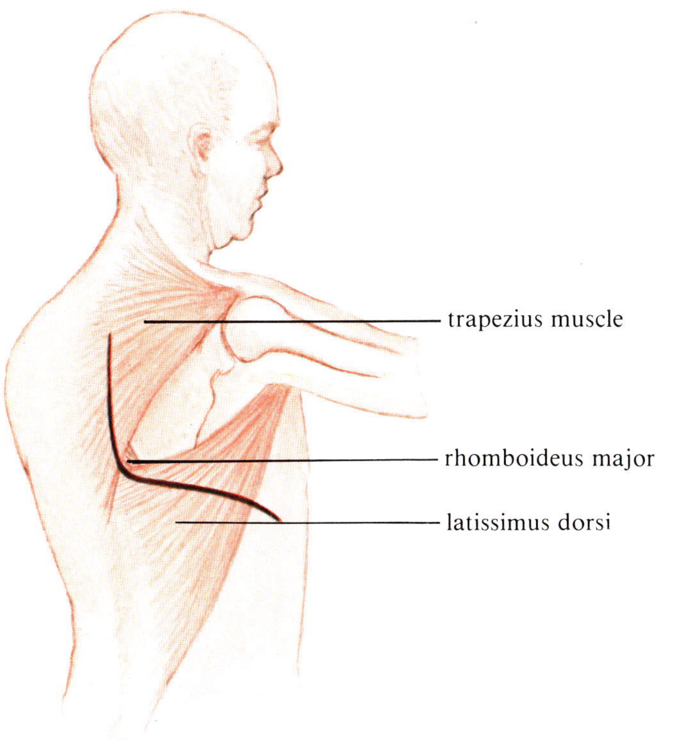

FIG. 6-7.

if the cancer is immediately adjacent to the vertebra, it has been my experience that a resection of even 20% of the vertebral body will not remove all the cancer if gross involvement of more than 5%–10% of its palpable circumference is present.

The approach to a combined chest wall and pulmonary resection varies with the location of the cancer. If the chest is invaded laterally near the level of the incision, it is difficult to visualize the hilus until the involved area of chest wall has been mobilized and can be retracted out of the way. Conversely, if the chest wall is invaded posteriorly near the spine, at the apex of the chest, or near the diaphragm, it is usually easier to complete the hilar dissection first and leave the involved lobe attached only to the chest wall so the limits of the tumor invasion may be more accurately determined.

The required pulmonary resection is performed as described in Chapter 4. The chest wall resection is usually started anterior to the cancer unless it involves the sternum. If necessary, detach the muscles of the shoulder girdle

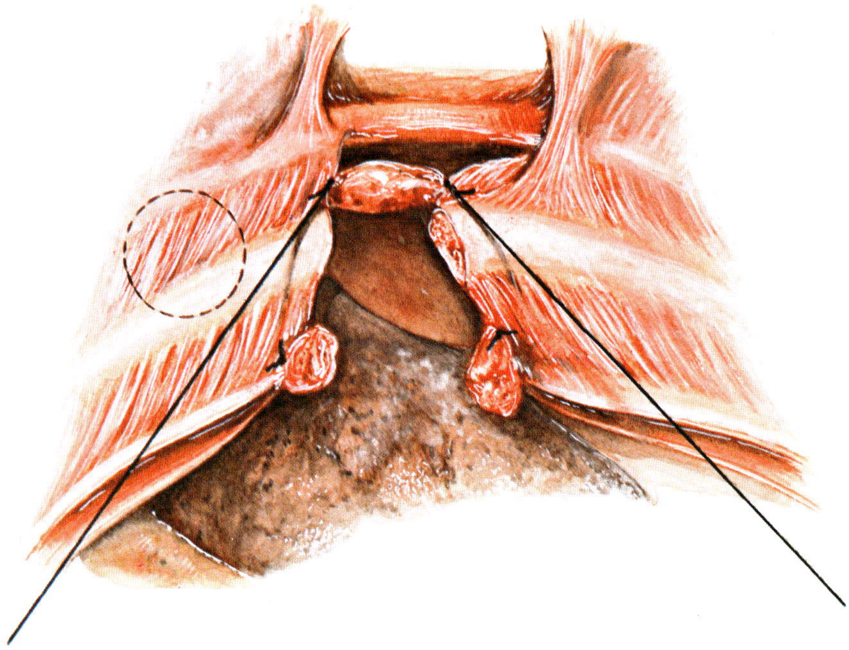

FIG. 6-8.

that take origin from the ribs to be resected. Beginning with the lowest involved rib, 3–4 cm from the gross margin of the tumor, resect a 2-cm subperiosteal segment of each involved rib. Incise the periosteum and pleura under each excised rib segment, ligate each intercostal bundle with two 2–0 nonabsorbable suture ligatures, and divide the bundles between the ligatures. Figure 6-8 depicts such a resection for a carcinoma of the right upper lobe invading the posterior chest wall over the area represented by the dashed circle; the fifth rib has been removed, a segment of the fourth rib has been removed anterior to the tumor, the periosteum has been stripped from a segment of the third rib, and the ligatures are around the third intercostal bundle.

The chest wall resection must include at least the interspace and possibly the rib above and below the gross extent of the cancer. After the necessary rib divisions have been made, make a longitudinal incision in the periosteum of the rib below the lowest intercostal bundle to be resected, from the anterior extent of the chest wall resection to a point 3–4 cm posterior to the gross margin of the tumor or to the transverse process of the vertebra if the cancer is close to the spine. Reflect the periosteum off both the superficial and deep surfaces of the superior half of the rib, but leave it attached to the inferior half of the rib. Incise the pleura and periosteum under the deep aspect of this rib, doubly ligate the intercostal bundle above the rib at the anterior extent of the chest wall resection, and divide it between the ligatures. In a similar fashion, reflect the periosteum off the inferior half of the rib above the highest intercostal bundle to be resected. Incise the pleura and periosteum along the deep surface of the rib, and ligate and divide the intercostal bundle below the rib at the anterior chest wall incision. At this point in the dissection, the chest wall will appear as depicted in Figure 6-9. The shaded area will be removed in continuity with the right upper lobe.

The involved area of chest wall is now free except for its posterior attachments. If the gross tumor is more than 3–4 cm from the spine, the ribs and intercostal bundles may be divided posterior to the tumor, using the same procedure described for the anterior division, and the diseased lung and chest wall removed. However, if the region of chest wall invasion is near the spine, the entire rib, the transverse process, and possibly a portion of the vertebral

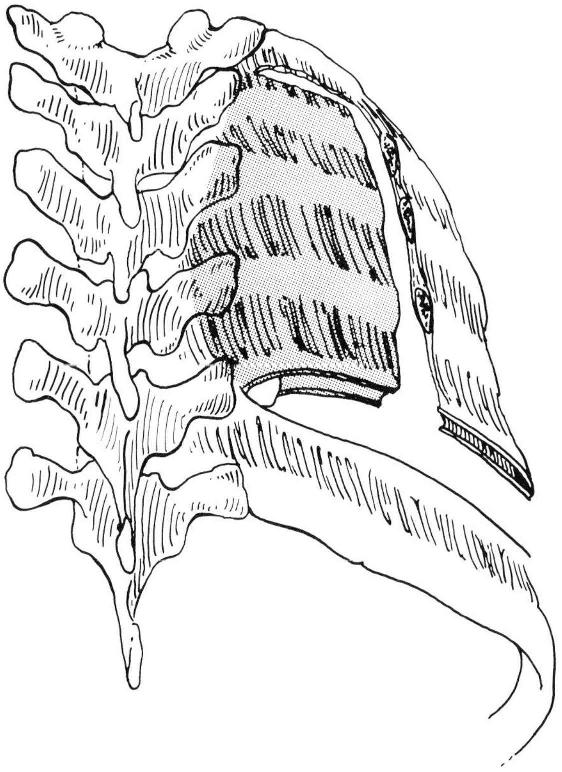

FIG. 6-9.

body of each involved segment must be resected. Incise the pleura overlying the vertebral bodies or the head of the rib anterior to the area of tumor invasion; ligate and divide the intercostal vessels on the vertebral bodies at this point to decrease hemorrhage during the subsequent resection. With an Alexander periosteal elevator, reflect the lumbodorsal fascia and the sacrospinalis muscles off the posterior portions of the ribs and transverse processes to be resected for least 1 cm past the articulation of the rib with the transverse process (Fig. 6-10). The transverse process can be palpated as a 4–5 mm prominence on the posterior surface of each rib. Adequate exposure of the transverse processes often requires the partial transection of the lumbodorsal fascia at the upper and lower limits of the resection.

The method for freeing the rib from the vertebra is depicted in Figure 6-11. Using an osteotome and a hammer, transect the transverse processes lateral to the articular facets, about 1 cm from the tip of the transverse process, as shown in the illustration. With these divided, the edge of the osteotome is placed against the posterior surface of that portion of the rib between the transverse process and the vertebral body; directed by the surgeon at the pleural incision anterior to the head of the rib, it is driven by the surgical assistant through the intervening tissue in the plane represented by the dashed line next to the vertebral body in Figure 6-11. During this procedure it is helpful to have inward pressure placed on the anterior end of the rib segment (represented by the arrow). Complete the resection by dividing the intercostal nerves and any remaining soft tissue. The resected right upper lobe with the attached segments of ribs 2, 3, and 4 is illustrated in Figure 6-12. The bleeding points may be controlled with bone wax, ligatures, or cautery, but cautery must be used cautiously in this region because of the risk of damage to the spinal cord from the cone of heat released.

After the chest has been irrigated with warm saline, examine the raw area over the vertebra for a spinal fluid leak. If one is found, it may be

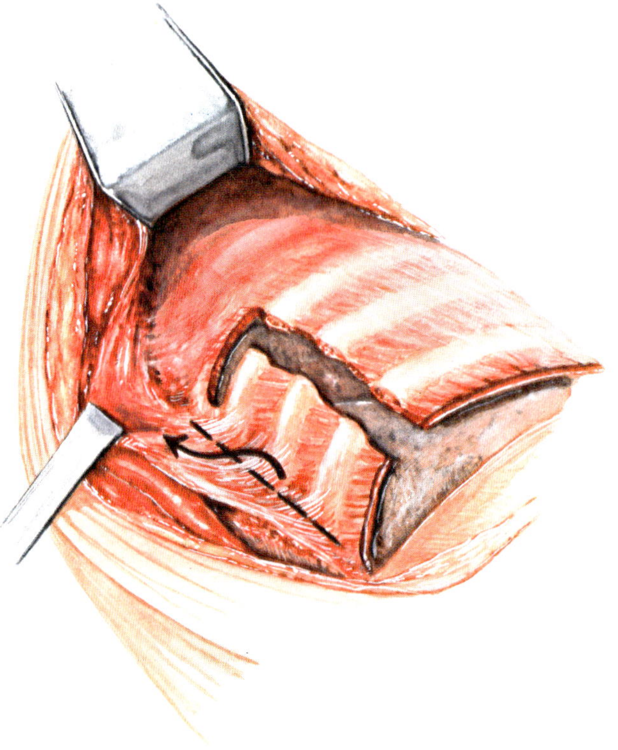

FIG. 6-10.

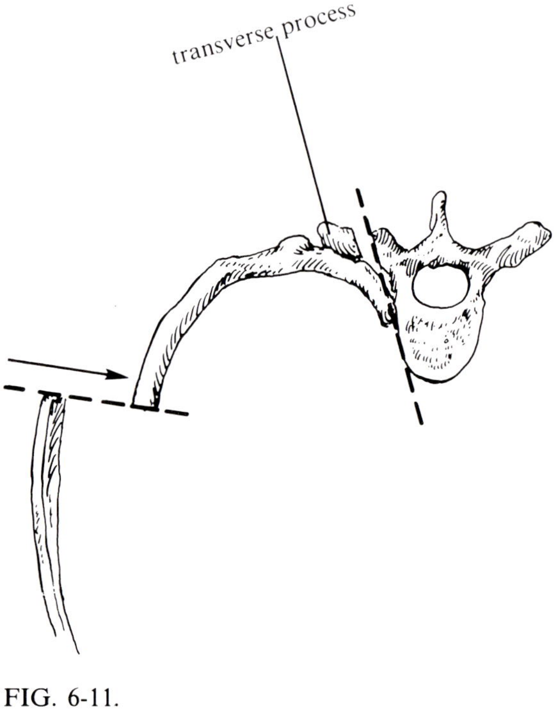

FIG. 6-11.

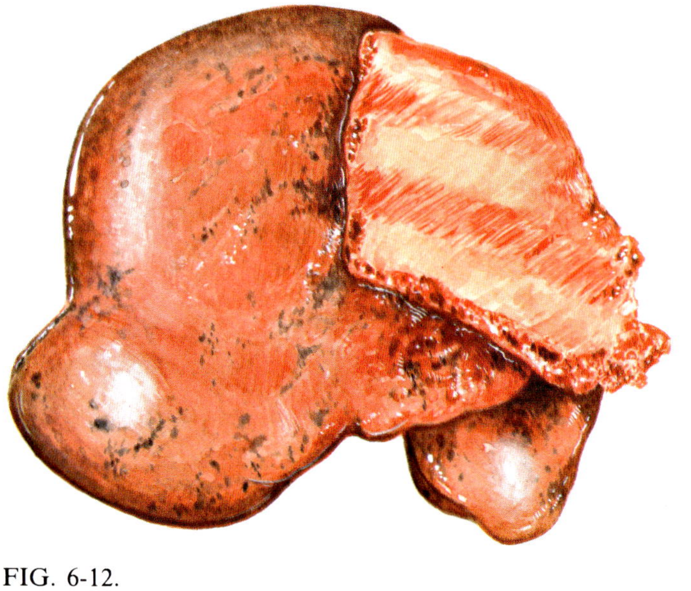

FIG. 6-12.

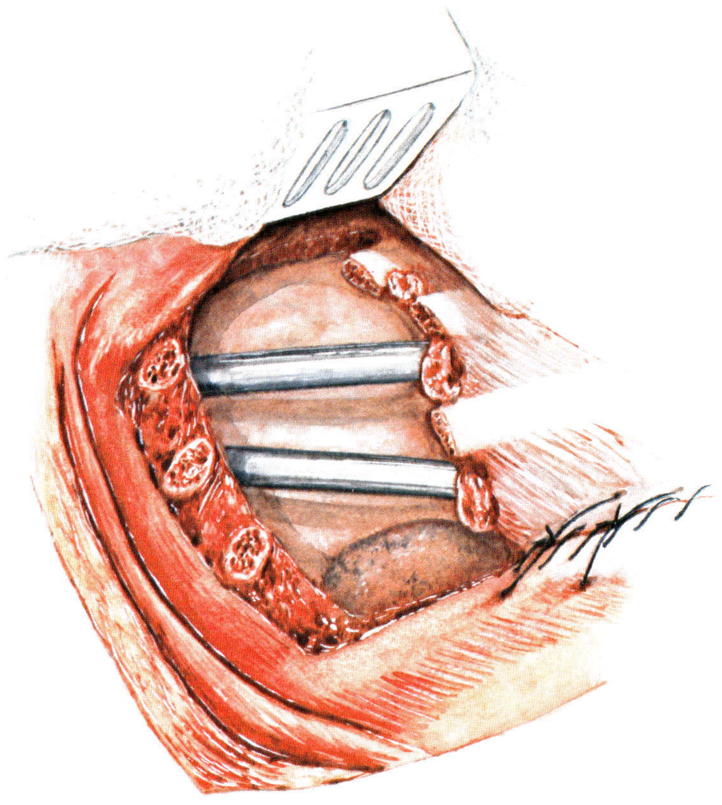

FIG. 6-13.

stopped, as suggested by Paulson (2), with an excised piece of muscle sutured into the intervertebral foramen. The chest wall at the end of the procedure is pictured in Figure 6-13. The periosteal bed of the fifth rib has been sutured closed anterior to the chest wall defect. The areas of articulation of the vertebral bodies with the heads of the ribs are apparent on the left, and two intrapleural catheters can be seen in the chest. Because this remaining chest wall defect is posterior and will be covered by the scapula, no further effort will be made to close it. The muscles of the shoulder will be reapproximated in the usual manner.

Superior Sulcus Carcinomas

Carcinomas invading the superior sulcus of the chest with or without an associated Pancoast syndrome, are resected using much the same method as that previously described for a pulmonary resection with resection of the chest wall. However, the more complex anatomy of the apex of the chest justifies a separate description of its resection.

The incision and the findings contraindicating a resection are the same as those previously described. If a resection is possible, the hilar dissection of the upper lobe is completed first, leaving the lobe attached to the apex of the chest by the area of tumor invasion. The removal of this area of tumor invasion will usually require a resection of the first two or three ribs with the surrounding tissue. Divide the mediastinal pleura anterior–medial to the tumor from a point below the tumor to the region above the first rib past the origin of the internal mammary artery and vein. Dissect out the subclavian artery and vein as far laterally as possible from this approach, taking care on the right side not to injure the recurrent laryngeal nerve as it loops around the subclavian artery (visible in Fig. 6-14 just under the forceps).

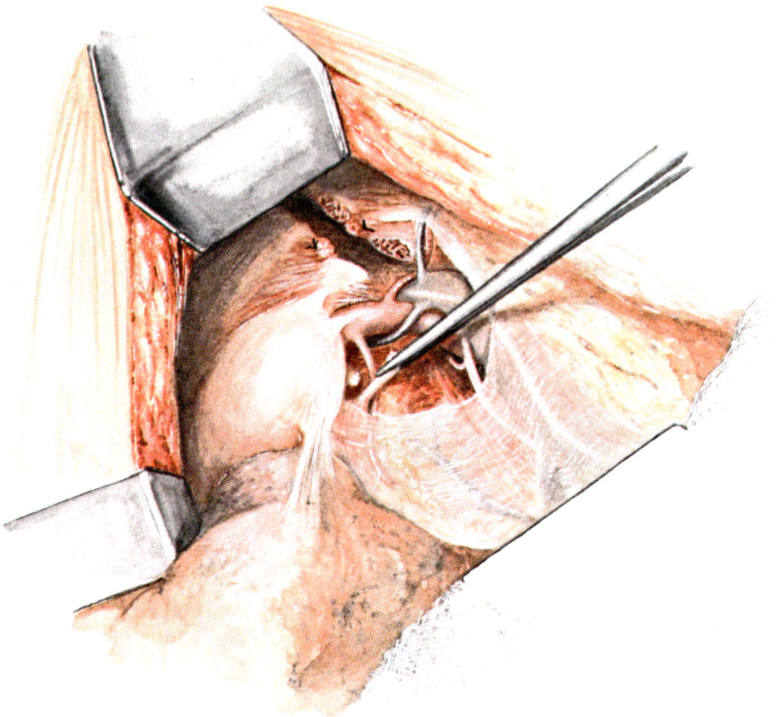

FIG. 6-14.

If a segment of the subclavian artery is resected to remove the carcinoma completely, continuity of the artery must be restored by an interposed graft after the chest wall resection has been completed, or loss of the hand is likely. The dissection of the cupula may be done either before or after dividing the upper ribs anterior to the tumor. In Figure 6-14 the apex of the right pleural cavity is shown after the first and second ribs have been divided. The tumor has extended out of the right upper lobe to involve the posterior portions of the first and second ribs. The subclavian artery disappears above the first rib just at the limit of tumor extension. The internal mammary vessels are immediately anterior to the site of division of the first rib. The phrenic nerve can be seen descending on the superior vena cava, and the superior intercostal vein is visible on the bodies of the vertebra. Continue the dissection inferiorly along the bodies of the first two or three thoracic vertebra, ligating the superior intercostal artery and vein where they are encountered.

The dissection of the external surface of the ribs should begin by detaching the serratus anterior muscle from the first three ribs. This allows increased mobility of the scapula and better exposure of the apex of the chest. Divide the attachments of the scalenus posterior and the serratus posterior superior from the second rib. In Figure 6-15, the upper hemostat is holding the scalenus posterior that has just been divided from its site of attachment on the second rib; the lower forceps is holding a portion of the serratus posterior. By palpation, identify the location of the subclavian artery and vein above the first rib, where they are shown in the illustration. Divide the scalenus anterior and scalenus medius muscles above the first rib at the level of the dashed line in Figure 6-15; connect this external field of dissection with the dissection of the subclavian vessels started inside the chest to completely free these vessels from the first rib and from the tumor.

Reflect the lumbodorsal fascia and the sacrospinalis muscles from the posterior part of the ribs to be resected. If it has not been done previously,

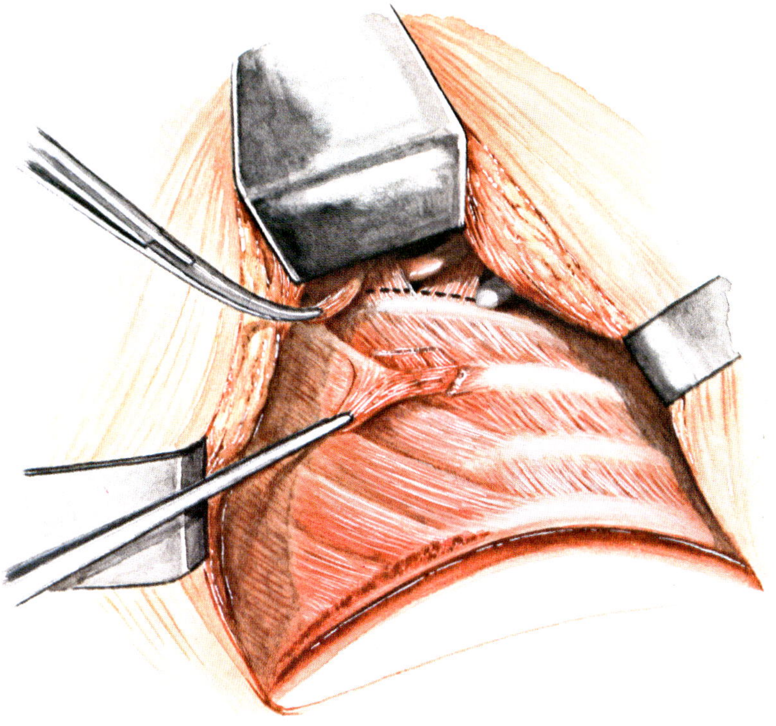

FIG. 6-15.

divide the periosteum from the transverse process to a point 3–4 cm anterior to the gross margin of tumor invasion, on the external surface of the lowest rib to be removed and reflect the periosteum off both the inner and outer surfaces of the lower half of that rib. Divide the rib at the anterior end of the periosteal incision, then incise the periosteum and the pleura in the bed of that rib back to the transverse process.

In succession, each superior rib, including the first, should be divided anterior to the tumor and the intervening intercostal vessels and muscle bundle should be doubly ligated and divided between the ligatures (Fig. 6-8). With downward traction on the anterior end of the first rib, complete the separation of the rib and tumor from the subclavian vessels and brachial plexus (Fig. 6-16). In this figure the area of tumor attachment is being dissected off of the subclavian artery after the anterior end of the first rib has been divided and the attachments of the scalenus anterior and medius muscles to the first rib have been cut.

Divide the anterior ramus of the first thoracic nerve in two places: 1) above the first rib lateral to the tumor and medial to its junction with the lower trunk of the brachial plexus, and 2) within the chest near the intervertebral foramen. The forceps in Figure 6-14 is holding the medial end of this nerve in the chest; the distal end of the nerve is visible at the edge of the tumor. If necessary, also divide the lower trunk of the brachial plexus, formed from C-8 and T1 nerve roots.

Continue this dissection above the first rib past the point of articulation with the transverse process so the segment of chest wall to be resected is attached only by the costovertebral articulations and their associated ligaments. Divide the transverse processes about 1 cm from the tip, and using the osteotome as previously described (and illustrated in Fig. 6-11), divide the costovertebral articulations, including portions of the vertebral bodies if necessary. After the bleeding points have been controlled, the chest irrigated with warm

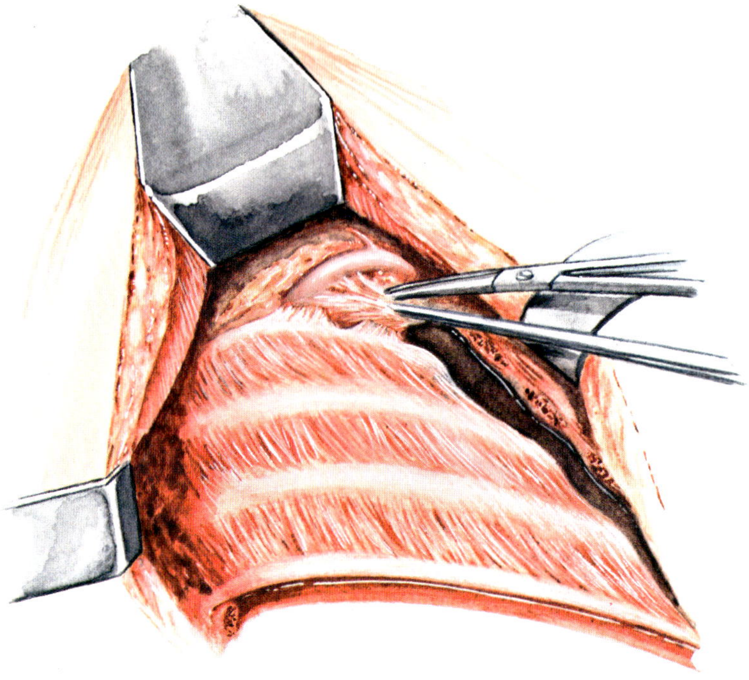

FIG. 6-16.

saline, and the raw area of the vertebra examined for a spinal fluid leak, the intercostal catheters are inserted. The chest wall defect is usually left without a plastic mesh closure because it is under the scapula and is filled by the muscles of the shoulder girdle.

Osteoradionecrosis and Costal Chondritis

Osteoradionecrosis of the chest wall most commonly follows postoperative irradiation for carcinoma of the breast. It is often associated with infection and with local recurrence of the cancer, resulting in a large, foul-smelling ulcer with ischemic costal cartilage and rib exposed. The closure of such an ulcer requires the excision of all necrotic tissue and tumor, as well as coverage by healthy tissue carrying its own blood supply. The patient's estimated life expectancy must be considered when planning such therapy. If it is on the order of 2–3 months, an expedient procedure, such as the use of the opposite breast to cover the defect, may be advisable. However, this procedure is cosmetically unacceptable to many women, even though they have evidence of distant metastasis, and little indication for its use now exists. For most patients the use of a latissimus dorsi myocutaneous flap (Figs. 6-29–6-31) should be considered.

Costal chondritis commonly develops either as an extension of an infection, such as tuberculosis, from the internal mammary lymph nodes, or as a complication of a surgical procedure in which denuded cartilage is left in a wound or in which an abscess is drained through a region of cartilage. It may present as an area of localized swelling with pain and erythema or as a persistently draining sinus after a surgical wound infection. The course of this condition, especially for infections of the cartilaginous web of the fifth through the tenth ribs, may be inordinately prolonged because hyaline cartilage is essentially avascular and because drainage or local excision results in spread of the infection to adjacent regions of previously healthy cartilage.

Successful treatment of costal chondritis requires the complete removal of all infected and ischemic cartilage and the protection of uninvolved cartilage.

Infections of the first through the fourth costal cartilages may be adequately treated by a complete excision of the entire infected cartilage plus 1–2 cm of the rib, but the fusion of the costal cartilages of ribs 5 through 9 requires an additional action to prevent spread of the infection to adjacent regions of cartilage by the surgical procedure. In such patients, an isolated incision should be made through healthy tissue over connected cartilages 4–5 cm away from the area of chondritis. Figure 6-17 depicts such chondritis (the stippled area) in the costal cartilage of ribs 5, 6, and 7. As illustrated, remove a 2-cm segment of healthy cartilage, close the incision, and wait approximately 3 weeks for a barrier of connective tissue to form between the ends of the divided cartilage. All of the cartilage from the region of chondritis to the connective tissue barriers should then be removed and the wound left open.

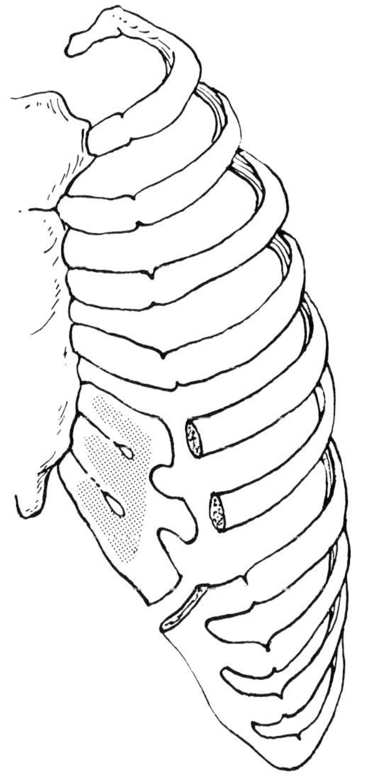

FIG. 6-17.

Reconstruction of the Chest Wall

Effective ventilation depends upon a rigid bony thorax and a sealed pleural cavity. When a significant area of one chest wall loses its rigidity either from multiple fractures of the ribs or from a defect in the bony thorax caused by a chest wall resection, a flail chest will occur and ventilation will be impaired, although the degree of impairment depends to some extent on the mobility of the mediastinum. If the defect in the chest wall is covered by the scapula, it may be left without fear of a flail chest developing, but if the defect includes more than two ribs and is not covered by the scapula, the chest wall must be stabilized. A special problem may occur if an extensive chest wall defect includes the posterior portion of the sixth rib, and the seventh rib is left intact: The scapula can then move inward and catch underneath the seventh rib. Although this condition has been treated by removing the posterior portion of the seventh and eighth ribs or by resecting the inferior angle of the scapula, I have found it more satisfactory to repair the defect with a synthetic mesh as described below.

At present, stabilization is most commonly done by reconstructing the defect in the chest wall with a synthetic fiber mesh. Fascia lata has been utilized for this purpose in the past, but it has not been as satisfactory as synthetic fibers because the fascia has strength in only one dimension while the chest wall undergoes strain in two dimensions. Marlex Mesh, a polypropylene cloth, has been the most widely used material. It is strong and well tolerated by the body, it does not fray easily, and even in an infected wound it is often not extruded.

The mesh must be drum-head tight when the chest wall closure is completed. To achieve this, drill holes in the ribs forming the superior and inferior edges of the defect at about 1-cm intervals; using interrupted nonabsorbable 2–0 sutures, such as Ethabond™, suture the mesh to the underside of the superior rib. The edge of the mesh should be doubled over so that the rough edge is outside and not against the lung, and the sutures should be placed 7–8 mm from the edge (Fig. 6-18). After the superior suture line has been tied, pull down on the mesh strongly and mark the level of the mesh that is opposed to the holes in the lower rib. Place the row of interrupted sutures from the lower rib to the chosen level of the mesh in a manner that puts the mesh underneath the rib. Tie the sutures as an assistant pulls the superior and inferior edges of the chest wall defect closer together. Complete the closure by suturing the mesh with interrupted mattress sutures to the intercostal muscles and rib ends on the anterior and posterior margins of the defect. The completed closure is shown in Figure 6-19.

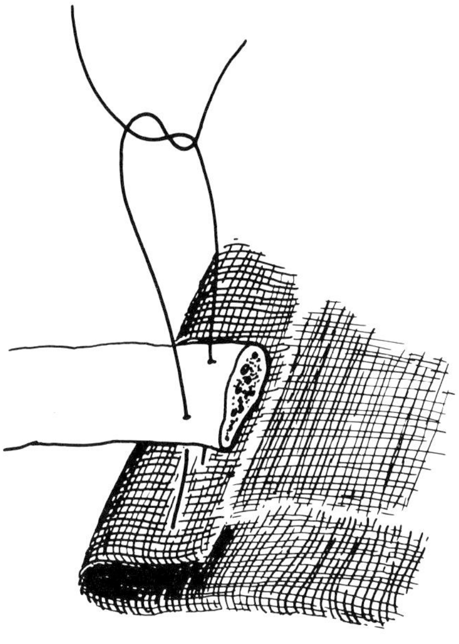

FIG. 6-18.

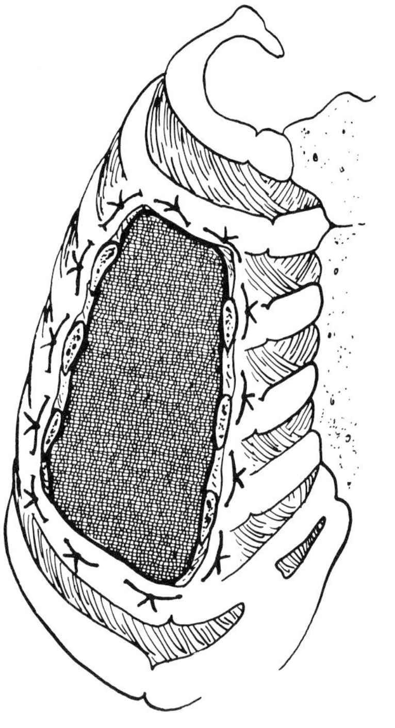

FIG. 6-19.

Chest wall defects following resection of the sternum may also be repaired successfully with Marlex mesh. If a portion of the sternum, particularly the manubrium, can be left intact, the problem of repair is simplified and the risk of respiratory insufficiency is less. However, in a patient with adequate muscle strength, the resection of the entire sternum or any portion of it with repair and adequate pulmonary function should be possible if the lengths of adjacent ribs that are resected is not great over the entire length of the anterior chest wall.

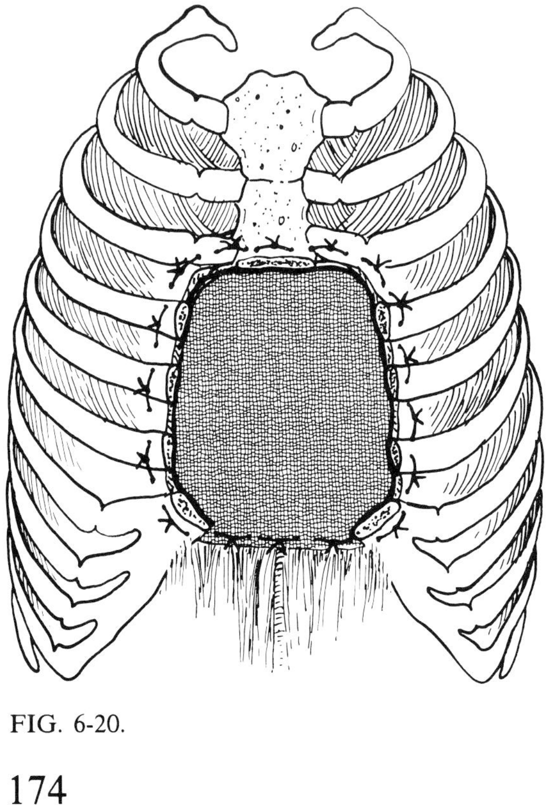

FIG. 6-20.

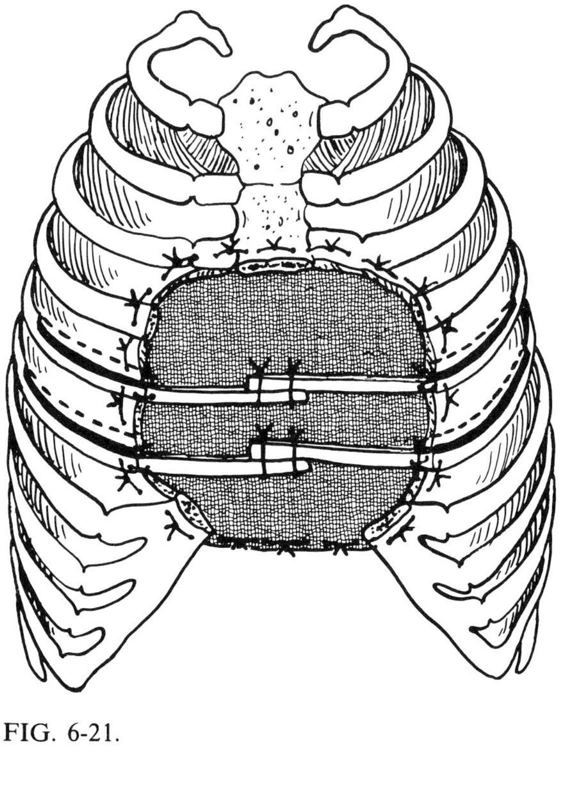

FIG. 6-21.

In the manner depicted in Figure 6-20, the defect caused by the sternal resection should be closed by suturing the mesh to the remaining sternum, to the ends of the ribs, to the intercostal muscles, and if indicated, to the diaphragm and the rectus sheath. This mesh must be sutured into place while the ribs on both sides are pushed together anteriorly so that when finished, it is tight, with no slack areas resulting from any maneuver. If the lower sternum and the pericardium are removed, I reflect the greater omentum superiorly and suture it to the cut edge of the pericardium prior to covering the chest wall defect with Marlex mesh. When the body of the sternum plus long lengths of adjacent ribs are removed, the heart is unprotected from external trauma. If the patient's age or occupation makes this a significant risk, some protection can be obtained by splitting one or two adjacent ribs longitudinally and moving the superior half of the rib across the defect, suturing it to the ribs on both lateral margins and to a similar split rib from the opposite side (Fig. 6-21). The coverage of a large defect that includes the skin and full thickness of the thoracic wall requires the use of a myocutaneous flap.

Cutaneous and Myocutaneous Flaps for Chest Wall Reconstruction
Alan R. Shons M.D.

When a planned chest wall resection will result in a large defect that includes the skin and full thickness of the thoracic wall, reconstruction, employing a muscle or musculocutaneous unit, should be planned before the resection. The two muscles found to be most useful are the pectoralis major muscle and its posterior counterpart, the latissimus dorsi muscle.

The area of coverage of the muscle or musculocutaneous unit is dependent upon an arc of rotation about a pivot point. The pivot point is the insertion of the muscle or the vascular pedicle if the insertion is divided. In the use of the secondary medial blood supply for an inferior transposition of either the pectoralis major or the latissimus dorsi muscle, the pivot point is the most superior attachment of the muscle. A defect can be covered by muscle or by skin and muscle that is equidistant from the pivot point, that is, within the arc of rotation of the musculocutaneous unit.

The expanse of the pectoralis major muscle is shown in Figure 6-22. It arises from the medial one-half of the clavicle and from the sternum down to the seventh rib and inserts into the lateral lip of the bicipital groove of the humerus. The pectoralis major is an adductor and medial rotator of the arm, so some disability will result from loss of its function. It has a dual blood supply (Fig. 6-23). The major pedicle is the thoracoacromial artery, which arises from the axillary artery, but a secondary blood supply is provided by perforating branches of the internal mammary artery. The muscle is innervated by the medial and lateral pectoral nerves, which are direct branches of the medial and lateral cords of the brachial plexus.

The pectoralis major muscle and all or part of the overlying skin can be transposed, based on either the primary or secondary blood supply. Based on its major vascular pedicle, the musculocutaneous unit can be used to cover the entire sternum and medial clavicular area as well as the opposite costochondral cartilage. Laterally it will cover the axilla and upper half of the chest wall. Based upon its medial blood supply, it can be used to cover the lateral and inferior half of the chest wall.

When used as an island musculocutaneous flap, the skin island is first outlined. Primary closure of the donor site can be accomplished if limited areas of skin are used with the underlying muscle. If a major portion of the

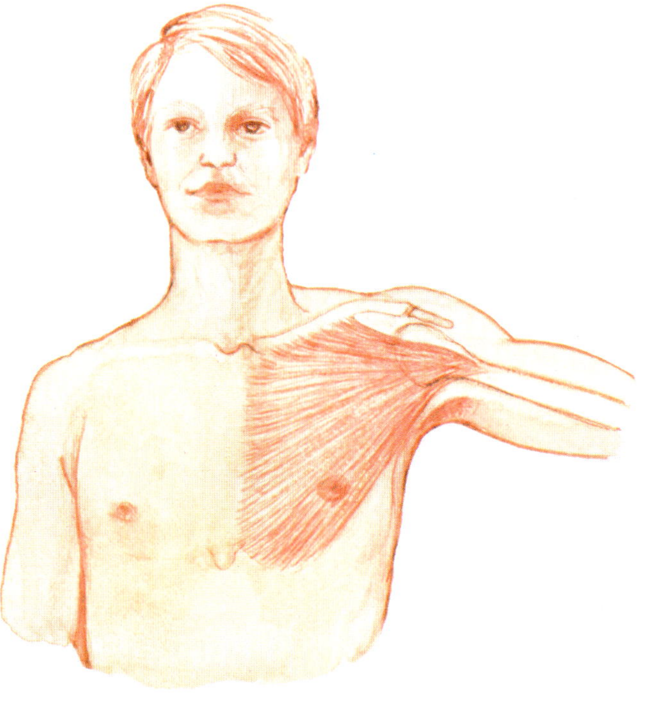

FIG. 6-22.

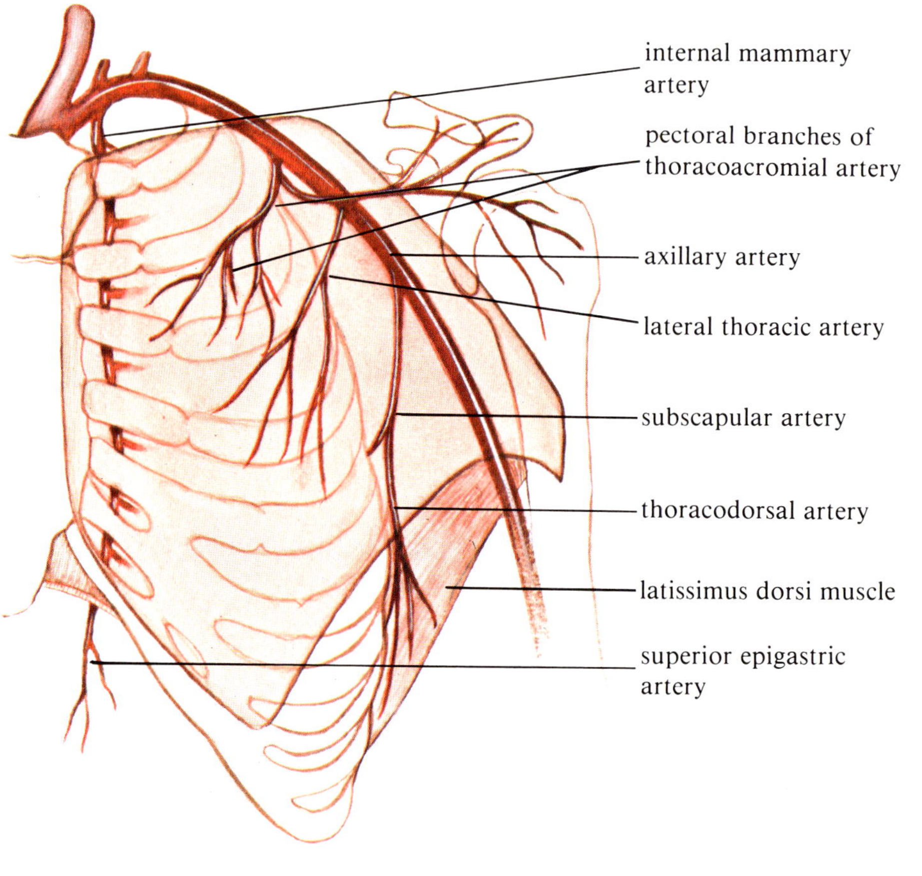

FIG. 6-23.

overlying skin is to be used with the underlying muscle, a split thickness skin graft will be necessary for coverage of the donor site. The dissection begins with an incision in the anterior axillary fold over the pectoralis major muscle. The muscle is divided close to its insertion at the lateral lip of the bicipital groove. The major vascular pedicle entering the muscle at the level of the upper medial border of the pectoralis minor muscle must be identified and carefully preserved. Additional length of the vascular pedicle can be achieved by ligation of branches to the pectoralis minor muscle. The skin island is formed and sutured to the underlying muscle with a dermis–muscle stitch of 4–0 Vicryl to prevent disruption of the skin–muscle attachment during subsequent manipulations. Skin flaps should be raised to expose the origin of the muscle, and the sternal and clavicular origins divided. With this preparation, the myocutaneous flap can be transposed medially (Fig. 6-24) or laterally (Fig. 6-25). In these figures, the defect to be covered by a split-thickness skin graft, is a light stippled area. By division of both the insertion and the major vascular pedicle, the muscle or musculocutaneous unit can be transposed inferiorly, based upon the secondary blood supply from the branches of the internal mammary artery. The muscle used in this fashion can cover lower anterior thoracic wall defects (Fig. 6-26).

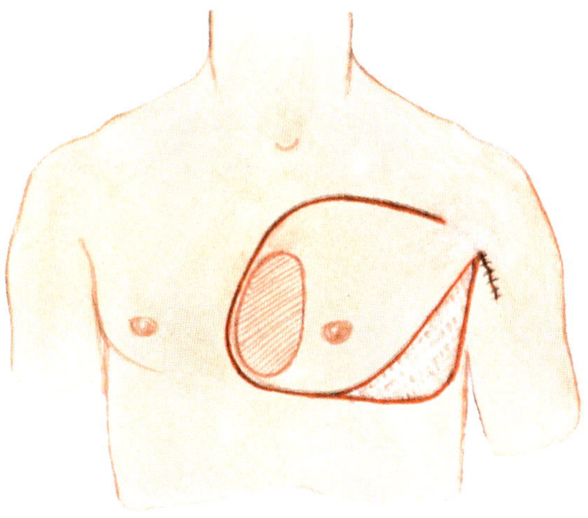

FIG. 6-24.

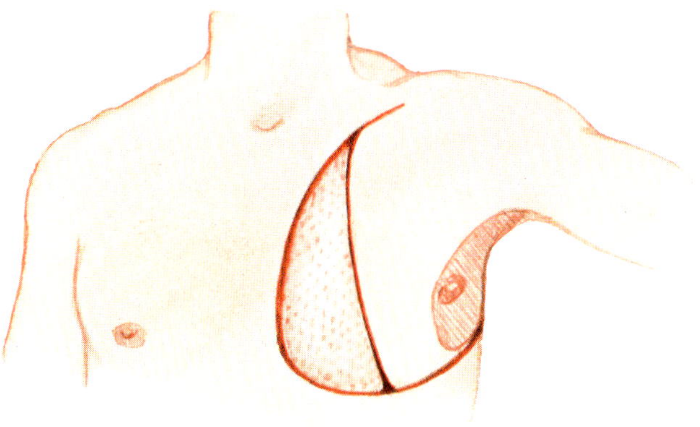

FIG. 6-25.

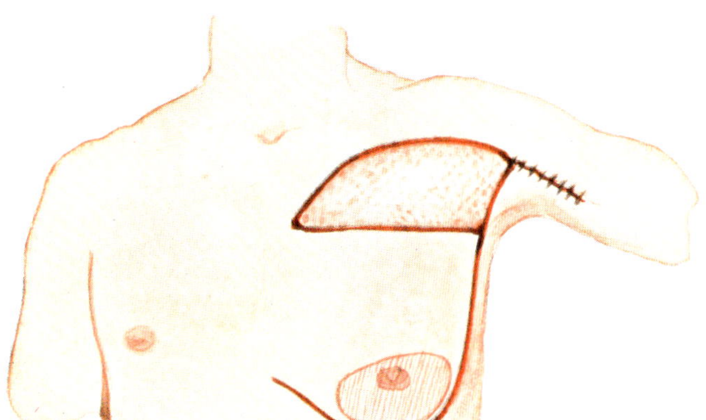

FIG. 6-26.

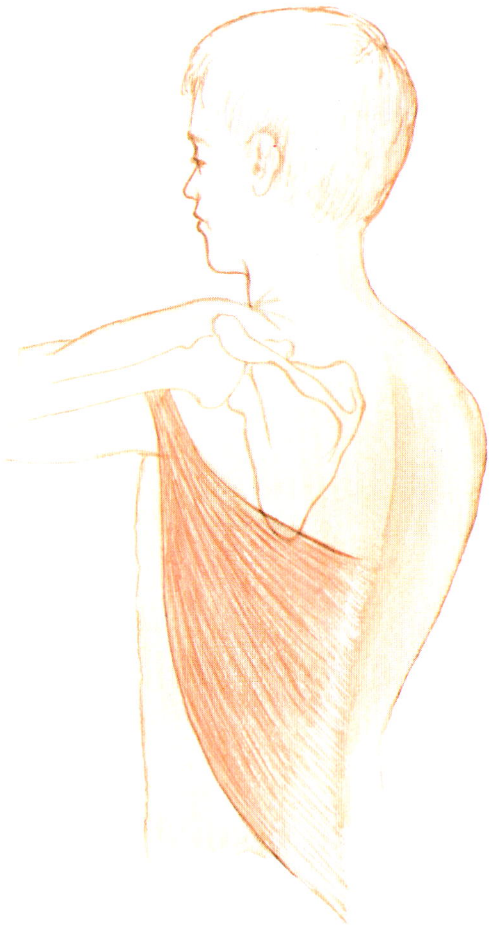

FIG. 6-27.

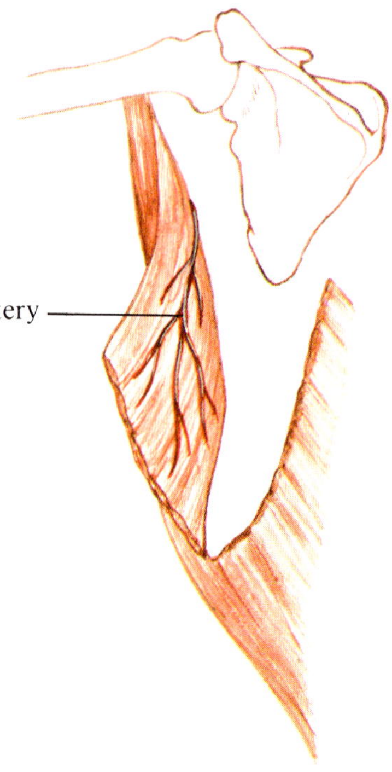

FIG. 6-28.

The extent of the latissimus dorsi muscle, which together with the teres major muscle forms the posterior fold of the axilla, is shown in Fig. 6-27. It arises from the spines of the lower six thoracic vertebrae, the spine of the lumbar and sacral vertebrae, and the posterior crest of the ilium; it inserts into the intertubular groove of the humerus. The muscle is an adductor, extender, and medial rotator of the humerus, but little or no functional disability is noted from loss of its functions. The latissimus dorsi muscle also has a dual blood supply. In Figure 6-28, the muscle has been partially divided and turned over to expose the major vascular pedicle, the thoracodorsal artery, a terminal branch of the scapular artery that supplies the anterior two-thirds of the muscle and courses on the undersurface of the muscle anteriorly. This creates an independent myocutaneous zone of the anterior 12 cm of the muscle, which can be raised without delay. The muscle is also supplied by perforating branches of the intercostal and lumbar arteries that pierce it medially. It is innervated by the thoracodorsal nerve, a branch of the posterior cord of the brachial plexus that enters the muscle with the thoracodorsal artery approximately 10 cm from its insertion.

The muscle, all or in part, can be transposed with all or part of the overlying skin. With division of its origin, the muscle or musculocutaneous unit can be transposed to cover defects in the lateral or anterolateral chest wall. With division of both the origin and the insertion of the muscle, additional medial transposition can be achieved with coverage of the upper half of the anterior chest wall possible to the lateral border of the sternum and the medial aspect of the clavicle. Based on its major vascular pedicle the musculocutaneous unit will cover the lower three-fourths of the anterior chest wall and will reach to the sternum. Posteriorly it will cover the thoracic vertebrae and will reach the neck. Based upon its medial blood supply it will reach the lower posterior chest wall.

Figures 6-29A–6-31 illustrate the use of a latissimus dorsi myocutaneous flap to repair an anterior chest wall defect (Fig. 6-30A) caused by osteoradionecrosis that developed following radiotherapy after a mastectomy for carcinoma of the breast. The skin island to be transposed is first outlined (Fig. 6-29A). It is generally oriented obliquely, beginning at the anterolateral free border and extending inferiorly and medially. The donor defect can be closed primarily if the skin island does not exceed 18–20 cm in length and 8–10 cm in width. Larger skin islands will require split thickness skin graft coverage of the defect. The skin island is formed and the skin edges sewn to the underlying muscle. Form superior, inferior, and medial skin flaps to expose the muscle and elevate it away from the serratus anterior without injuring the long thoracic nerve. The thoracodorsal artery is identified and carefully preserved in the transposition of the muscle or musculocutaneous unit. Divide the muscle from its origin on the iliac crest and split it vertically about 12 cm from its anterior margin. The prepared musculocutaneous unit is shown from the posterior in Figure 6-29B, with the donor site closed, and from the anterior in Figure 6-30A. If the muscle alone is used, exposure can be achieved by an incision 3 cm anterior to the anterolateral free border of the muscle with the elevation of skin flaps medially, superiorly, and inferiorly. Elevate the skin between the anterior chest wall defect and the anterior margin of the muscle to produce the skin bridge illustrated in Figure 6-30B, and create a subcutaneous pocket surrounding the chest wall defect (the dashed lines in Fig. 6-31) that will be adequate to accept the muscle. Transpose the muscle and its skin island under the intervening skin bridge (Fig. 6-30B) and into position to cover the defect.

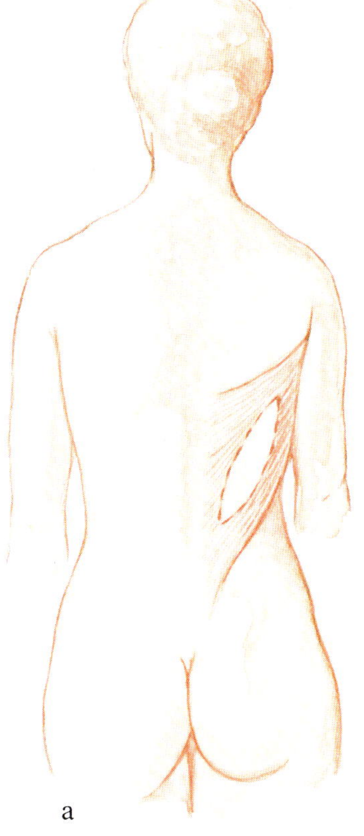

a

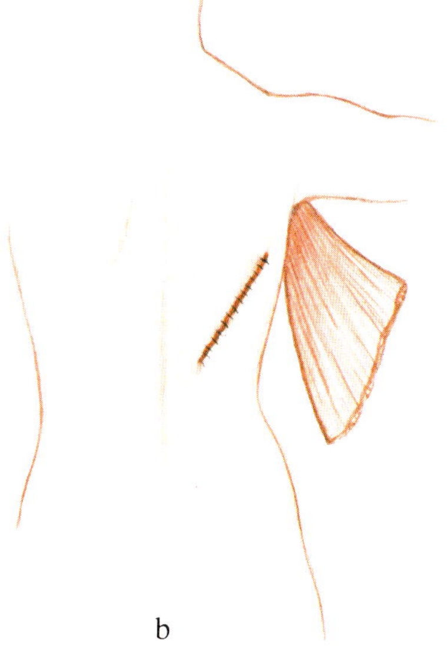

b

FIG. 6-29A,B.

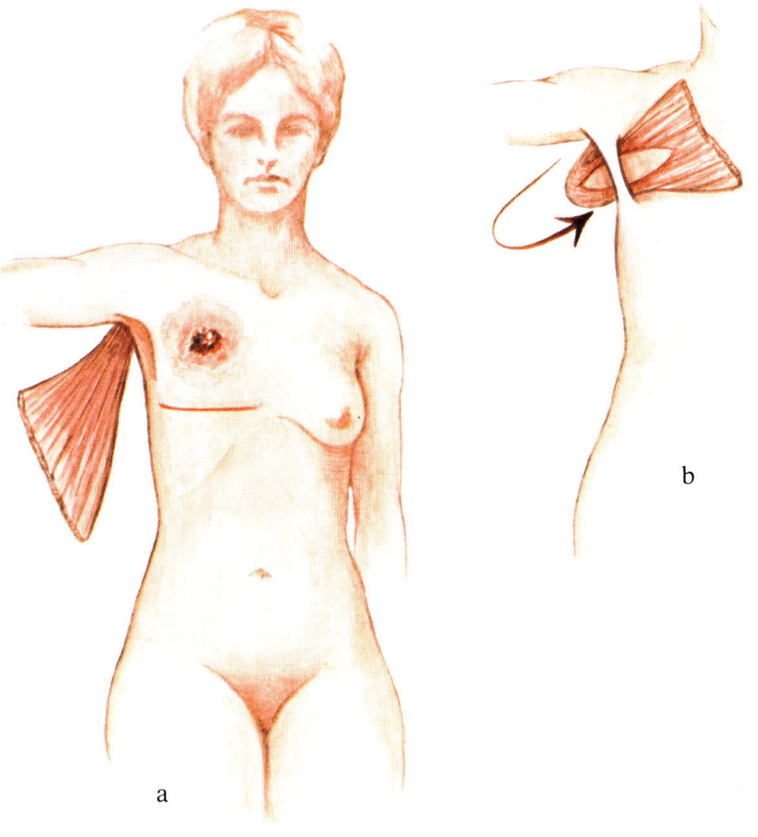

FIG. 6-30A,B.

The transposed muscle is sutured to surrounding soft tissue or periosteum using 2–0 Vicryl sutures, and the transposed skin island is sutured to surrounding skin using subcutaneous and subcuticular sutures of 4–0 Vicryl. The completed operation is illustrated in Figure 6-31. If the skin island donor site is closed primarily, a 10-mm Jackson Pratt drain is placed in the donor area. Drains are not used in the recipient area.

The entire muscle can be transposed based upon the secondary blood supply of the perforating branches of the intercostal and lumbar arteries. As in the use of the secondary blood supply of the pectoralis major muscle, the latissimus dorsi muscle and overlying skin can be transposed inferiorly following division of the insertion of the muscle and major vascular pedicle. If muscle alone is used to cover defects, skin coverage is provided by immediate split thickness skin grafts to the muscle surface.

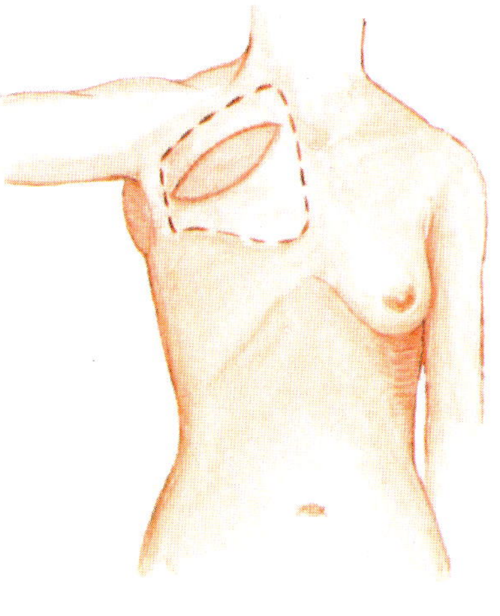

FIG. 6-31.

Split thickness skin grafts, 15/1000 in. thick and meshed 1.5 to 1, are used to cover large skin island defects and transposed muscle. The skin grafts are stapled in position or sutured with 4–0 Vicryl. They should be covered with gauze kept moist with 0.25% neomycin solution and changed each day for 5 days. Following this, all dressings are removed and the area is allowed to dry. Compression dressings should not be used.

The use of the musculocutaneous unit, as described for the pectoralis major and latissimus dorsi muscles, has largely eliminated the need for the more complex full thickness skin flap reconstructive procedures. The reliability and versatility of the musculocutaneous flap has been far superior to skin flap reconstructive procedures.

Thoracoplasty

Extrapleural thoracoplasty was initially designed to cause a collapse of underlying diseased lung, but at the present time it is used almost exclusively to obliterate an intrapleural space. This usually involves reducing the volume of one thoracic cavity from 25%–30% by an intraperiosteal resection of the upper three to five ribs. Regeneration of bone from the periosteum of the resected ribs maintains the chest wall in its collapsed position. The rib resection should include the entire length of the first three ribs. It is usually not necessary, however, for present purposes, to also resect the transverse processes of the corresponding vertebra. The fourth rib is resected from the transverse process to the anterior axillary line and if necessary, the fifth rib is resected to the midaxillary line.

If in the surgeon's opinion, a residual pleural space will be present after a given pulmonary resection, a thoracoplasty to obliterate that space may be performed 1–5 weeks prior to the pulmonary resection or 2 weeks or more after the resection. It should not be done concomitantly with the pulmonary resection because of the risk of atelectasis and pneumonia in the remaining lobe, with the development of pulmonary insufficiency. The thoracoplasty should not be done more than 5 weeks prior to the pulmonary resection since by that time the regenerating ribs become so stiff that further collapse will not occur after the resection.

The patient is placed in an approximately 45° prone position with the upper arm internally rotated, the elbow flexed, and the hand fixed near the patient's hip (Fig. 6-6). The incision extends from the anterior axillary line, horizontally under the inferior angle of the scapula, then superior to the level of the scapular spine, staying midway between the vertebral border of the scapula and the spinous processes. Divide the latissimus dorsi, the rhomboideus major, and the portion of the trapezius below the spine of the scapula, and retract the scapula anteriorly. Detach the serratus anterior from the first three ribs and divide the attachments of the scalenus posterior and the serratus posterior superior from the second rib. Expose the transverse processes articulating with the first four ribs by reflecting the erector spinae muscle groups and the lumbodorsal fascia medially (Fig. 6-10).

Usually the costectomy begins with the removal of the fourth rib, because the fifth rib either has been or will be removed in the performance of the pulmonary resection. With cautery, divide the periosteum of the fourth rib from the anterior axillary line to the transverse process, and with an Alexander periosteal elevator, remove the periosteum from the lateral surface of the rib. Strip the periosteum from both edges of the rib by working from anterior to posterior on the inferior edge and from posterior to anterior on the superior edge. With a Hedblom periosteal elevator (Fig. 6-32), separate the periosteum

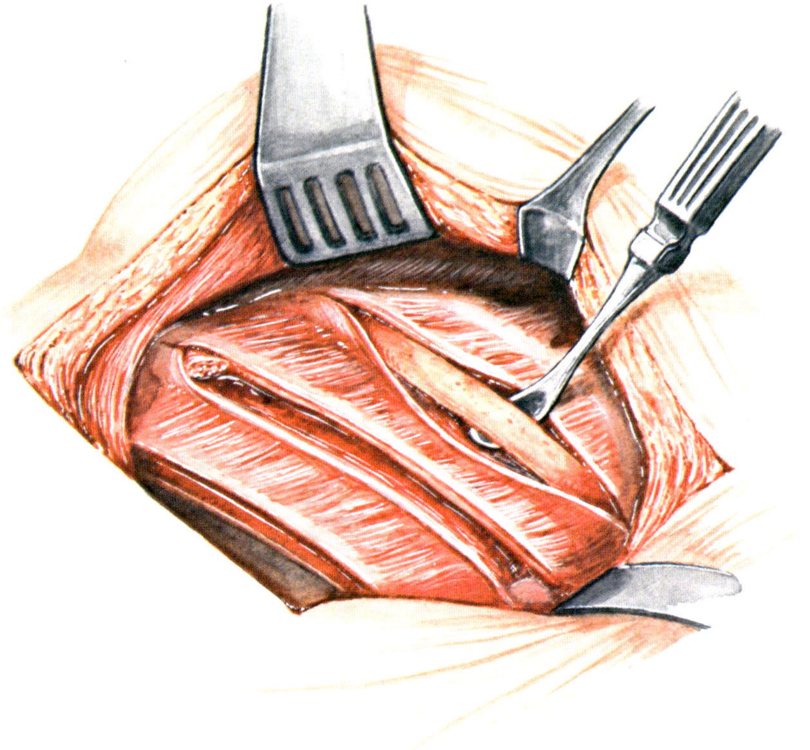

FIG. 6-32.

from the inner aspect of the rib. Divide the rib anteriorly at the anterior axillary line, and posteriorly, flush with or medial to the end of the transverse process. The same procedure is used to remove the third rib and then the second rib, except the point of anterior division for these ribs should be the nipple line for the third rib and the costochondral junction for the second rib. In Figure 6-32, the fourth rib has been removed, and the periosteum is being separated from the inner aspect of the third rib.

Notice in Figure 6-33 that the configuration of the first rib differs from that of the other ribs in that the two surfaces of the rib body face cranially and caudally rather than medially and laterally. Therefore, in removing this rib, first incise the periosteum on the lateral border of the rib by scraping the border with an Alexander periosteal elevator, then reflect the periosteum off the caudal surface of the rib. In stripping the periosteum from the cranial surface, care must be taken not to injure the subclavian vessels. Usually the easiest method is first to strip the periosteum from the posterior part of the cranial surface. Then, with a finger on the subclavian vessels to locate and protect them (Fig. 6-33), remove the periosteum from the remaining portion of the cranial surface. Use the curved end of the Hedblom periosteal elevator to remove the periosteum from the medial border of the posterior part of the rib, and divide the rib at its articulation with the transverse process. With lateral traction on the rib, separate the periosteum from the rest of the rib and divide it at the costochondral junction. After hemostasis has been secured and the wound irrigated, it is closed without drainage tubes. Figure 6-34 is a graphic presentation of the bony thorax after a left four rib thoracoplasty that followed a thoracotomy through the bed of the resected fifth rib. Notice the different levels for the anterior division of each rib.

For those patients in whom the pleural space is the site of a chronic empyema and in whom a decortication is not indicated, the thickness of the peel on the parietal pleura often necessitates a modification of the standard

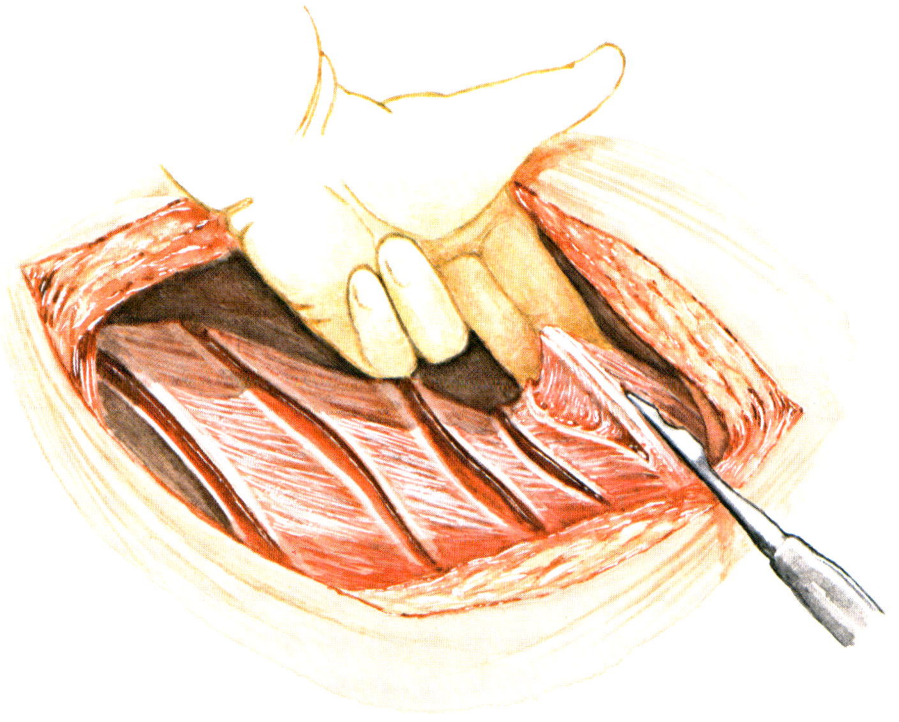

FIG. 6-33.

thoracoplasty technique in order to collapse the chest wall. The original operation for this condition was described by Shede, but the procedure as he described it is rarely performed today because it results in extensive denervation of the chest and abdominal wall. After the required costectomy is complete, if it is apparent that the chest wall has not collapsed sufficiently to obliterate the pleural space, make an incision into the cavity through the bed of one resected rib and open the space over the length of the rib bed. Grasp the cut edge of the periosteum with Allis forceps (Fig. 6-35), use the tip of a closed scissors as a blunt dissector, and separate the thick parietal peel from the intercostal muscles, preserving the intercostal nerves and vessels, then

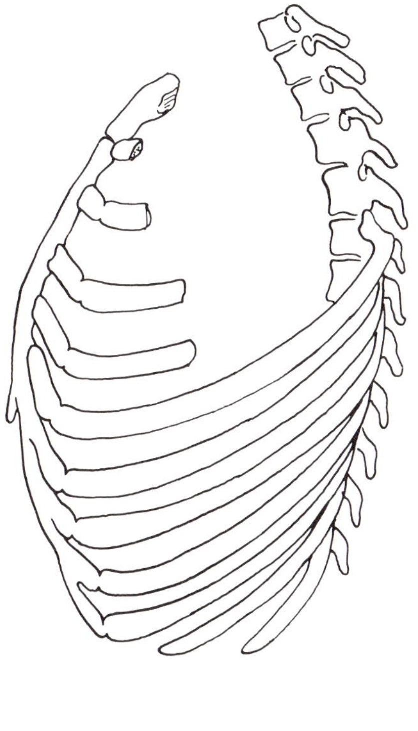

FIG. 6-34.

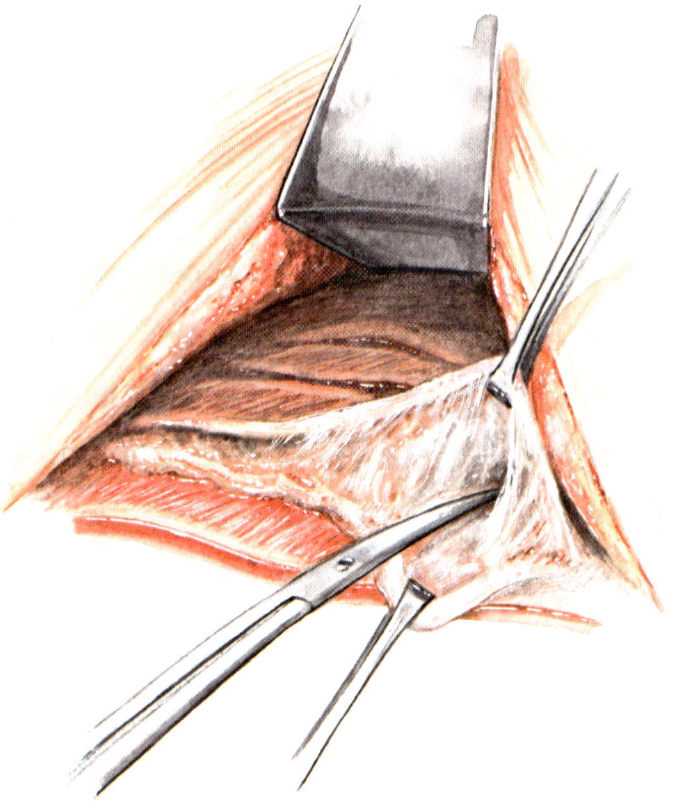

FIG. 6-35.

resect the peel. This dissection should free the entire lateral wall of the empyema pocket from the sternum to the vertebra. It is usually not necessary to decorticate the mediastinum. When completed, the intercostal bundles will lie as ribbons across the space. Prior to closing the wound, insert two #28 suction catheters into the intrapleural space from a skin site other than the incision. This procedure entails a slight risk of producing a subscapular abscess, but if the empyema cavity has been well drained and irrigated with an appropriate antibiotic solution prior to surgery and if the suction catheters keep the pocket empty after surgery, the risk is small.

Thoracic Outlet Syndrome

This syndrome is the result of the various mechanisms that compress one or more trunks of the brachial plexus, the subclavian artery, or the subclavian vein; it comprises the symptoms thought to result from this compression. In a majority of patients, the symptoms are neurologic, i.e. pain or paresthesias, but in 4%–12% significant vascular problems are seen. These symptoms are quite nonspecific and may also occur with angina pectoris, Pancoast syndrome, cervical disc syndromes, nonspecific neuromuscular disease, cervical radiculitis, and vasospastic disease. A history of trauma is present in 25%–50% of patients. The diagnosis is usually made from the physical findings or from an abnormal ulnar nerve conduction velocity, but even in the best hands, errors in the assignment of cause may occur; these errors are probably responsible for the significant number of patients that have less than excellent results from surgery.

The neural or vascular compression is due to a cervical rib in 5%–9% of patients, but in most, it is ascribed to abnormal fascial or tendinous bands, or to the muscles that insert on the first rib. No matter what the cause, the surgical treatment is the removal of the first rib, and a cervical rib, if present. It is generally agreed that most patients with this syndrome may be adequately treated without surgery. If vascular changes or bony abnormalities, such as cervical rib, are present, surgery is usually indicated, but beyond this, no consensus exists. If the patient's symptoms are truly disabling, if no other conditions are present that could explain them, if the characteristic physical abnormalities are found, and if the ulnar nerve conduction velocity is significantly impaired, then surgery is probably indicated. In recent series, 8%–10% of patients with this syndrome have required surgery, although in older series, 30%–40% of patients were operated on. Reported excellent relief of symptoms from surgical therapy has varied from 57% to 80%. Usually, the smaller the percentage of patients operated on, the better are the surgical results.

Axillary Approach For Resection of the First Rib

Although the first rib can be resected through a standard posterior–lateral incision, through a posterior paraspinous approach, or by the supraclavicular transcervical route, the transaxillary approach of Roos (3) has become most popular because no muscle is divided in approaching the rib and because the incision is cosmetically more pleasing than are the others. The patient is placed in a straight lateral thoracotomy position and the arm is prepared and draped in the operative field so that it can be held up by an assistant (Fig. 6-36).

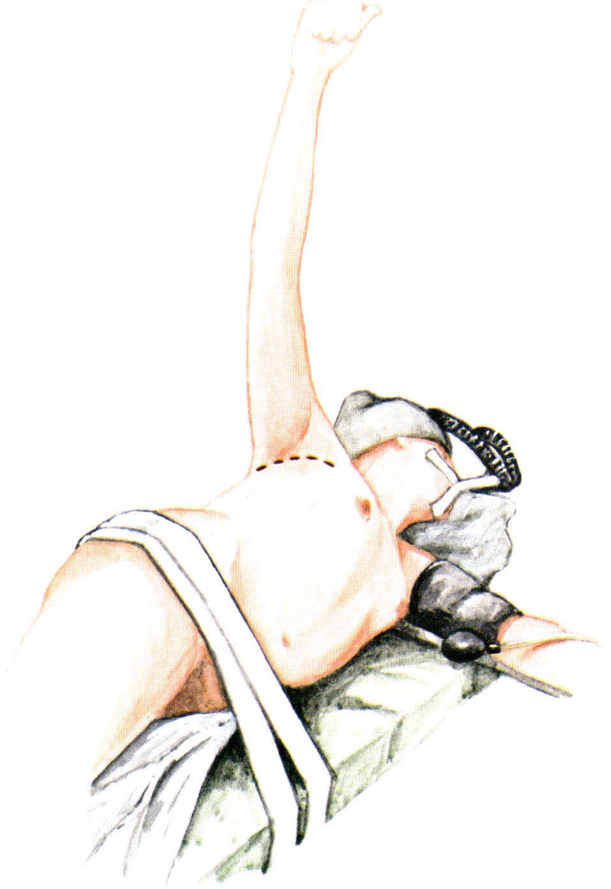

FIG. 6-36.

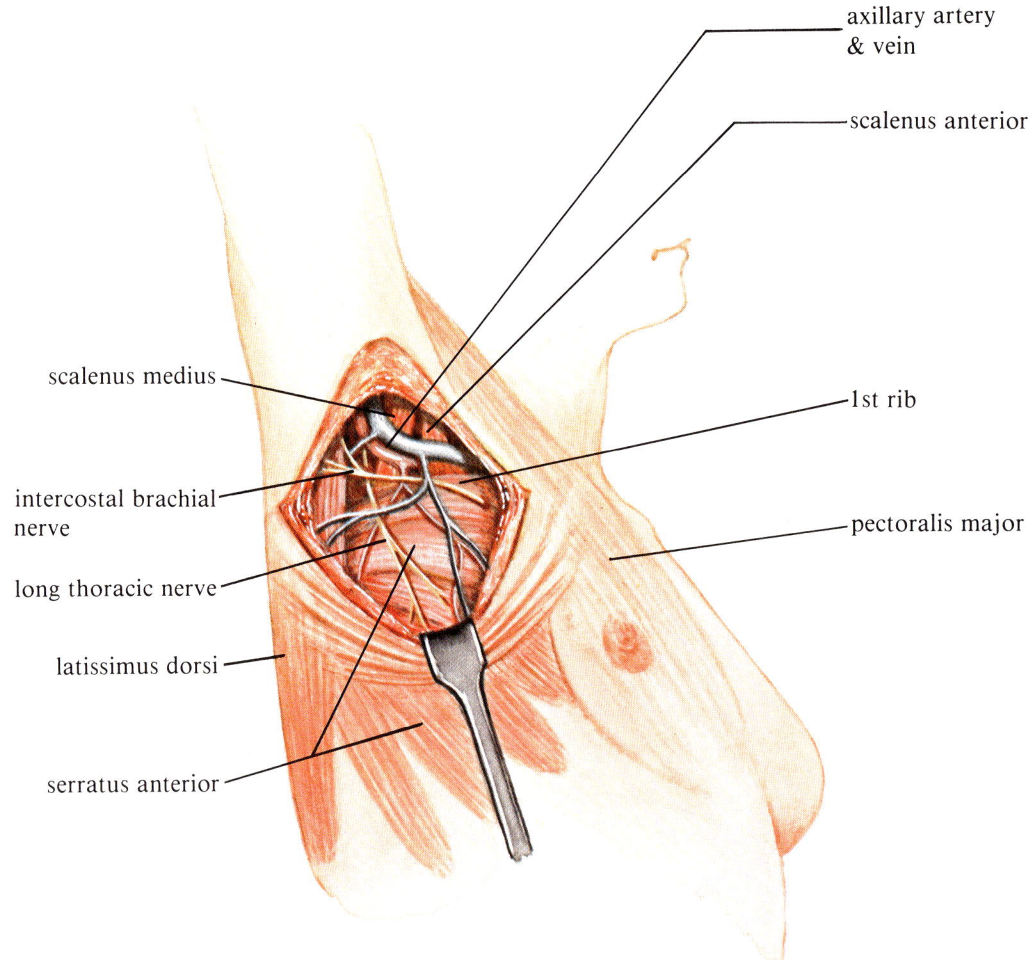

FIG. 6-37.

Make a horizontal 10–12 cm incision from the anterior to the posterior axillary fold just below the axillary hairline (the dashed line in Fig. 6-36). Dissect directly down to the chest wall; do not make the dissection obliquely upward through the axillary fat pad. Expose the chest wall from the latissimus dorsi to the pectoralis major. The anatomy of this region is shown in Fig. 6-37. Identify and preserve both the long thoracic nerve lying on the serratus anterior muscle and the intercostobrachial nerve running from the second or third interspace through the axilla to the arm. Dissect upward along the chest wall until the axillary blood vessels are identified. The assistant should raise the shoulder girdle by pulling vertically up on the arm with the elbow bent; this lifts the subclavian vessels and the brachial plexus off the superior surface of the first rib. Although this traction must be strong, it must not be excessive and must be interrupted at intervals to prevent permanent damage to the brachial plexus. Such damage is more likely during reoperation or during surgery following trauma to the area, in which case scar tissue may prevent easy exposure, resulting in excessive use of traction on the brachial plexus.

Expose the first rib and identify the scalenus anterior muscle inserting on its superior surface with the subclavian vein anterior to the muscle and the subclavian artery and brachial plexus posterior to it (Fig. 6-38). Also identify the scalenus medius muscle posterior to the brachial plexus and to the subclavian artery, but avoid unnecessary or excessive retraction of the brachial plexus. The first rib should be removed extraperiosteally to prevent regeneration and recurrence of symptoms. Divide the intercostal muscle at the lateral edge of the rib and reflect the pleura and areolar tissue off the

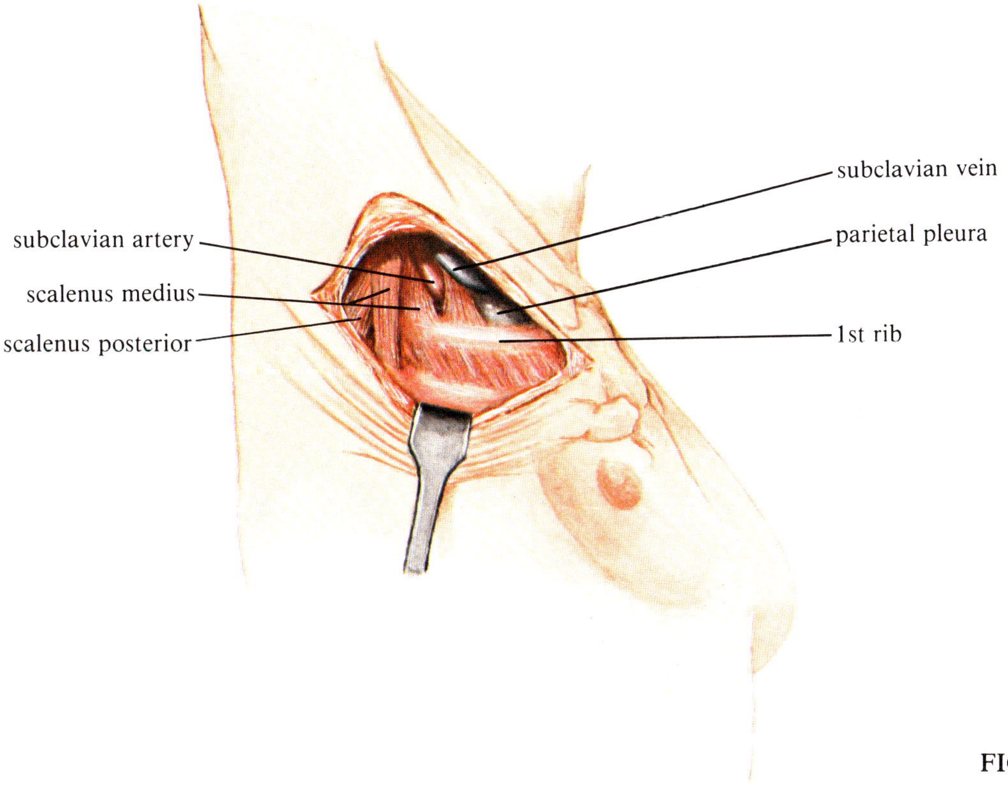

FIG. 6-38.

entire inferior surface of the rib. This may require ligation of the intercostal vessels below the rib. Divide the scalenus anterior muscle above its insertion on the first rib, and reflect the pleura and the subclavian vessels from the superior surface and medial edge of the rib. Divide the rib in the middle, and retract the anterior segment downward and outward (as depicted in Fig. 6-39, in which the severed insertion of the scalenus anterior muscle can be seen on the superior aspect of the anterior rib segment being held by the

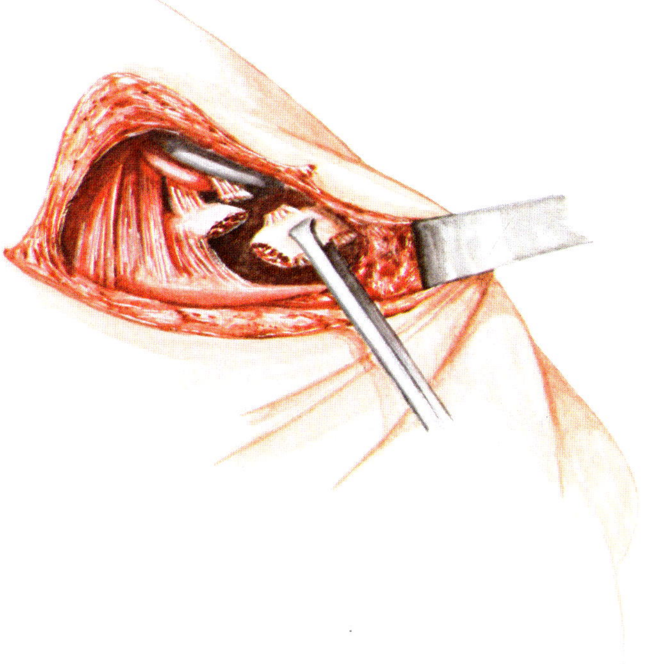

FIG. 6-39.

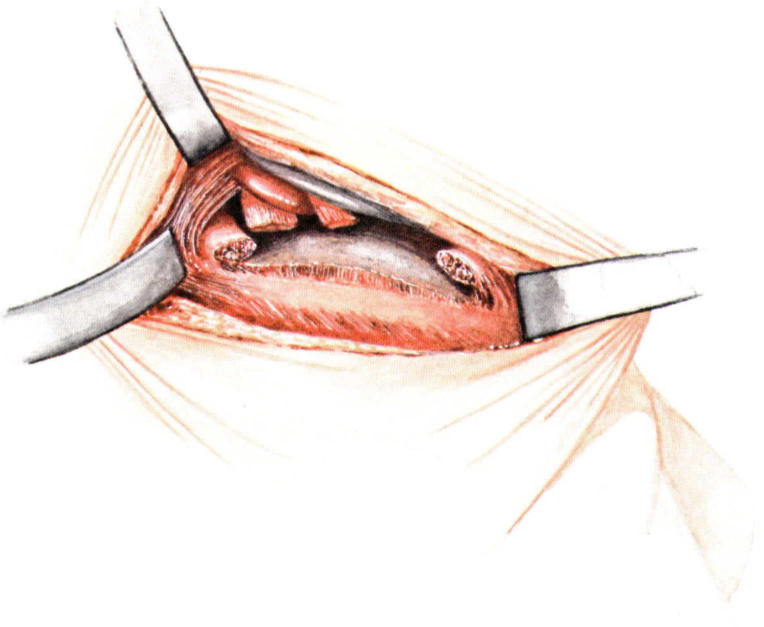

FIG. 6-40.

Allis forceps). Complete the dissection and divide the rib anteriorly at its costochondral junction. Complete the dissection of the posterior portion of the rib by freeing it from the brachial plexus and dividing the scalenus medius muscle above its insertion; then divide the posterior part of the rib at its junction with the transverse process of the vertebra. Palpate the posterior cut end of the rib and remove any bony spicules that could damage the brachial plexus. The completed dissection is shown in Figure 6-40. The anterior and posterior ends of the first rib are visible at the limits of the incision.

If a cervical rib is present, it can usually be removed with a rongeur after the first rib has been removed. When this proves difficult, it should be removed through a separate supraclavicular incision. No drain is used unless the pleura was entered. If this entry was small and closed immediately before a pneumothorax developed, drainage is still not necessary, but if a significant pneumothorax developed, an intrapleural suction catheter is placed in the chest through a separate site some distance from the operative field.

Congenital Disorders of the Sternum and Contiguous Chondroosseous Structures

Richard L. Varco, M.D.

The most common deformity of this anatomic complex is a depression of the sternum distal to the second rib. The attached cartilages and, at times, adjacent rib segments participate in the dorsal incurvation. The defect is usually referred to in English literature as funnel chest or pectus excavatum; it is called trichterbrust, schusterbrust, thorax en entonnir, or tórax en embudo by German, French, and Spanish writers. The surgical attempts at its treatment are more modern. In fact, few patients were operated upon to revise this birth defect until the past few decades. A greater contemporary willingness to operate upon this condition is revealed by the much larger numbers reported in relatively recent publications. It is probably more than coincidence that generally the frequency of cosmetic procedures has simultaneously risen.

What are the indications for recommending an operation for treatment of pectus excavatum? At best they are limited; and for many patients with limited involvement, they are nonexistent. Between those extremes, the majority are operated upon with faith in the assumption that the eventual result will be cosmetically preferable. To some thoracic surgeons this is a dubious proposition; given the inevitable and lengthy scar, which may be associated with degrees of keloid formation over a portion of its length, and the inherent imperfection of the correction, these doubts appear to this writer to have some merit. The American male's preoccupation with, and acclaim for, ever more cleavage makes it rather anomalous for surgeons to devise operations that minimize this aspect of female charm. Documentation indicates that significant and serious physiologic consequences created by the pectus were remediable by its correction. This sequence, however, is quite uncommon, at least as confirmed by appropriately derived cardiopulmonary function tests and similar analyses. The decision to recommend (or not) the procedure turns on a belief in its desirability from a cosmetic perspective. The observation is made that fewer publications about surgical treatment of this condition are to be noted in the literature of countries with a National Health Service.

A decision to operate should always be linked with a firm commitment by the parents and, if old enough, by the child to work diligently at reshaping the postural defects that are invariably intertwined with this problem. To fail to enlist the family's allegiance in that cause is to prejudice adversely the cosmetic result. The associated postural problems that deserve this attention, and even over-correction by "bending the green bough," are 1) sloping (round or stooped) shoulders, 2) protuberant (pot-bellied) abdomen, and 3) lordotic (sway) back. To rehabilitate the child's posture, have the individual stand upright, with heels together, calves touching an upright such as a doorjamb. Have the hips "tucked in" and also held against the vertical line, along with a few upper thoracic vertebral spines and the occiput. Now coach the patient to walk from that stance. Periodic return to these check positions is part of the training exercise. Together with properly conceived and utilized incentive programs, the results in a few weeks can be quite reassuring. A failure to win this rehabilitation contest is likely to assure loss of much of any operative benefits. For resumption, post-operatively, of the typically rounded shoulders, pot-bellied, sway-back posture is to insure defeat of much of the corrective attempt, including a tendency to resumption of the declivity in the mid sternal area. On the positive side, if the postural challenge is soundly managed, the post-operative result rests firmly and solely on the operative accomplishments.

Let us assume that a cooperative and dedicated patient achieves the desired postural improvements and we can, thereafter, proceed to examine the technical aspects of the operation.

A serious wound infection, in particular for "clean" elective cases, is always disturbing both to patient and to surgeon. This procedure involves de-vascularization, wide dissection, and extensive creation of pockets and flaps. Thus, any serious invasion with virulent pathogens can seriously prolong and complicate the convalescence. This elective procedure should be delayed until any and all local cutaneous infections (pimples, acneform lesions, folliculitis, etc.) are treated and healed. For the healthy skin, preparation the night before with a cleansing soap which contains an antibacterial product, seems a wise precaution. Routine preoperative skin care should *NOT* include shaving any lengthy period before the operation. Rather, this is best delayed until just before starting the intra-operating room cleansing, followed by the surface application of a bactericidal disinfectant.

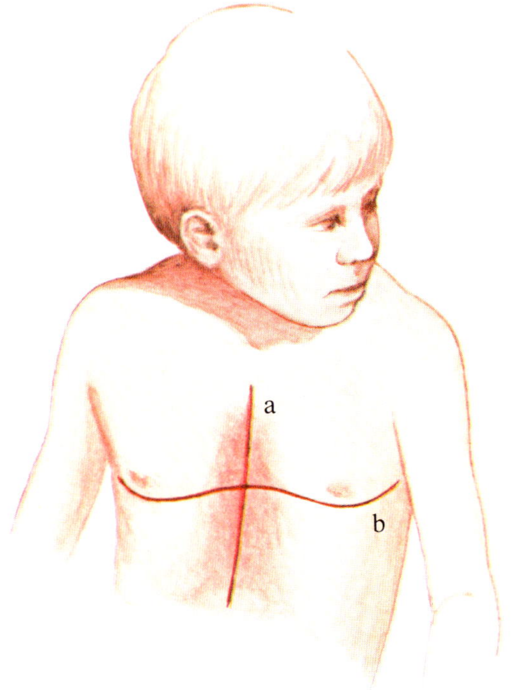

FIG. 6-41.

Either of the two skin incision placements depicted in Figure 6-41 can provide a satisfactory exposure. For males, the vertical midline cut, (*a*), which begins just below the sternal notch and proceeds caudally to the tip of the xiphoid, provides reasonable access to the required deeper dissections. For females, an inframammary placement, (*b*), nipple to nipple, upward curved in the midline and at about the level of the fifth rib, is probably more felicitous. However, the central portion of this cut has, at times, an awkward predisposition towards exuberant keloid formation. Any segment of the vertical one can also develop this unattractive blemish. Carry the skin opening, regardless of location, vertically through the soft tissues to the fascia which lies on the pectoral muscles. The underlying fat, superficial fascia and other structures should *NOT* be "shaved" back, or sloped. Achieve mobility of the skin flaps and exposure of the depths by developing full-thickness flaps to include all tissue, specifically the breast mass down to the anterior aspect of the pectoral fascia. Develop the undercut laterally, in that plane, for several centimeters in the case of the vertical incision and superiorly and inferiorly for the infra mammary approach, until the opening created is deemed adequate. In each circumstance its extent can be increased if required for greater exposure. An opening of lesser dimensions, which can easily be enlarged, has something to commend it while one is acquiring an experience with the procedure. The extent of dissection essential to provide the exposure needed for the proposed operative revision of the deformed sternum, cartilages, and at times ribs, can be evaluated through periodic palpation of the extent of the underlying deformity.

Expose each malformed strut by incising the overlying pectoral fascia. With minimal blood loss, separate the fibers of the pectoralis major in the direction of their attachments to the midline and to the lateral structures. Retract these fibers for a nice exposure (Fig. 6-42). Next, cut linearly the subjacent perichondrium and, to the extent that the rib participates in the posterior bowing, deal with its periosteum in a similar manner. The site and extent of this division is represented by the dashed line in Figure 6-42. Divest

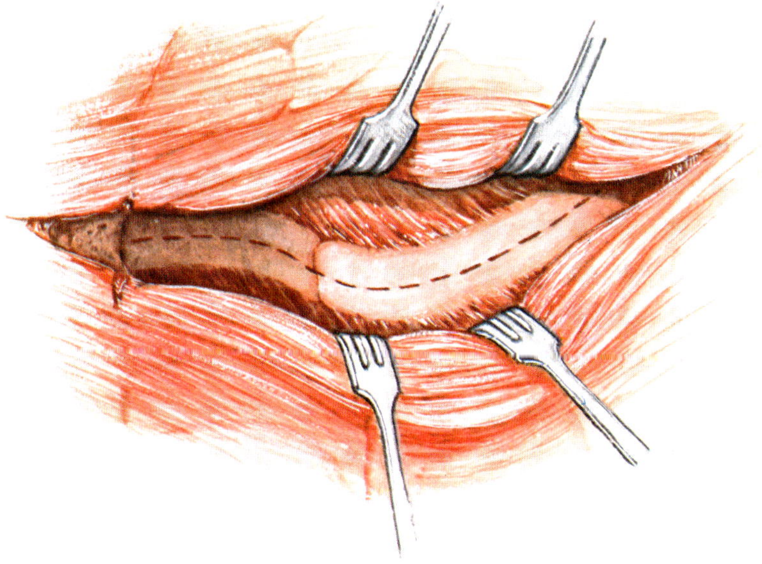

FIG. 6-42.

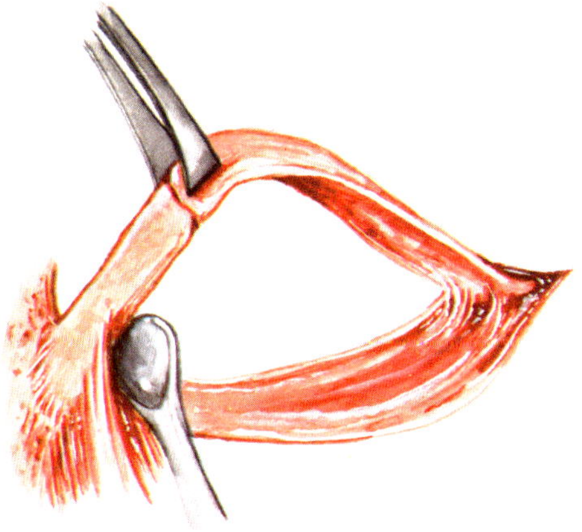

FIG. 6-43.

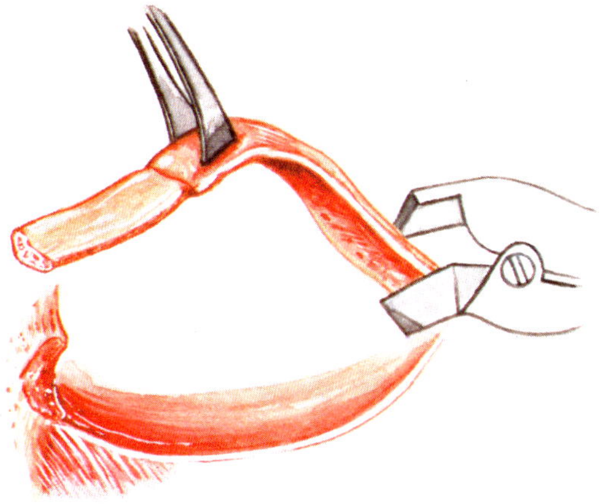

FIG. 6-44.

each cartilage and rib of its sheath (Fig. 6-43). Divide and remove the deformed chondrocostal elements (Fig. 6-44). The lateral end of the residual stump should point anteriorly. Care is necessary, particularly in the case of young children, if the surgeon is to avoid instrumental puncturing of the thin lamellae of the perichondrium and pleura during dissection and removal of the cartilage. Pediatric equipment, rather than adult-sized tools, is strongly recommended for such circumstances. This technique, initiated over any convenient site of a deformed cartilage and rib, is now repeated over all other abnormal struts on one side and then on the other. The pectoral fascia and its muscle are not detached; rather the surgeon works between muscular fasicles (Fig. 6-42), while excising the underlying struts. Cartilages which require removal usually include, as well, those that attach to the xiphoid.

Next, expose the loose areolar tissue-filled compartment deep to the sternum by careful division of the perichondrium immediately adjacent to the sternum. The pleural reflection is usually then visible. With care, some skill, and a modicum of good fortune, one can avoid injuring the internal mammary artery and adjacent vein. Circulation to surrounding tissues, some of which have undergone devitalizing trauma, can thereby be better maintained. With the internal mammary artery visible and safely put aside, enlarge the pocket

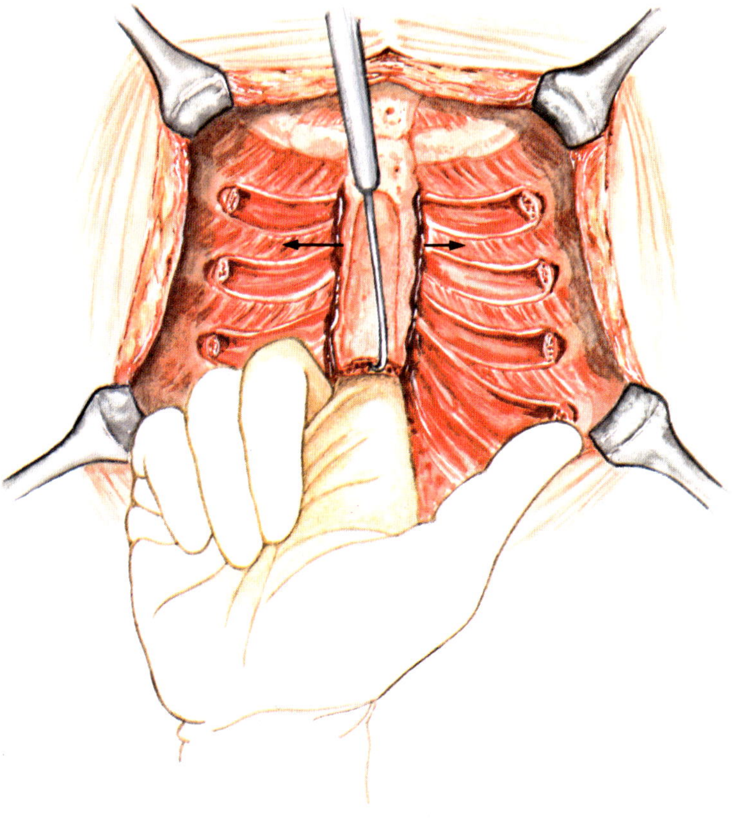

FIG. 6-45.

under the sternum (Fig. 6-45). With a hook in the under surface of the sternum as shown, create additional exposure by the application of external traction to the depressed gladiolus. Continue to cut away the perichondrial–intercostal muscular complexes adjacent to each deformed strut. Thus, the sternum will come to lie as a peninsula of bone freed of all attachments except to its continuum of the normally shaped upper portion. At this level, where the frontal plane of the sternum begins to veer from normal to assume a posterior declination, divide the sternal fascia–periosteal tissue in a transverse manner and carefully push it back for a few millimeters from the underlying bone, either on the front or on the back side. The decision to do an osteotomy in the anterior or in the posterior layer of the sternum hinges more on whim than unequivocal proof. For me, the anterior wedge osteotomy shown in Figure 6-46A permits satisfactory correction. One can use an osteotome or a narrow nosed, Cushing type, neurosurgical rongeur. With the latter, nibble away the outer table. Create a 1–2 mm cleft. Carefully, infract the intact posterior table by anterior bending of the sternum and thus create a "green stick" fracture. Support it in a slightly over-corrected (anteriorly protuberant) position by the insertion of vertical through and through, sturdy, nonabsorbable stitches that pierce the sternum and are started above and then come out below the cuneiform osteotomy (Fig. 6-46B). Suture the sternal fascia–periosteal layer with similar material. If the xiphoid juts out too prominently, bevel or excise it as shown to meet the cosmetic need.

With the sternum firmly positioned in a protuberant configuration and with a definitely over-corrected tilt, reattach each perichondrial-intercostal muscle bundle to the sternum with suitable size, nonabsorbable stitches. These repositioned structures customarily come to lie at sites different from those of their origin, in the deformed state. This should cause no concern; rather a new-found symmetry is the goal. Any minor defect in the area formerly

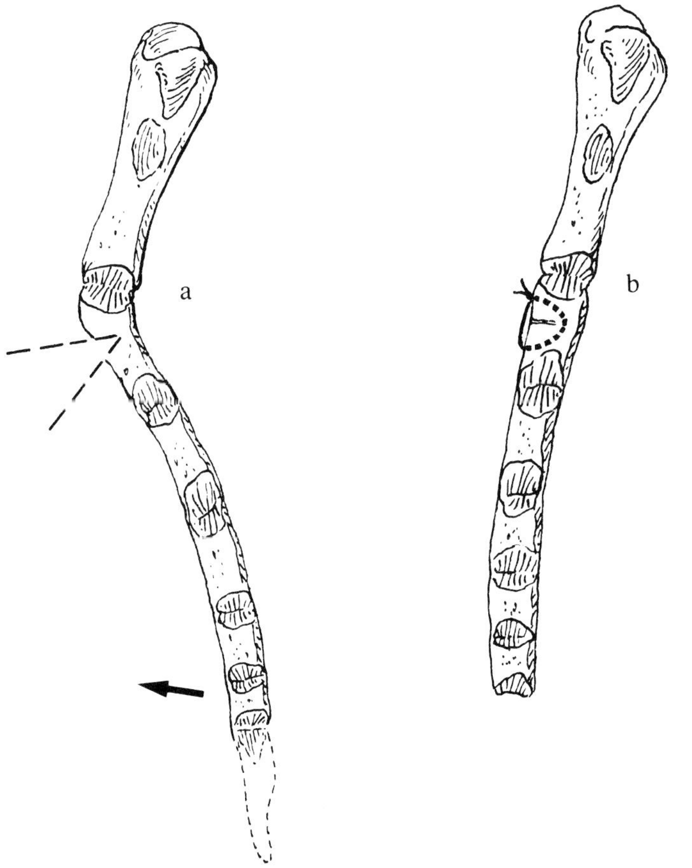

FIG. 6-46A,B.

occupied by the xiphoid can usually be closed by midline approximation, or realignment, of the adjacent perichondrial sheaths. Figure 6-47 is a graphic illustration of the reconstructed bony thorax at the conclusion of the procedure.

At times the pectus deformity is rather asymmetrical with a component of sternal rotation. In such a circumstance create an oblique sternal osteotomy of one table to permit the necessary correctional untwisting. Thereafter, maintain it in the desired configuration by the same type of suturing of the bone and separately of the fascia. Two separately placed osteotomies can be required, occasionally, for unusual configurations.

In my experience, it has not been necessary to remove routinely the second costal cartilage since it usually does not participate in the deformity. However, if the level required for sternal osteotomy is that high, deal with it in the same fashion as required to overcome any other deviation of the sternum.

Prior to closure of the skin and subcutaneous layers, place one or two polyethylene catheters, with multiple holes that spiral around it, under the flaps and in sites of potential pocketing. Bring these out through inferolateral stab wounds and fasten each carefully to the skin with nonabsorbable material (Fig. 6-48). Apply continuous low pressure suction to this system in the postoperative period. Maintain it until the drainge is but a few milliliters per day.

If, perchance, the pleura is punctured but without incurring significant bleeding or pneumothorax (for instance, the lung can be seen to remain expanded), no intrapleural drainage is required. However, if there is any doubt as to the significance of an induced pneumothorax, take the precaution of placing an intrathoracic catheter for decompression in the postoperative period. Also, when the operative field continues to ooze, despite serious efforts to control it, it is wiser and safer to open the pleural space generously. Cut

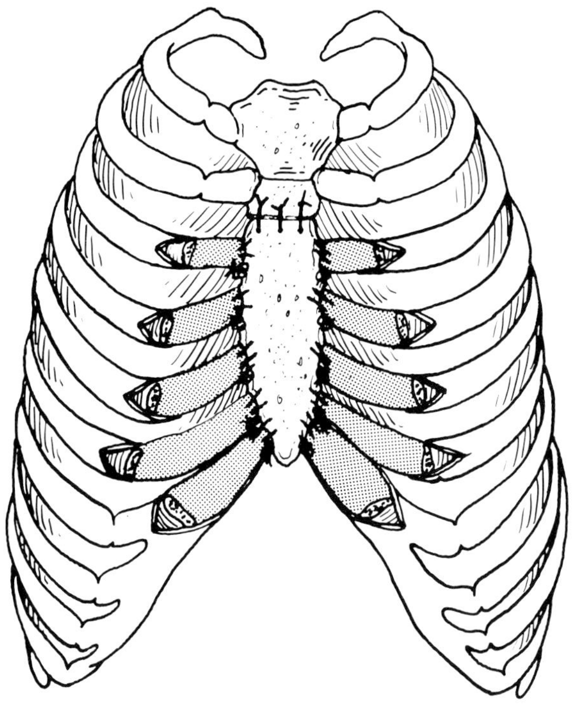

FIG. 6-47.

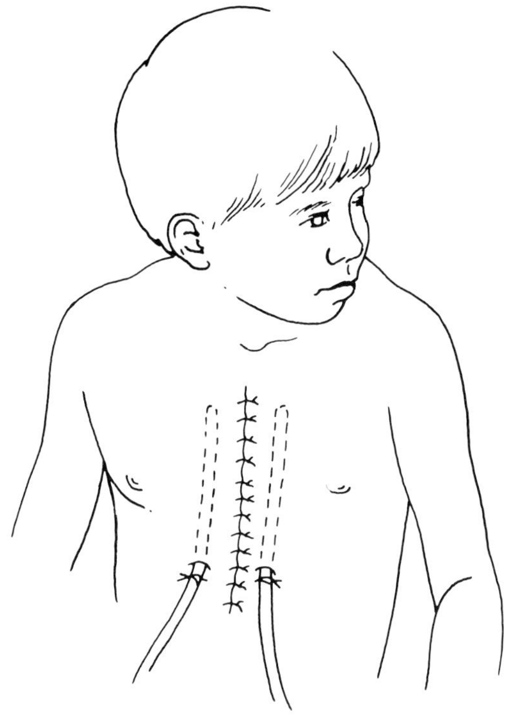

FIG. 6-48.

through several centimeters of the rib bed to create this internal avenue of drainage. Do this in a dependent (inferoposterior) area of the dissection. Then place a multiple-holed catheter in the lower posterior thorax. Bring it out through a separate intercostal stab wound and fix it firmly to the adjacent skin. Take care to avoid injury to an intercostal artery in this step.

A particularly careful wound closure is required. During the negative pressure phase, avoid any air leakage, either of inspiration or from suction applied through catheters to the subcutaneous space, through the incision. Close the subcutaneous tissues in a solid layer with interrupted stitches. Then, coapt the skin precisely in a separate procedure. With proper closure technique, air and bacteria will not be sucked into the depths of the wound.

It is not customarily necessary to use either an internal strut or external support for the newly positioned sternum. But, when required, as perhaps for a large adult, or under circumstances in which the tissues do not provide the sound internal fixation previously described, traction can easily be used to maintain the sternal tongue in place. Insert a wire through a small caliber polyethylene tube; with an absorbable suture, fasten this unit at a suitable site beneath the sternum. Bring out each end through a lateral stab wound and attach it to the skin as for any other catheter. Join rubber bands to this unit; they will give any desired amount of traction. When this system is hooked up, as to the body bow (Fig. 6-49), the patient can be ambulatory. After the sternum is acceptably firm, snip the wire and the device will slide out easily.

In summary, the principles of this operation are:

1. Completely free the captive sternum. This includes:
   a. Excision of all deformed cartilaginous and costal elements along with preservation of their respective perichondral and periosteal sheaths
   b. Division of the corresponding perichondral and intercostal muscle attachments from their sternal attachments

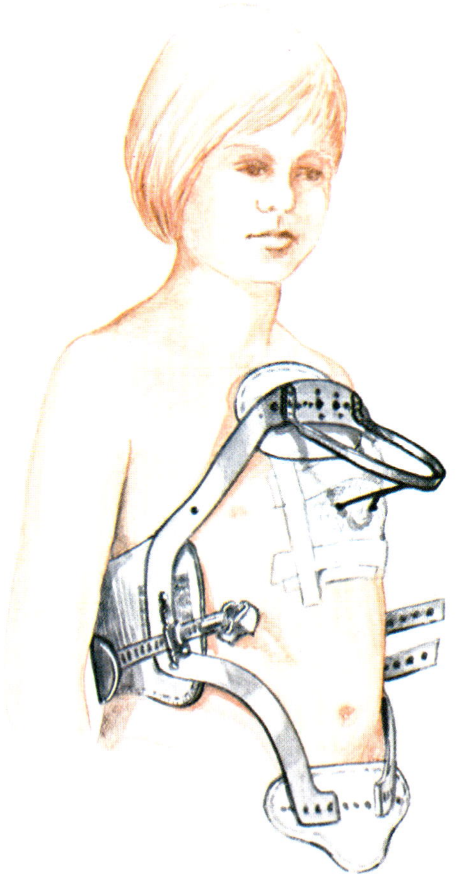

FIG. 6-49.

2. Osteotomy of one table of the sternum in a fashion that allows it to be bent and rotated as required into full correction of the deformity
3. Reattachment of the perichondral–intercostal muscle complexes to the repositioned sternum at sites that will best meet the cosmetic configuration desired

Other deformities of the sternum (pectus carinatum, sternal cleft, and fissure) are rather uncommon. Their management can probably best be dealt with by particular reference to each specific problem in the relevant literature, should the occasion arise to attempt its correction. In general, however, one can utilize above-outlined principles i.e., free and excise any deformed cartilage and bone, while preserving their surrounding sheaths; adapt osteotomy to restore shape to disfiguring bony elements; cover with native tissues or synthetic fabric any important residual defect in the chest wall. Give each wound painstaking care lest an always serious and potentially devastating invasive wound infection arises.

Surgery of the Diaphragm

Traumatic rupture of the diaphragm is discussed in the *Manual of Trauma Surgery* by Shires et al., 1983. As our understanding of the pathophysiology of patients with an esophageal hiatus hernia has increased, it is apparent that the symptoms are due to abnormalities of the gastroesophageal sphincter and not primarily to an abnormality of the diaphragm; this subject is discussed in the *Manual of Upper Gastrointestinal Surgery* by ReMine et al., 1983.

Tumors

Primary tumors of the diaphragm are rare and include benign mesotheliomas, lipomas, fibromas, and neurolemmomas. The malignant tumors are primarily of muscle or connective-tissue origin. Secondary invasion of the diaphragm by malignant tumors of neighboring structures, such as lung, chest wall, stomach, esophagus, colon, pancreas, or retroperitoneum, is not rare, however.

Whenever possible, the tumor, with a rim of normal diaphragm, should be excised. If the diaphragmatic disease is an area of invasion from an adjacent structure, the involved area should be excised in continuity with the original tumor.

Hernias

Excluding esophageal hiatus hernias, the nontraumatic diaphragmatic hernias that commonly occur in adults are those through the foramina of Morgagni. These foramina are bilateral, parasternal potential spaces through which the internal mammary arteries pass to become the superior epigastric arteries. A sac is usually present, and although it may contain abdominal viscera, it more commonly contains only omentum; at times the hernia may contain preperitoneal fat that has enlarged as the patient gains weight. Ordinarily these hernias are asymptomatic, but occasionally a patient will complain of low anterior chest or upper abdominal discomfort, and rarely a loop of bowel, usually colon, in the sac may become obstructed. If it seems that the patient's symptoms are caused by such a hernia, it should be repaired.

This repair is most easily done from the abdomen utilizing a subcostal incision, although if the hernia is discovered incidentally during a thoracotomy, its repair can be performed from the chest. After the contents of the hernial sac have been reduced into the abdomen, the diaphragmatic defect is closed with interrupted 2–0 nonabsorbable mattress sutures. If no anterior margin of the diaphragm is present, the posterior margin should be sutured to the chest wall, including the posterior surface of the sternum, and to the posterior layer of the rectus sheath (Fig. 6-50). The defect, visible just above the liver, is being closed by mattress sutures, which include the anterior chest wall. Rarely, the diaphragmatic defect is so large that it cannot be closed without

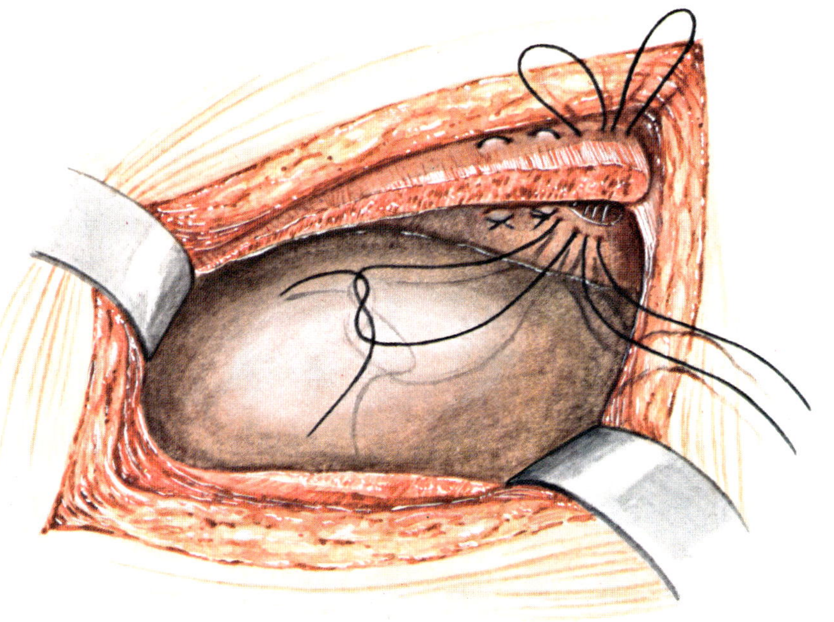

FIG. 6-50.

excess tension. In these situations a piece of Marlex mesh should be used for the closure. Unless the pleural cavity is accidentally entered, pleural drainage is unnecessary.

Eventration of the Diaphragm

The term eventration is used to describe an abnormally high position of the intact diaphragm that is due to a lack of diaphragmatic muscular strength. It may be congenital or acquired and may be unilateral or bilateral. Congenital eventration is caused by a lack of, or incomplete development of, diaphragmatic muscle; it may be partial or complete. Acquired eventration is caused usually by paralysis of the phrenic nerve.

A large eventration in the neonate may be life threatening and require immediate repair; however, if it remains asymptomatic for the first week of life, it is unlikely to cause difficulty later. Although such symptoms as dyspnea, cardiac arrythmias, epigastric pain, meteorism, and constipation have been attributed to an eventration, most patients with this condition are asymptomatic. Indeed, the evidence that any particular symptom in an adult with a unilateral eventration can be ascribed to the eventration is very unsubstantial, and the indications for repair of this condition in an adult are few or nonexistent. Varpela et al. (4) reported on nine patients operated on for acquired diaphragmatic eventration and repaired by transthoracic plication of the affected diaphragmatic leaf. None were asymptomatic postoperatively. Four of the seven patients who were dyspneic before surgery were also dyspneic after surgery. No statistically significant changes were found between the pre- and postoperative values of any lung function tests.

If one found an abnormality that could be improved by lowering the position of the diaphragm without restoring its function, the repair should be done through a thoracotomy incision by the use of Marlex mesh stretched from the anterior to the posterior chest wall. Numerous reports have shown that plication of the diaphragm results in a very temporary correction of its position, and the eventration recurs in a large percentage of patients followed for more than two years.

Repair of the Diaphragm

The diaphragm can be thought of as a truncated cone consisting of a central tendon connected to the chest wall by muscle. The apex of this cone is directed toward the sternum, so the anterior muscle fibers are the shortest and the posterior fibers are the longest. It is important to remember this shape when considering the type of repair to utilize after a partial diaphragmatic resection. If the defect is small, a simple closure of the defect is possible using interrupted, 2–0, nonabsorbable mattress sutures, as described in the section on thoracoabdominal incisions. When the defect is posterior or lateral and is too large for simple closure, or if an area of chest wall has been resected adjacent to the diaphragmatic defect, the insertion of the diaphragm on the chest wall can be raised to shorten the length of diaphragm needed and to make use of the longer posterior surface of the diaphragm. In these situations, suture the diaphragm to the chest wall above the chest wall defect or above its original site of insertion at a level that will produce little tension on the suture line. In Figure 6-51, the edges of a posterior–lateral diaphragmatic defect, which resulted from the excision of a localized mesothelioma, are being sutured to the chest wall through an intercostal space above the original insertion line. Pledgets of teflon wool are used to buttress the sutures. Large defects in the diaphragm and even moderate-sized defects situated anteriorly can often not be closed or can be closed only with excessive tension that

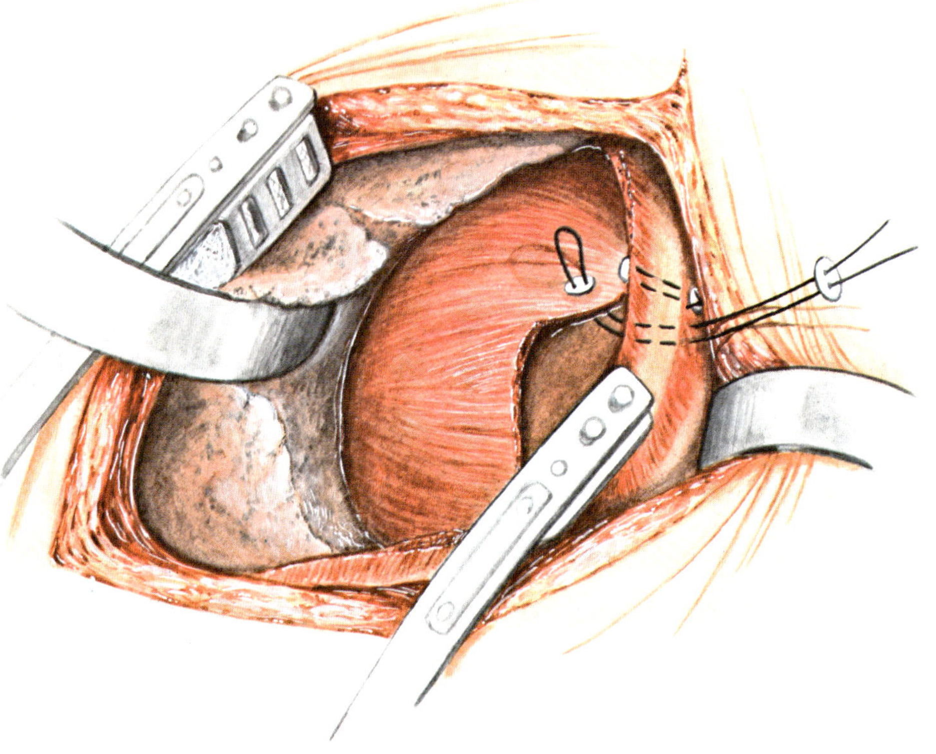

FIG. 6-51.

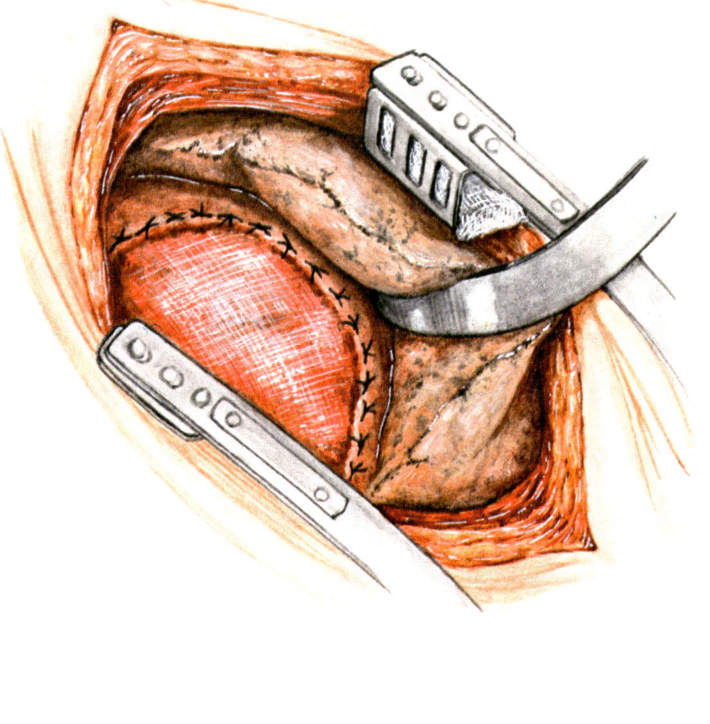

FIG. 6-52.

will eventually cause a dehiscence. In such circumstances it is advisable to repair the diaphragmatic defect using a piece of Marlex mesh sutured to the diaphragmatic margin and to the chest wall with interrupted nonabsorbable mattress stitches (Fig. 6-52). If inadequate tissue for the repair is found medially, the mesh can be sutured directly to the pericardium.

References

1. Huvos AG: Bone tumors: diagnosis, treatment and prognosis. Philadelphia, Saunders, 1979.
2. Paulson DL, Urschel HC Jr: Superior sulcus carcinomas. *In* Gibbon's Surgery of the Chest, Ed. Sabiston, D.C. and Spencer, F.C. Philadelphia, Saunders, 1976.
3. Roos DB: Transaxillary approach for first rib resection to relieve thoracic outlet syndrome. Ann Surg 163:354–358, 1966.
4. Varpela E, Laustela EV, Viljanen A: Acquired eventration of the diaphragm—Results of surgery. Ann Chir Gynaecol 66:284–289, 1977.

Emphysema and Disorders of the Pleural Cavity

7

Bullous Emphysema

Bullous emphysema is a disorder in which the lungs contain bullae that are not associated with an intrinsic disease of the airways or with pulmonary scarring from a disease such as tuberculosis. For surgical purposes, a bulla is defined as an emphysematous space, not lined by epithelium, with a roof formed by visceral pleura. Most single bullae that occupy less than one-third of a thoracic cavity and that are situated in otherwise normal lungs do not cause symptoms. A large bulla, however, can compress and compromise the function of the rest of the lung. In addition, a bulla can cause a relaxation of the adjacent lung, thereby decreasing the radial tension on airways and causing an increased resistance to airflow. A bulla can become infected; the lung can bleed into a bulla, occasionally causing life-threatening hemoptysis; and a bulla can rupture, producing a pneumothorax.

Surgery for bullous emphysema is performed for two reasons: to improve dyspnea or to treat or prevent the complications of bleeding or pneumothorax. The selection of patients for surgery to improve dyspnea is based on the following criteria: 1) the dyspnea is disabling, 2) a bulla occupies more than one-third of a hemithorax, and 3) the compressed lung is adequate to fill the space previously occupied by the bulla.

The first criterion implies that the dyspnea is largely due to the presence of the bulla. The more normal the remaining lung, the greater will be the improvement following surgery. The surgeon should be particularly wary of patients in which the degree of dyspnea is out of proportion to the size of the bulla. If the dyspnea is due primarily to underlying bronchitis or emphysema, little improvement following removal of a bulla can be expected. FitzGerald et al. (8) reported no significant improvement following removal of a bulla in patients with severe panacinar emphysema and an $FEV_{1.0}$ less than 30% of predicted. Patients with rapidly progressive pulmonary disease, such as that caused by an α-1-antitrypsin deficiency, are not good candidates for surgery.

The evaluation of patients for the third criterion is based on finding bronchial and vascular crowding on the chest radiograph. This criterion is used to exclude patients with a "disappearing lung syndrome" [Reid's type three bulla (13)]. Such patients have large, poorly defined spaces that are a local accentuation of generalized disease rather than a bulla as previously defined. Because lung tissue has been destroyed rather than displaced, an attempt to remove such areas leaves parenchyma inadequate to fill the thoracic cavity. In borderline patients, a pulmonary angiogram can be helpful in determining the presence or absence of vascular crowding. Perfusion scans, on the other hand, have not been helpful. A bronchogram should not be done in these patients because of the risk of an iatrogenic pneumonia.

The operative procedure should preserve all possible lung tissue; consequently a bulla should not be removed by a lobectomy. It should be unroofed, that is, the portion of the bulla wall composed of only visceral pleura should be removed. The operation is performed through a posterior–lateral thoracotomy. Usually many bullae of varying sizes will be encountered, but no attempt should be made to remove all of them. Rather, select for unroofing those areas of bullae that are chiefly responsible for distorting the lung. Because the junction between the visceral pleural roof of the bulla and the lung parenchyma is easier to distinguish when the bulla is inflated, mark this junction around the circumference of the bulla base with a series of small hemostatic clamps before opening the bulla. Leaving 1–2 cm of the pleural roof attached to the lung, incise the bulla distal to the hemostats around 25% of its circumference and oversew the cut edge of the lung using a continuous suture of 3–0 Vicryl with a taper point needle (Fig. 7-1). The suture should be placed no greater than 1 cm deep because the lung in this condition has very little

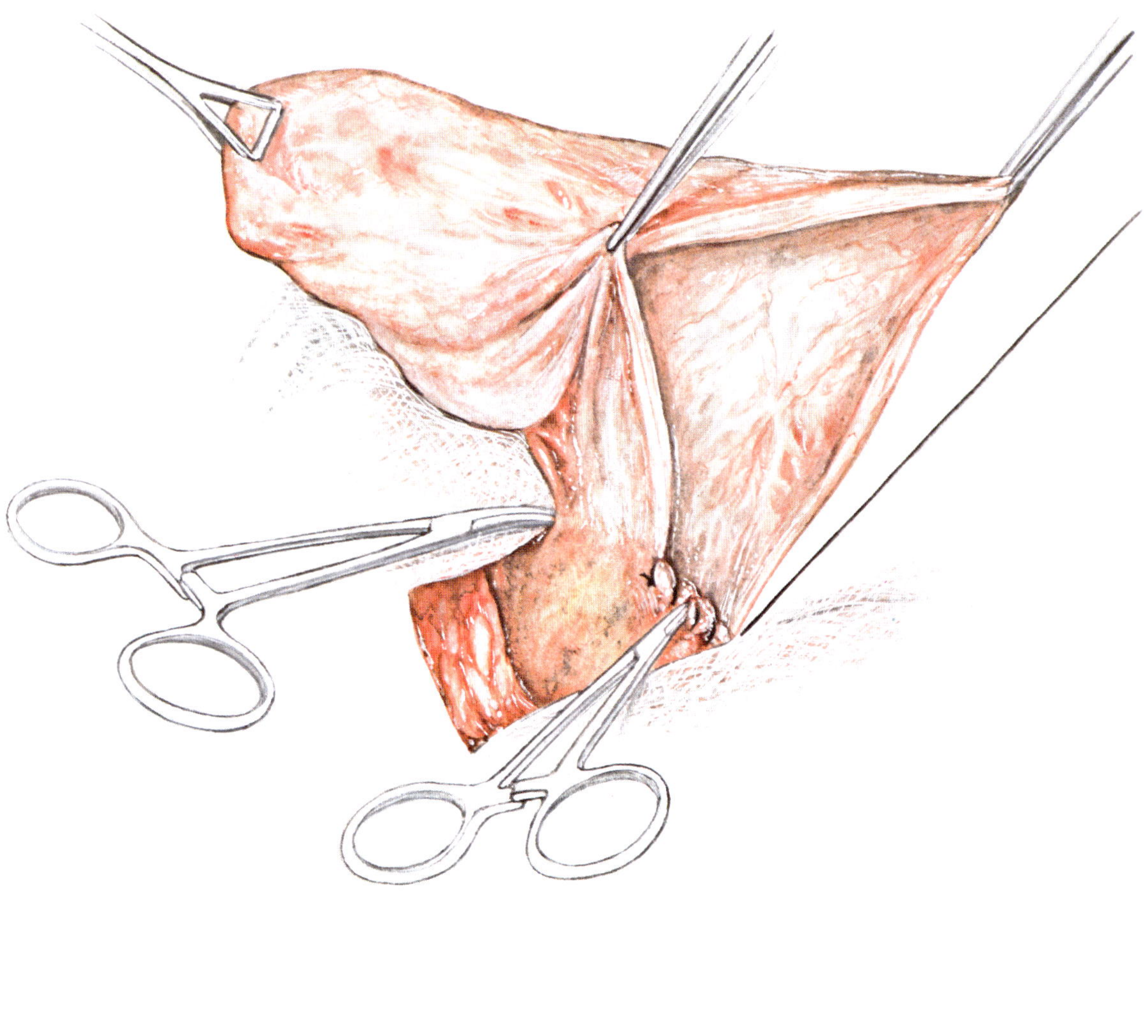

FIG. 7-1.

tensile strength. Large bites will tear the lung and increase the air leak. Continue incising the bulla and oversewing the edge until the entire pleural roof has been removed. After the bulla has been opened, the circumference of its base will gradually shrink as the rest of the lung expands. A bulla with a base 12–14 cm in diameter when the chest was first entered may have a diameter of only 6 cm when the procedure is concluded. The air leak is often surprisingly small, but any significant leak or any bleeding point in the base of the bulla should be sutured using the technique illustrated in Figure 4-35. Just before closing the chest a pleural abrasion should also be done to prevent a future pneumothorax.

Prolonged air leaks are relatively common after this operation. Do not cut in the intercostal catheters any extra holes that would limit the amount the catheters could be withdrawn without completely removing them from the pleural cavity. If the catheters are slowly withdrawn, the lung will adhere to the parietal pleura behind the catheter, thus obliterating the tube track and sealing any air leak coming from adjacent lung.

Spontaneous Pneumothorax

A spontaneous pneumothorax is defined as a pneumothorax not due to a traumatic or iatrogenic cause. Two types are described: primary, if the patient has no clinically evident pulmonary disease, and secondary, if a specific underlying disease is present. The overall incidence of spontaneous pneumothorax is approximately 5 per 100,000 per year, but it is 4–6 times more common in men than in women and has a peak incidence in the third and fourth decade of life. The incidence in young men has been estimated to be 1 in 500.

Primary pneumothorax is most commonly due to rupture of small bullae or pleural blebs in lungs that otherwise appear normal. These blebs, which are probably congenital, frequently occur in groups at the tip of the apical segment of the upper lobe or at the tip of the superior segment of the lower lobe; they often resemble a cluster of grapes on a relatively narrow pedicle. On the other hand, solitary blebs that can rupture occur at any position on the visceral pleura. Secondary pneumothorax may be associated with pulmonary emphysema, eosinophilic granuloma, tuberculosis and some fungal diseases, carcinoma of the lung, scleroderma, idiopathic pulmonary fibrosis, staphylococcal pneumonia, and rarely with menses (catamenial pneumothorax).

Usually, primary spontaneous pneumothorax is a relatively benign condition, but rarely it can cause a serious, even life-threatening situation. Significant hypoventilation can occur in two situations. With a large pneumothorax, the intrapleural pressure will rise above the pressure of the opposite pleural cavity and a shift of the mediastinum toward the normal side with a decrease in the ventilation of the normal lung can occur. Hypoventilation will also be present in the 1% of patients in which simultaneous bilateral pneumothoraces occur. If either of these two conditions are extreme or happen to a patient with a limited ventilatory reserve, serious hypoxia will result.

The presence of a fluid level in the pleural cavity is reported in 13%–20% of patients with a spontaneous pneumothorax. When it occurs, a thoracentesis should be performed to determine the character of the fluid. Usually the fluid will be blood, but if a black-colored fluid is obtained, a ruptured esophagus, not a primary spontaneous pneumothorax, should be suspected. Of patients with a spontaneous pneumothorax, 4%–5% will bleed significantly into the pleural cavity from torn adhesions. Usually this bleeding will stop with the placement of a thoracostomy tube as soon as the intrapleural blood has been evacuated, the lung is reexpanded, and the parietal and visceral pleura are in contact. If it does not stop, a thoracotomy is indicated.

Subsequent to a pneumothorax, the lung may be trapped in a collapsed position. This rare occurrence is due to a fibrin peel that forms on the surface of the lung or to preexisting parenchymal disease that has significantly decreased the compliance of the lung. If in such instances the bronchopleural fistula closes, the pleural space will fill with fluid. If for a prolonged period the pleural space continues as an air filled pocket, a continuing bronchopleural fistula is present.

Sometimes a spontaneous pneumothorax will be associated with a pneumomediastinum and with subcutaneous emphysema. This finding in an adult is of no therapeutic consequence if a perforated esophagus or trachea has been ruled out. Although airway obstruction from mediastinal emphysema in young children has been reported, this complication does not occur in adults in spite of the grotesque appearance of the patient. If subcutaneous emphysema develops after the placement of a thoracostomy tube, either the tube has been positioned with one of the side holes outside the pleural cavity or the tube is obstructed. Air from a pneumothorax may pass through pores in the diaphragm to appear as free peritoneal air on a radiogram. Such an occurrence may be the source of considerable diagnostic difficulty, but if peritoneal signs and laboratory findings remain normal, this possibility should not be overlooked.

The diagnosis of a pneumothorax is usually made by a radiograph of the chest, but 100–200 ml of air must be present in the pleural cavity or the diagnosis will not be apparent. If a pneumothorax is suspected but cannot be confirmed by radiography, a film of the chest during expiration should be obtained to accentuate the pleural findings. Occasionally, it can be difficult or even impossible to differentiate between a pneumothorax and a large bulla from the chest radiograph. Such a distinction is important if the use of a thoracostomy tube is contemplated, because the percutaneous insertion of a tube into a bulla will result in a large air leak that may continue for many weeks and may produce a pneumothorax where one was not present initially. Computerized tomography has been of significant value in determining which of the two abnormalities is present.

The normal course of a spontaneous pneumothorax is the air leak seals and the lung reexpands. Because the rate of pleural air absorption is a function of the partial pressure of the gas and the area available for diffusion, both of which are relatively constant over a wide range of pleural air volumes, the rate of air absorption in an otherwise normal adult is relatively constant at 50–75 ml/day. If it is common for the lung to reexpand spontaneously, it is also common for a spontaneous pneumothorax to recur. The overall rate of recurrence in published series is about 10%, but the risk of developing a subsequent pneumothorax increases with each episode. Carr et al. (4) reported that of patients having one previous pneumothorax, 9.6% had a second, while of those who had two previous pneumothoraces, 18.2% had a third. Ransdell and McPherson (12) found that after two episodes of pneumothorax, 40% of individuals had a third.

The initial management of patients with a first primary spontaneous pneumothorax depends on the degree of pneumothorax present, on the unilaterality of the pneumothorax, and on the presence or absence of a hemopneumothorax. If blood is present in the pleural cavity, an intercostal catheter should be inserted and connected to water seal suction. This will expand the lung and remove the blood, hence minimize the risk of developing a trapped lung with a chronic pleural effusion. An intercostal catheter should also be used if bilateral pneumothoraces are found since this situation presents a significant risk to the patient's life. If neither of the above two indications exists and the pneumothorax occupies less than 10%–15% of the intrathoracic volume, I do not treat the patient, but continue following him until the pneumothorax is gone. If the pneumothorax is greater than 10%–15%, an intercostal catheter should be used to decrease the length of the patient's disability. The average time for reexpansion of the lung in this condition without the use of catheter suction has been reported to be 12–35 days.

Patients with a secondary pneumothorax will usually require the insertion of one or more intercostal catheters. In these patients the pulmonary air leaks do not close as readily and the compliance is often decreased. As a result, some of the decrease in the size of the pleural pocket must occur from elevation of the diaphragm or a shift of the mediastinum, changes that are facilitated by a decrease in the intrapleural pressure. If complete reexpansion does not occur following the placement of one intercostal catheter, a second should be positioned in the residual air space, which may have become sealed off from the original catheter.

In certain situations of limited duration, such as pneumothorax in a patient with atelectasis from far-advanced lung cancer in whom the lung could not be expected to reexpand to fill the thoracic cavity, the insertion of an intercostal catheter is contraindicated. A catheter could not improve the situation; it could only introduce an infection and produce an empyema. Permitting the pneumothorax to remain incurs less morbidity. When doubt exists about the ability of the lung to fill the thoracic cavity, as a trial, a catheter can be inserted and suction applied for 6–8 hours. If the lung cannot adequately reexpand in that period, the catheter should be immediately removed.

Rarely, unilateral pulmonary edema may be produced by the use of suction applied to an intercostal catheter, particularly in patients with a chronically collapsed lung or with decreased compliance. The risk of pulmonary edema developing increases with increasing negative pressure. Edema is usually evident within 2 hours, progresses for 24–48 hours, and then disappears in about 6 or 7 days.

The intercostal catheters used for treatment of a pneumothorax need not be larger than 18–22 gauge and should have no additional holes cut in them. Unless a significant amount of fluid is present, the optimum site for insertion of the tube is the anterior second interspace in the midclavicular line. This is the largest interspace, thereby minimizing the risk to the intercostal vessels. It is near the top of the chest, so it facilitates the positioning of the catheter near the apex of the lung, and by placing the catheter anterior, it decreases the risk of its kinking from the patient lying on it.

Using local anesthesia, an intercostal catheter may be inserted either using a trocar or by dissecting a tract with a curved hemostat, but the later method miminizes the risk of injury to a lung fixed to the anterior chest wall by adhesions. Make a small skin incision just below the second rib and tunnel the tube over the second rib and into the pleural cavity at the superior edge of that rib. The tube should be directed toward the apex of the chest as it is introduced, and should be inserted only far enough to position the last hole 2–3 cm into the pleural cavity. This distance can be estimated by measuring the distance from the skin to the pleural cavity with the needle used to anesthetize the chest wall. Mark off this observed distance on the catheter from a point 2 cm proximal to the last hole and place a hemostat on the catheter at the point selected to be at skin level. The catheter should be connected to water seal suction and fixed to the skin with a 2–0 nonabsorbable suture that also closes the skin incision tightly around the tube. A chest radiograph should always be obtained to verify the position of a catheter after its insertion.

The intercostal catheter should remain in the pleural cavity for 24 hours after the air leak has apparently stopped and the lung has completely reexpanded. During this time a check must be made for a slow air leak. Such a leak can be detected by fastening to the patient's bed in a horizontal position a segment of the tubing that connects the catheter and the water seal apparatus. If some fluid can be seen within this segment of tubing, make a mark on each edge of the fluid column and observe it over several hours for progression down the tube. If no such progression occurs, there is no air leak. If no fluid is found, a few milliliters of sterile water can be injected into the horizontal segment of tubing using a syringe with a 26 gauge needle.

In most patients, the pulmonary air leak will stop in 2–3 days. If a leak is still present after 4–5 days, a thoracotomy to obliterate the pleural space and stop the air leak should be considered. Other indications for a thoracotomy in the treatment of spontaneous pneumothorax are persistent intrapleural bleeding, recurrence of the pneumothorax, or one episode of a pneumothorax in a patient with an occupation in which a recurrent pneumothorax could be a hazard. A thoracotomy is also indicated in a patient with a chronic pneumothorax secondary to a pleural peel and a persistent bronchopleural fistula. This condition is discussed with the operation of decortication.

In an attempt to obliterate the pleural cavity, some authors have reported the use of various irritating substances, such as silver nitrate or talc. These substances have the disadvantages of being very painful and of frequently failing to completely obliterate the pleural cavity, although Larrieu et al. (10) have recently reported success from the intrapleural administration of quinacrine. Previously a parietal pleurectomy had been recommended for the treatment of recurrent spontaneous pneumothorax, but a consensus that this procedure should not be used has developed. It is associated with a significant blood loss, and it causes such solid adhesions to the chest wall that another thoracotomy on that side is impossible without significant, indeed, irreparable damage to the lung. Since the operation is commonly performed in young men, the probability of needing another thoracotomy during their lifetime is significant.

At the present, the method of choice to obliterate the pleural cavity in the treatment of spontaneous pneumothorax is a pleural abrasion. The operation is performed through a limited posterior lateral thoracotomy just large enough to insert a hand and examine the whole lung. During such an operation the anesthesiologist should be aware that the positive pressure ventilation might produce a pneumothorax on the previously uninvolved side and the patient should be monitored for this occurrence. If the location of the air leak is not immediately obvious, fill the chest with warm saline; as the anesthesiologist maintains an airway pressure of 20 cm H_2O, systematically submerge each lobe and examine it for a source of bubbles. Commonly an area of small bullae or blebs will be found at the apex of the upper lobe or at the apex of the superior segment of the lower lobe. Using the TA-55 stapler, a row of 3.5 mm staples should be placed below the bullae and the bullae amputated. If the air leak is from the side of a lobe instead of an edge, compress the region of the leak with a lung grasping forceps and close it with figure-of-eight sutures (Fig. 4-35).

When all air leaks have been stopped, the obliteration of the pleural cavity should be produced by systematically rubbing all surfaces of the parietal pleura with *dry* gauze sponges. This abrasion must include the diaphragm, the mediastinum, and also the interlobar fissures. The abrasion is adequate when small petechial hemorrhages can be seen on the pleura. Following the procedure, place three intercostal catheters in the chest to prevent the collapse of the lung from a nonfunctioning tube, an occurrence that could nullify any benefit of the operation.

Empyema

The meaning of the word empyema as it relates to the chest has been for generations a source of confusion to the medical profession. Prior to the early years of the nineteenth century it was used to describe both a serous and a purulent pleural effusion. Its meaning was even extended to the operation for draining the pleural cavity. Much of the confusion today in the treatment of empyema thoracis results from the multiple definitions implied by current medical writers. In the ensuing discussion, the word empyema is defined as pus in the pleural cavity, *not* pleural fluid from which bacteria can be cultured. Pus is a gross description meaning an opaque fluid of high specific gravity containing degenerating leukocytes, tissue debris, and living or dead bacteria.

Acute Empyema

At present a majority of patients that develop acute empyema have some significant underlying abnormality. In the series of Sherman et al. (17), 75% of the patients had a serious associated disease. Commonly reported conditions related to the development of empyema are pneumonia in a patient with a chronic debility, aspiration followed by the development and rupture of a septic lung abscess, rupture of the esophagus, extension through the diaphragm of a subdiaphragmatic abscess or a pancreatic abscess, and complications following an intrathoracic surgical procedure or trauma to the chest. These underlying conditions are to blame for a significant fraction of the mortality reported for empyema.

These underlying abnormalities are responsible for the wide spectrum of etiologic bacteria that can be isolated from patients with an empyema. In the preantibiotic era, *Streptococcus pneumoniae* was responsible for 50%–70% of all empyema, but recent reports, such as that from the Boston City Hospital by Finland et al. (7), indicate that the relative frequency of this organism is decreased but still significant in community-acquired disease. Finland found the most common organisms initially cultured during 1969 and 1972 were Gram-negative rods, *S. pneumoniae,* and *S. aureus;* 22.5% of patients had a mixed culture of aerobes. The incidence of anaerobes varies greatly with the institution reporting; Finland et al. found 15% but Bartlett et al. (1) isolated anaerobes from 75% of patients with an empyema not associated with previous surgery, and in half of these patients, only anaerobes were found. In infants and young children the predominant organism from several series has been *S. aureus,* often associated with a staphylococcal pneumonia.

Before the availability of antibiotics, the development of an empyema was often signalled by the onset of pleural pain and an increase in fever and toxicity. Now, the presence of an empyema is more often recognized by the persistence of fever and an elevated white blood cell count inspite of seemingly adequate antibiotic therapy. A chest radiograph usually reveals the presence of pleural fluid which must then be aspirated to confirm the diagnosis. A gram stain and both aerobic and anaerobic cultures should be done on the empyema fluid, even when an organism has been previously identified by a culture from some other source, such as sputum, because previous antibiotic therapy may have caused a rapid change in flora. Occasionally it may be difficult, on a chest radiograph, to distinguish between an empyema and a subpleural lung abscess or cyst. This distinction between intrapleural and intrapulmonary processes can often be made more accurately from computerized tomography.

Neglected cases of acute empyema may become complicated by the development of a bronchopleural fistula, or such a fistula may occur initially from the rupture of a lung abscess into the pleural cavity. If the fistula or the empyema is small, the greatest detriment may be the spread of the suppurative process to the opposite lung, but if an empyema of large volume suddenly erodes a sizable bronchus, the patient may drown from a sudden flooding of the tracheobronchial tree with purulent fluid. Other complications that can occasionally occur in neglected cases are brain abscess, pericarditis, empyema necessitatis, and most commonly, the development of a chronic empyema.

The goal of therapy for empyema is to sterilize the cavity and to *obliterate the cavity*. If lung tissue is present in the hemithorax, the former can rarely be permanently accomplished unless the latter is also achieved, and adequate drainage is the cornerstone for doing both. During the early stage of a pleuritis, in the presence of a thin exudative fluid containing bacteria but few leukocytes and little debris, the patient can often be managed by needle aspiration of the fluid and systemic antibiotic therapy. However, when an empyema as defined previously develops, needle thoracentesis is not adequate drainage. The healing of an empyema cavity was demonstrated by Carlson (3) to be due to the progressive adhesion of the opposed pleural surfaces. The continued presence of pus in the cavity delays or even prevents this healing. There are two potential phases of drainage for empyema: closed intercostal drainage and open thoracostomy drainage. Closed drainage utilizing an intercostal catheter connected to water-seal suction is used during the period before the parietal and visceral pleura are firmly adherent to one another and while the possibility of collapse of the lung from an open thoracostomy still exists. This procedure rapidly evacuates a large portion of the purulent material in the cavity, decreases the patient's toxicity, and starts the process of obliterating the cavity.

Select a site for placement of the intercostal catheter at the most dependent portion of the empyema pocket by referring to the chest radiograph and by aspirating with a large bore needle. If on the radiograph, the opacity of the empyema pocket is confluent with that of the diaphragm, care must be taken to locate the diaphragm exactly or the needle might lacerate the spleen or liver, or penetrate the diaphragm and seed the peritoneal cavity with bacteria. When the surgeon is uncertain of the proper location, fluoroscopy should be used to select a site for aspiration. If thin fluid, not pus, is encountered with the needle, additional aspiration attempts should be made at other sites, because in cases of loculated effusions, pus may exist in one area and serous fluid in another with no communication between. When the site has been chosen, insert a 22 or 24 French rigid plastic catheter directly into the empyema pocket, but away from the intercostal vessels. Do not tunnel the catheter under the skin as described for catheter insertion in a pneumothorax. Suture the catheter to the skin and connect it to water-seal suction. Occasionally loculations not drained by the first catheter will become apparent after 1 or 2 days, and the insertion of a second catheter will be necessary.

Many cases of empyema will be cured by closed drainage and antibiotic therapy, but some, because of the thickness of the pus or the presence of a pleural peel or a bronchopleural fistula, will require open thoracostomy drainage to permit complete obliteration of the pocket. After 10–12 days a decision should be made about the necessity for this second phase of drainage. If at that time it is apparent from the chest radiograph that the pocket has been obliterated, the intercostal catheter may be removed and no further therapy instituted. When the status of the empyema pocket is unclear, radiopaque contrast material should be injected through the catheter to permit a more accurate evaluation. If the pocket is still present and significantly larger than the tube track, open thoracostomy drainage should be established to completely evacuate all purulent debris from the pocket.

The thoracostomy should be made in the most dependent portion of the empyema pocket. The intercostal catheter, if it has been well placed, can serve as a guide to the proper site for the rib resection; otherwise posterior–anterior and lateral radiographs of the pocket should be obtained after outlining it with contrast material. Prior to making the incision, confirm the choice of site by a needle aspiration. If a bronchopleural fistula is present, the operation should be done with the patient in a sitting position to prevent the aspiration of purulent material into the opposite lung; otherwise the patient is positioned with the site for thoracostomy uppermost.

A thoracostomy can usually be made using local anesthesia. At the angle of the rib, inject 4–5 ml 0.5% Marcaine under the rib to be divided and under the two ribs above and the two below the chosen rib. The skin over the incision site should also be infiltrated with the anesthetic. Make an incision 5–6 cm long parallel to the rib and overlying its lower border. The fibers of the overlying muscle can be separated or divided as needed to expose the rib. Reflect the periosteum from a 4-cm segment of the rib using the technique illustrated in Figures 4.5 and 4.6; then resect this segment and make an incision with a scalpel into the empyema pocket through the thickened bed of the resected rib. With a finger or suction cannula, gently explore the interior of the pocket and break down any loculations encountered.

Occasionally, after the cavity has been entered, it will be discovered that the chosen rib is not the lowest. In such situations, a segment of the next lower rib should also be removed to permit good dependent drainage. A piece of the thickened parietal pleura should always be taken for a biopsy. If no bronchopleural fistula is present, irrigate the pocket thoroughly to remove all debris and purulent fluid, and record the volume of fluid required to fill the cavity. This volume can then be measured at weekly intervals and the change used as an estimate of healing.

A tube with an internal diameter of 1.5–2.0 cm should be placed into the pocket and securely sutured to the skin. The tube should be just long enough to extend about 3 cm into the cavity and to protrude about 3 cm beyond the skin. Cut some extra holes around its circumference within the chest so that no area of the cavity will be undrained; to pervent a subcutaneous collection of purulent fluid, do not close the skin tightly around the tube. The tube is not connected to water-seal suction, but is left open to drain freely. Cover the tube with a bulky dressing and obtain a chest radiogram to be sure that the lung has not collapsed.

When the volume of the residual pocket is no greater than the volume of the tube, the tube should be removed. A short 22 or 24 French catheter is substituted for a few days, after which the catheter is removed and the pleurocutaneous sinus permitted to heal.

Chronic Empyema

Chronic empyema by definition is an empyema that will not heal with drainage and antibiotics alone. Some of the common causes for this condition are listed in Table 7-1. In addition to the complications listed for acute empyema, chronic

TABLE 7-1 Causes of Chronic Empyema

1. A poorly treated case of acute empyema
2. A persistent bronchopleural fistula
3. A foreign body in the pleural cavity
4. Tuberculosis of the pleura
5. Actinomycosis of the pleura
6. A fungal infection, such as blastomycosis or coccidioidomycosis
7. A proximal carcinoma of the lung

empyema may also be a cause of secondary amyloidosis. The goal in the treatment of chronic empyema is the same as that for acute empyema, i.e., sterilization of the cavity and obliteration of the cavity. The method chosen depends upon the condition of the lung and the debility of the patient.

Decortication of the Lung

Decortication is a procedure to remove a restrictive membrane or peel from the surface of the lung and the chest wall to permit the lung to expand completely and fill a persistent pleural space. The sole indication for the operation is the presence of a persistent intrapleural pocket; it is not indicated for the removal of thickened pleura without a space. No evidence exists that the function or mobility of the chest wall undergoes any significant improvement from this procedure. A criterion for the performance of this operation is that the lung must be able to expand to fill the pleural cavity. In some patients with preexisting pulmonary fibrosis, far-advanced tuberculosis, or other chronic lung disease, such expansion is not possible. These patients can usually be selected out on the basis of their history and radiographic findings. More enigmatic are the patients with long-standing chronic empyema, but otherwise relatively normal appearing lungs in which the fibrotic process has extended from the peel into the lung parenchyma, making the operation technically difficult and the resulting expansion unsatisfactory. Prior to a decortication, the patient should undergo bronchoscopy to rule out bronchial obstruction as a cause for any lack of expansion.

The chest should be entered through a posterior lateral incision centered over the empyema pocket. The empyema pocket is entered and opened widely from anterior to posterior. With a scalpel carefully make an anterior–posterior incision, 2–3 cm long, in the visceral peel, separating the edges as one progresses down toward the lung. Usually a cleavage plane will be encountered at or just under the superficial layer of visceral pleura. This can be recognized by the minute black streaks of anthracosis on the pleura. Grasp the edges of the peel with hemostatic forceps, and using a closed scissors as a blunt dissector, develop the plane in all directions from the incision. Usually the peel is least adherent to the lung over the anterior and mediastinal aspects of the lung, so as the cleavage plane is developed, the incision in the visceral peel should be extended anteriorly to the point at which the peel is reflected off the chest wall onto the lung. The parietal peel will separate from the chest wall in the plane of the endothoracic fascia. This separation should be continued anteriorly, extending the incision in the parietal peel until the incision in the visceral peel is reached. During this dissection of the anterior and mediastinal aspects of the peel, care must be taken to identify and spare the phrenic nerve, which may be incorporated in the peel or adherent to it.

After the peel has been separated from the lung for several centimeters above and below the incision, grasp the hemostat holding the edge of the peel with the left hand and evert the freed area of peel over the third and fourth fingers of that hand. Using a Küttner dissector, continue freeing the lung by wiping the lung away from the peel. It is important in doing this to put the pressure on the peel overlying one's fingers, not on the lung itself, or the lung parenchyma may be torn and large air leaks result. If the dissection enters the lung in one area, quit that area and dissect around it, leaving a small piece of peel to sew over the laceration in the parenchyma. The entire lung including the fissures should be released. This includes removing the fine film of connective tissue that often encompasses the lung so that full expansion can be obtained.

As much of the peel as possible should be removed from the diaphragm and chest wall, but because the peel is often quite adherent to the diaphragm, it may be necessary to leave patches of it attached, for without a clear cleavage plane, it is easy to dissect through the diaphragm. If the surgeon finds the dissection on the lung to be very difficult and to result in numerous air leaks, the procedure should be discontinued and some other operation employed. This situation can arise from a long-standing empyema or from an empyema associated with continuing inflammation in the lung, but it can also be caused by mesothelioma.

In addition to the usual cultures and pathology examination, the peel should be cultured for mycobacteria and for fungi. The use of three intercostal catheters as well as early bronchoscopy for retained secretions is advisable after this operation, because obstruction of the catheters or atelectasis of a lobe may easily jeopardize the final result.

Other Operative Procedures For Chronic Empyema

If it is important to preserve the lung associated with a chronic empyema, but if the lung is diseased to the extent that it cannot fill the thoracic cavity, or if an adequate decortication is technically impossible, the empyema cavity can be obliterated by a partial thoracoplasty or by a combination of a decortication and a thoracoplasty. In the past this situation indicated a Schede thoracoplasty, but this operation, in which the overlying bony thorax, ribs, periosteum, intercostal muscles, and parietal pleura were resected as a whole, is mutilating and results in a large ventral hernia from denervation of the abdominal wall. A less extensive thoracoplasty, described in Ch. 6, in which the intercostal bundles are preserved, is now used.

If the underlying lung is totally destroyed and requires excision, an extrapleural pneumonectomy, described in Ch. 4, is indicated. In this procedure the intact empyema cavity with the peel and the underlying lung are all removed as a whole. Because this procedure is commonly performed in patients with disease of long duration, extensive calcification of both the parietal and the visceral peel may be present. This calcification commonly extends into the chest wall as well as into the lung and may necessitate resecting a portion of the chest wall to remove the empyema cavity intact.

Many patients with a chronic empyema are severely debilitated from an underlying disease and would be at considerable risk from any of the previous operative procedures. However, to leave the empyema untreated would condemn the patient to the probability of developing amyloidosis or any of the other complications associated with continuing sepsis. A useful alternative procedure for such patients is the creation of a permanent pleurocutaneous fistula into the empyema cavity by the use of an Eloesser flap (6). After emptying the cavity, a well-designed permanent fistula will drain only small amounts and require only a simple dressing, even in the presence of a bronchopleural fistula. But such a fistula will keep the cavity clean and prevent the complications of continuing sepsis.

The placement and construction of such a fistula is similar to that described for creation of a thoracostomy for open drainage of an acute empyema. Measure the distance from the skin to the inside of the empyema cavity with a syringe and needle, and raise a full-thickness rectangular-shaped skin flap that is 2.5 cm longer than the distance measured by the needle. In most patients the skin flap should be about 6–7 cm long and 4–5 cm wide. It is centered over the rib to be resected and based either medial or lateral to the proposed site of rib resection. Using the technique described for a rib resection (see p. 208), remove a 5–6 cm length of rib. The transected end of the rib under the base of the skin flap should be cut back 1–2 cm from the base so the rib does not impinge on the flap. Incise through the thick parietal peel into the empyema cavity over the length of the resected rib bed and enlarge the height of the opening to equal the width of the skin flap by resecting an area of the peel. Using interrupted absorbable 2–0 sutures, tack the free end of the skin flap to the inside of the parietal peel, thus creating a tract partially lined by epithelium. This fistula will need dilatation for several months following surgery until it becomes completely covered with epithelium.

Chronic Pleural Effusions

The etiology of a chronic pleural effusion in most patients can be determined from the clinical evaluation and from a study of the pleural fluid and tissue. Some of the causes are listed in Table 7.2. The last three entities in the table are discussed elsewhere in this chapter or in Ch. 3 in the sections on tuberculosis and fungal disease. When the etiology of the pleural effusion is obscure, a thoracotomy and an open pleural biopsy are not uncommon.

Many of the patients who require a thoracotomy for diagnosis will be found to have a trapped lung, a lung in which one or more lobes is encased in a thin organized peel that prevents the lung from completely expanding. This trapping results in a persistent pleural space that will fill with fluid because of the negative pressure relative to the microvasculature that develops if a pulmonary air leak is not present. Once the peel is removed by a decortication (described on page 209), the lobe can reexpand to fill the pleural cavity and prevent a recurrence of the effusion.

Histologically the peel is usually interpreted as showing only chronic inflammation. It may be caused by an organizing fibrin clot secondary to a pneumothorax or to some previous trauma; more commonly, the etiology may never be determined. Ryan and colleagues (15) reviewed the course of patients from the Mayo Clinic who underwent a thoracotomy for a pleural effusion whose etiology was obscure and in whom no underlying disease was discovered at surgery. In 60.8% there was no recurrence of the effusion and

TABLE 7-2 Causes of Chronic Pleural Effusion.

1. Pleural metastasis from a neoplastic tumor
2. A trapped lung
3. Cardiac abnormalities
4. A pancreatic pseudocyst that has burrowed through the diaphragm
5. Ascites that enters the chest through diaphragmatic pores
6. Connective tissue disease
7. Yellow-nail syndrome
8. Meigs syndrome
9. An infectious process
10. Chylothorax
11. Mesothelioma

no cause became apparent. In 35.3% the cause did become apparent in time: 25% had a malignancy and the other 10% had a collagen–vascular disease or the yellow-nail syndrome.

A pleural effusion in association with advanced cancer can cause significant respiratory distress in patients who may already have compromised pulmonary function. Any patient who has an exploratory thoracotomy for a carcinoma of the lung and is found to be unresectable should have a pleural abrasion performed at the time of the thoracotomy to obliterate the pleural cavity and prevent the development of a pleural effusion later in the course of the disease.

Of patients who do develop an effusion secondary to pleural metastasis, 35%–45% can be helped by obliterating the pleural cavity with some sclerosing solution such as nitrogen mustard or tetracycline. For this procedure to be successful, the lung must be capable of fully expanding to fill the pleural cavity. After the chemical has produced an inflammation, the parietal and visceral pleura must abut and adhere together; if they do not, the procedure is without benefit.

Insert a 20–24 French catheter into the pleural cavity and remove all of the pleural fluid. If the fluid cannot be removed and the lung completely reexpanded in 8 hours, remove the catheter and discontinue the procedure. In such cases, either because of parenchymal disease or a pleural peel, the lung will be unable to expand enough to fill the pleural cavity. Permitting the catheter to remain longer in the vain hope of further expansion only increases the risk of an empyema, a catastrophic occurrence in these patients. If all the fluid can be removed, dissolve either nitrogen mustard (0.4 mg/kg body) or tetracycline (500–1000 mg) in 30–50 ml saline and inject it into the pleural cavity through the intercostal catheter. Clamp the catheter for 6–8 hours and turn the patient frequently during this period. Return the catheter to suction and maintain continuous aspiration for an additional 3–4 days to permit the lung's adherence to the parietal pleura.

Chylothorax

The two predominant causes for an accumulation of chyle in the pleural cavity are traumatic injury to the thoracic duct and obstruction of the mediastinal lymph nodes and lymphatic channels by a neoplastic disease. Iatrogenic injury during esophagectomies, resection of thoracic aortic aneurysms, or cardiovascular operations on infants or young children are the most common forms of trauma. The most common neoplastic disease associated with a chylothorax is a lymphoma. A chylothorax following surgery will usually become apparent from the third to the tenth postoperative day. It may present as an enlarging mediastinal mass that later ruptures into the pleural cavity, or it may be manifest by a continuing high volume of fluid draining from the chest catheters.

The diagnosis of a chylothorax is often made by the discovery of a milky-appearing fluid in the pleural cavity after an intake of cream, but not all milky-appearing fluid removed from the pleural cavity originates from the thoracic duct. For example, a perforation of the esophagus into the pleural cavity may also result in a milky-appearing pleural effusion. On the other hand, not all chylous effusions appear milky. Staats et al. (18) found that the gross description of pleural fluid was consistent with chyle in fewer than 50% of patients with a chylous effusion. In doubtful cases, two methods may be used to confirm the diagnosis: a lymphangiogram or an analysis of the fluid for triglyceride concentration. Staats concluded that triglyceride concentrations greater than 110 mg/dl were highly suggestive of a chylous effusion and values below 50 mg/dl were rarely chylous. Equivical cases between these two values require a lipoprotein analysis, as recommended by Seriff et al. (16).

Most chylous fistulas caused by neoplastic diseases, especially those associated with a lymphoma, will close with antineoplastic chemotherapy or with radiation therapy to the mediastinum. In such patients, a prolonged period of nonoperative management is indicated. This management must include adequate drainage and good nutrition, plus parenteral therapy as needed to prevent a metabolic deterioration or the development of abnormalitics in fluid and electrolyte concentration. A diet low in fat has been recommended by some authors; although this will change the character of the pleural fluid, its value in increasing the rate of fistula closing has not been demonstrated. Many fistulas secondary to trauma will also close with nonoperative management. However, the volume of lymph flow from such a fistula, while usually 1–2 liters/day, can exceed 8 liters/day in some patients, and immunologic depletion can occur rapidly.

Patients with a high-flow fistula or patients that continue to drain after 2–3 weeks of nonoperative management should undergo a transthoracic ligation of the thoracic duct. The duct originates from the cisterna chyli and is commonly a single trunk from the level of the inferior pulmonary vein to the diaphragm. In the lower part of the thorax, it lies to the right of the midline between the aorta and the azygos vein and is immediately dorsal to the esophagus. At about the level of the carina, it crosses to the left and ascends behind the aortic arch and adjacent to the left subclavian artery. Usually the location of the injury can be suspected from the nature of the previous operative procedure. The actual site of the laceration can sometimes be identified more easily during thoracotomy if the patient is given 150–200 ml of cream to drink 2 hours before call to the operating room. If the site is identified, the duct should be closed with two or more nonabsorbable suture ligatures placed both above and below the laceration. If the site of injury cannot be discovered, the duct should be ligated below the level of the inferior pulmonary vein by reflecting the esophagus anteriorly and identifying the duct, which may be 6–12 mm in diameter, between the aorta and the azygos vein. Do not dissect the duct out, but determine its lateral boundaries and ligate it in place with two or three suture ligatures. These patients should be followed for a protracted period, because occasionally these chylous fistulae will recur several months after surgery.

Oleothorax

The intrapleural instillation of mineral oil to induce pulmonary collapse for the treatment of tuberculosis was popular during the 1930s and early 1940s. Unless removed, this material remains in the pleural cavity, and even after 40 years it poses a constant threat to the patient. In patients in whom the pocket of mineral oil forms a fistula to a bronchus, over 50% will die, either from a widespread lipoid pneumonia or from a bacterial pneumonia and an empyema within the rigid intrapleural cavity.

The development of a bronchopleural fistula is signalled by the onset of a cough productive of a yellow, oily sputum that is often associated with a daily fever. By the time such an event is brought to the attention of a physician, widespread permanent destruction of the lung parenchyma may have already occurred. A chest radiograph at this time will usually show either an air–fluid level or an oil–water interface within the cavity. However, radiographic changes are not necessary to make the diagnosis. Any patient who has an oleothorax and begins to cough up oil must be assumed to have a fistula and must have the pleural pocket emptied of oil immediately to prevent the progression of the lipoid pneumonia. The quickest way to do this is by the insertion of a 24 French intercostal catheter into the pocket and the application of suction.

Once a bronchopleural fistula develops, an infection is inevitable and the pleural pocket must be obliterated by an apical thoracoplasty (described in Ch. 6). It may also be necessary to divide the insertion of the pectoralis major and move the muscle in to fill the space and close the bronchial opening. Prior to doing this, the pocket must be drained of all oil and any infection must be eliminated.

A mortality rate in excess of 50% after the development of a bronchopleural fistula warrants a surgical intervention in these patients prior to the development of such a fistula. It is my opinion that any patient with a continuing oleothorax, even though it has been present and asymptomatic for many years, should be advised to have the oil removed. This can be done by inserting a 24 French intercostal catheter into the pleural pocket and positioning the patient so that the region of the pocket containing the catheter is uppermost. Alternately aspirate the oil and inject a saline solution containing 0.5%–0.25% neomycin until no further oil can be aspirated and no oil–water interface can be seen on a chest radiograph. The pocket is left filled with the neomycin solution; the catheter is removed, and the entry site is closed.

Pleural Tumors

Mesotheliomas

Pleural mesotheliomas are relatively rare tumors that are thought to have a mesothelial origin, in contrast to malignant tumors that arise in the lung or at some other distant site and subsequently metastasize to the pleura. These primary pleural tumors occur in two forms: localized and diffuse. The latter are associated with exposure to asbestos; the former are not.

Localized Mesothelioma

In addition to pleural mesothelioma, localized tumors of the pleura have also been called pleural fibroma, benign fibrous mesothelioma, or if malignant, fibrosarcoma. Localized pleural mesothelioma may be either benign or malignant. Of the patients with a localized primary pleural tumor described by Okike and colleagues (11), 87% were benign, but 13% were malignant. This is similar to the statement by Briselli et al. (2) that 12% of these localized fibrous pleural tumors were responsible for the patient's death and to Dalton et al. (5) that 20% behaved in a malignant fashion.

These tumors are usually firm and encapsulated. They vary in size from 1-cm nodules to tumors that occupy an entire hemithorax. They may arise from either the parietal or visceral pleura, but are more common on the visceral pleura. Sites of origin from the pericardium, the diaphragm, and the interlobar fissures have been described. Localized mesotheliomas may be pedunculated or sessile, or they may be partially or totally within the substance of the lung. Rarely, both the benign and malignant tumors may be associated with a pleural effusion.

From 25%–50% of the patients with these localized pleural tumors are asymptomatic, but if symptoms are present, the most common are nonpleuritic chest pain, cough, dyspnea, and fever. Okike reported that benign tumors larger than 7 cm in diameter were invariably associated with the symptoms and findings of pulmonary osteoarthropathy. These symptoms usually regressed after removal of the tumor. Both the benign and malignant localized tumors are diagnosed by thoracotomy and pathologic examination. The indication for a thoracotomy is the finding of a nodule or a mass on the chest radiogram. Bronchoscopy is useful only to rule out the presence of an intrabronchial tumor when a large mass or pleural effusion is present. The cytologic examination of the pleural fluid has not been helpful, but a thoracentesis should be done in a febrile patient with an effusion in order to obviate the diagnosis of an empyema.

Because there is a significant possiblity of thesc tumors' being malignant and of their recurrence even when histologically benign, their resection should also include an adequate tumor-free margin. If the tumor is on a pedicle, the pedicle should not be transected, but the entire tumor with a small area of the underlying lung should be resected using the GIA stapler (discussed in Ch. 4). If the tumor is partially or totally intrapulmonary, it may require a lobectomy for adequate removal. Tumors on the parietal pleura should be removed with an area of surrounding pleura. If invasion through the parietal pleura is suspected, an area of the chest wall should be included in the resection. Sessile tumors arising from the diaphragm will require removal of an area of the diaphragm and its reconstruction (described in Ch. 6).

Diffuse Mesothelioma

Diffuse mesotheliomas are malignant pleural tumors with a dismal prognosis. Although uncommon, they occur more frequently than do localized mesotheliomas. The disease is characterized by a pleural cavity lined with sheets of tumor cells and filled with a gelatinous, hemorrhagic fluid. The initial symptom is typically an aching, nonpleuritic chest pain. This pain, often in association with increasing dyspnea, continues unabated for the duration of the disease. As the disease progresses, it will spread to the opposite pleural cavity, and hematogenous metastasis will occur in half of the patients. Survival has averaged about one year after diagnosis.

The chest radiograph usually shows a unilateral pleural effusion, often associated with a thickened pleura. Thoracentesis commonly yields a bloody fluid. The histologic diagnosis of diffuse mesothelioma is often difficult. In the past some cases of mesothelioma have not been recognized, while other patients diagnosed as having mesothelioma with a long survival after therapy have not had the disease. The reason for this problem is twofold: first, metastatic adenocarcinoma may closely mimic the appearance of mesothelioma, and secondly, the well-differentiated nature of the cells in certain cases make them difficult to distinguish from reactive hyperplasia. Because of this difficulty, pleural fluid cytology and needle biopsy of the pleura are not helpful in establishing the diagnosis. A thoracotomy with removal of an adequate sample of tissue is usually required.

Although resectional surgery is not indicated for a diffuse mesothelioma, the disease may be encountered by a thoracic surgeon either during a thoracotomy for biopsy or for a decortication of a presumed trapped lung from another cause. The presence of a mesothelioma can be suspected from the lobulated nature of the peel and by the inability to find a plane of dissection between the peel and the lung. A large amount of the peel should be removed for pathologic examination, but a deep biopsy of the lung that results in an air leak should not be done. Such air leaks are very difficult to stop because the lung is stiff and immobilized. Sutures tear through the lung parenchyma rather than compress it. There is no evidence that radiotherapy or current chemotherapy significantly prolong the life of patients with this disease.

Pleural Plaques

Pleural plaques are smooth, white or light yellow, raised areas of firm hyaline and fibrous tissue that occur on the parietal pleura most commonly over the vertebral column, over the lower chest wall, and on the diaphragm. The plaques have sharp borders and do not adhere to the lung. They may be less than 1 cm in diameter or extensive enough to cover the entire parietal pleura. Pleural plaques occur relatively commonly. Robinson (14) found plaques over 5 cm wide in 2.7% of male autopsies. If thick enough, they may be seen on a chest radiograph, but Hillerdal and Lindgren (9) reported that only 12.5% of all pleural plaques found at autopsy were visible by x-ray. Some investigators (9) have related their presence to asbestos exposure, but others (14) have failed to find such a correlation.

They are of no known clinical significance. The only importance lies in their being confused either with metastasis from a carcinoma or with mesothelioma. The distinction from appearance alone, however, is usually not difficult. Pleural plaques are typically smooth and of uniform thickness, while pleural metastasis have a rough or granular appearance. Mesothelioma, if localized, is usually thicker, lobulated, and irregular.

References

1. Bartlett JC, Gorbach SL, Thadepalli H, Finegold SM: Bacteriology of empyema. Lancet 1:338–340, 1974.
2. Briselli M, Mark EJ, Dickersin R: Solitary fibrous tumors of the pleura. Cancer 47:2678–2689, 1981.
3. Carlson HA: Acute empyema thoracis. J Thorac Surg 5:393–433, 1936.
4. Carr DT, Silver AW, Ellis FH Jr: Management of spontaneous pneumothorax: With special reference to prognosis after various kinds of therapy. Proc Mayo Clin 38:103–109, 1963.
5. Dalton WT, Zolliker AS, McCaughey WTE, Jacques J, Kannerstein M: Localized primary tumors of the pleura. Cancer 44:1465–1475, 1979.
6. Eloesser L: An operation for tuberculous empyema. Surg Gynecol Obstet. 60:1096–1097, 1935.
7. Finland M, Barnes MW: Changing ecology of acute bacterial empyema: Occurrence and mortality at Boston City Hospital during twelve selected years from 1935 to 1972. J Infect Dis 137:274–291, 1978.
8. FitzGerald MX, Keelan PJ, Cugell DW, Gaensler EA: Long-term results of surgery for bullous emphysema. J Thorac Cardiovasc Surg. 68:566–587, 1974.
9. Hillerdal G, Lindgren A: Pleural plaques: Correlation of autopsy findings to radiographic findings and occupational history. Eur J Respir Dis 61:315–319, 1980.
10. Larrieu AJ, Tyers FO, Williams EH, O'Neil MJ, Derrick JR: Intrapleural instillation of quinacrine for treatment of recurrent spontaneous pneumothorax. Ann Thorac Surg 28:146–150, 1979.
11. Okike N, Bernatz PE, Woolner LB: Localized mesothelioma of the pleura. J Thorac Cardiovasc Surg 75:363–370, 1978.
12. Ransdell HT Jr, McPherson RC: Management of spontaneous pneumothorax. Arch Surg 87:1023–1028, 1963.
13. Reid L: The Pathology of Emphysema. Chicago, Year Book, 1967.
14. Robinson JJ: Pleural plaques and splenic capsular sclerosis in adult male autopsies. Arch Path 93:118–122, 1972.
15. Ryan CJ, Rodgers RF, Unni KK, Hepper NGG: The outcome of patients with pleural effusion of indeterminate cause at thoracotomy. Mayo Clin Proc 56:145–149, 1981.
16. Seriff NS, Cohen ML, Samuel P, Schulster PL: Chylothorax: Diagnosis by lipoprotein electrophoresis of serum and pleural fluid. Thorax 32:98–100, 1977.

17. Sherman MM, Subramanian V, Berger RL: Management of thoracic empyema. Amer J Surg 133:474–479, 1977.
18. Staats BA, Ellefson RD, Budahn LL, Dines DE, Prakash VBS, Offord K: The lipoprotein profile of chylous and nonchylous pleural effusions. Mayo Clin Proc 55:700–704, 1980.

Disorders of the Mediastinum

8

The mediastinum is a complex region of the thorax between the two pleural cavities. It extends from the thoracic inlet to the diaphragm and from the posterior surface of the sternum to the articulations of the ribs with the vertebral bodies. Because many of the primary disorders of the mediastinum tend to occur in distinctive regions, it is convenient to divide the mediastinum into the three divisions illustrated on the lateral chest radiogram (Fig. 8-1). The anterior–superior mediastinum is that region anterior to the esophagus, anterior and superior to the pericardium, and posterior to the sternum; it contains the thymus, the trachea, and the great vessels above the base of the heart. The posterior mediastinum is that region posterior to the pericardium; it contains the esophagus, the sympathetic ganglia, and segments of the intercostal nerves and blood vessels. The middle mediastinum contains the heart, the hilus of each lung, the carina, and numerous lymph nodes.

The common etiologies of the masses that occur in each of the three mediastinal regions are listed in Table 8-1. Conditions not listed, such as a parathyroid adenoma, may also involve surgery on the mediastinum. However, a lesion such as a parathyroid adenoma does not present as a mediastinal mass, nor is a mediastinal exploration the primary treatment. Other disorders that have not been included in this discussion are primary disease of the esophagus or airways, and disease which has spread to the mediastinum from some other anatomic site.

Many mediastinal abnormalities are discovered on a routine chest radiogram in asymptomatic patients, so reasons other than symptomatology must be used to decide on the need for surgery. The diagnostic procedures used to evaluate these abnormalities should contribute directly to such a decision and should permit the surgeon to decide on the best operative approach. The condition that is most important to exclude in many cases, since it changes the operative approach, is an aneurysm or congenital abnormality of the great vessels at the base of the heart. Computerized tomography has been of great help in differentiating between a vascular and a nonvascular lesion, but if any question remains, thoracic aortography should be performed. At the present, computerized tomography is the most useful modality for evaluating the

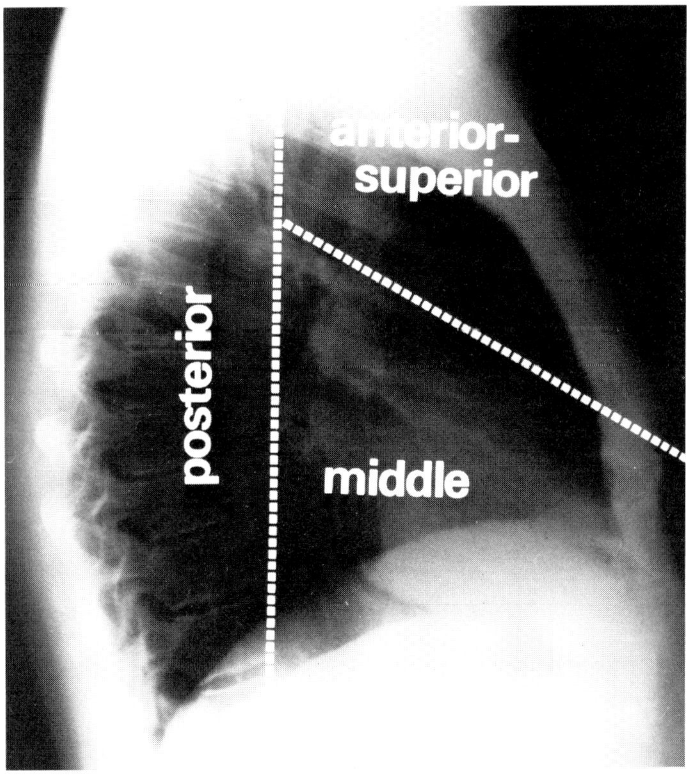

FIG. 8-1.

mediastinum. In addition to determining if a lesion is vascular or nonvascular, it may be used to decide whether a mass is in the lung or in the mediastinum, to determine if a mass is composed of fat, and to discover small tumors within the thymus. Radioisotope scans can be used to detect thyroid tissue. Sonography has been helpful in diagnosing cysts. No place remains now for a therapeutic trial of radiotherapy in evaluating any mediastinal lesion.

TABLE 8-1 Common Etiology of Masses in the Mediastinum

	Anterior–superior mediastinum	Middle mediastinum	Posterior mediastinum
Primary mediastinal tumors and cysts	Thymoma Germ cell tumors Malignant lymphoma Thyroid lesions Mesenchymal tumors Thymic cyst Cystic hygromas Carcinoid	Malignant lymphoma Pericardial cyst Bronchogenic cyst Mesenchymal tumors	Neurogenic tumors Esophageal, gastric, and enteric cysts
Other conditions	Aneurysm Granulomatous disease of lymph nodes	Granulomatous disease of lymph nodes	Diaphragmatic hernia Aneurysm Paravertebral abscess

Myasthenia Gravis

Myasthenia gravis is a disease characterized by weakness and easy fatigability of voluntary muscles. It especially affects younger women and older men. The muscular weakness occurs from the failure of neuromuscular transmission, probably due to a decrease in the number of acetycholine receptors. Recent investigations have suggested an autoimmune basis for the disease and have significantly altered the diagnostic procedures used. The reader is referred to a review on this subject by Drachman (5).

The thymus has long been implicated in the etiology of myasthenia gravis, but although the thymic abnormalities are usually the most apparent, the disease may sometimes be part of a generalized glandular failure or other systemic illness. Of patients with myasthenia gravis, 5% will have some thyroid disorder, commonly Grave's disease or Hashimoto's thyroiditis. The disease may also occur in association with other autoimmune diseases, such as rheumatoid arthritis, lupus erythematosis, and polymyositis.

Thymic abnormalities are found in 75%–90% of patients with myasthenia gravis, but the nature of this association is unknown. From 8%–10% of patients with the disease will have a thymoma, and of patients that have a thymoma, 20%–30% will have myasthenia gravis. Thymic follicular hyperplasia, which is not true hyperplasia, but a condition characterized by the presence of germinal centers in the thymus, is seen in 65%–70% of patients with myasthenia gravis; follicular hyperplasia, however, is also commonly seen in patients with hyperthyroidism, Addison's disease, lupus erythematosis, and other autoimmune disease.

Along with the better understanding of the disease mechanism in the last decade, an improvement in the treatment has also occurred. Anticholinesterase drugs still remain the choice for initial therapy: pyridostigmine bromide is the most commonly used of the oral anticholinesterases. These agents are not without risk, because excessive amounts can increase weakness and prolonged use may decrease the available acetylcholine receptors. The recognition of myasthenia gravis as an autoimmune disease has led to the use of corticosteroids for its treatment when the weakness is not well controlled by anticholinesterase drugs or thymectomy. Steroid therapy is reported to give good to excellent results in 50%–100% of patients (5), and it has been especially useful in the treatment of older men. It must, however, be continued indefinitely, and such a long-term regimen has a significant incidence of serious side effects. In addition, there is often a worsening of the patient's symptoms for a short time after the onset of steroid therapy, so such treatment cannot be undertaken in the absence of experienced personnel.

Despite conflicting reports on the value of thymectomy, since its introduction by Blalock, it has been used sporadically for the treatment of myasthenia gravis. Recurrently, statements have been made that many patients will obtain sustained remissions after a thymectomy, but these reports have been difficult to evaluate because of the great variability in the natural history of myasthenia gravis and because of the finding that spontaneous remissions also occur. No randomized, controlled study on the role of thymectomy has ever been done, but recent studies have confirmed that 57%–86% of patients undergoing a thymectomy will show improvement. In a retrospective study from the Mayo Clinic (3), 80 patients over 17 years of age without a thymoma who had undergone a thymectomy for myasthenia gravis were matched with 80 medically treated patients. The postoperative mortality was 6%, but at an average follow-up of almost 20 years, 21 of the 80 surgical patients were dead compared to 47 of the 80 in the medically treated group. A complete remission occurred in 27 of the patients treated by a thymectomy, compared to 6 of those treated medically. The improvement in survival was independent of age or duration of symptoms, but because of the more unfavorable survival of women in the medically treated group, the study indicated that thymectomy resulted in a greater improvement for women than for men.

Although most authors report a complete remission rate of about 30% after thymectomy in patients without a thymoma, the results in patients with a thymoma are not as favorable. Wechsler and Olanow (11) quotes a remission rate of 10% in patients with a benign thymoma, and less if the tumor is invasive.

No consensus exists regarding the indications for a thymectomy in myasthenia gravis, although general agreement is found that a thymoma should be removed. Because all thymomas are not visible on a chest radiogram, every patient with myasthenia gravis should have computerized tomography of the mediastinum to detect small tumors. Many surgeons believe a thymectomy should be offered to most patients with generalized symptoms early in the course of the disease. A thymectomy is not recommended for patients with only ocular symptoms, unless a thymoma is found. Wechsler and Olanow (11) and Buckingham et al. (3) do not use the age of the patient as a reason for refusing surgery, but Drachman (5) recommends a thymectomy only for those patients whose age is less than 50. In general, as the reports of significant improvement from thymectomy have increased in frequency, the indications for the operation have also expanded significantly.

In large part the preoperative preparation of patients with myasthenia gravis will determine the difficulty they will have in the postoperative period. Because respiratory problems constitute the greatest threat, every effort should be made to restore the pulmonary function to optimal condition. In addition to the regimen described in Chapter 2, all drugs that interfere with neuromuscular transmission, such as the aminoglycoside antibiotics and certain of the antiarrhythmic drugs, should be discontinued. The patients should be on the lowest dose of pyridostigmine and prednisone that will maintain a stable neurologic status.

Bolooki and Schwartzman (2) have recommended high-dose corticosteroid therapy in the perioperative period for all patients. They begin an intravenous infusion of methylprednisone as soon as the patient arrives in the operating room, and give 200 mg prednisone during the hour prior to induction, plus 200 mg/hour for the first 2 hours after induction. The infusion is then continued at the rate of 20 mg/hour for a total amount of 1 g in the 24-hour period.

Wechsler and Olanow (11), on the other hand, use plasmapheresis to obtain the best clinical condition prior to surgery; they report that in most cases this permits the surgery to be performed without the administration of antimyasthenic medications. Anesthesia for the thymectomy should *not* include any muscle-relaxing agents.

Postoperatively, most patients experience increased weakness for 1–2 weeks, followed by a gradual improvement. During this early period the patients must be monitored closely because respiratory failure can occur after several days of adequate ventilation. Clark et al. (4) reported that 13 of his 20 patients less than 35 years of age required ventilator support for an average of 5 days in the postoperative period. Bolooki, however, encountered no episodes of postoperative respiratory failure in his patients treated with high-dose corticosteroids.

A thymectomy is only one facet of the treatment of patients with myasthenia gravis. The patient should be followed postoperatively by a clinical group interested in the disease. Corticosteriod therapy is an important part in the treatment of patients who do not develop a complete remission, but because the maximum improvement may take 1–10 years after thymectomy, constant adjustment of the corticosteroid dose may be necessary.

Thymectomy

The thymus is a bilobed, roughly H-shaped organ that is located primarily in the anterior–superior mediastinum, but extends slightly into the base of the neck. It is in the same fascial compartment as the thyroid, and each lobe of the thymus is connected to the corresponding lobe of the thyroid by a delicate fascia termed the thyrothymic ligament. Anteriorly the thymus is covered to a greater or lesser extent by reflections of both pleural cavities. Laterally the thymus is often quite adherent to the pleura along the course of the phrenic nerve, so during a thymectomy the nerve is quite susceptible to laceration or injury from cautery. Posteriorly, the thymus overlies the pericardium, the trachea, and the great vessels above the base of the heart. It may extend over the arch of the aorta to lie on the left pulmonary artery. The upper portion of the gland lies on the left innominate vein, and an enlarged gland may sometimes surround the vein or extend across the superior vena cava. The arterial supply of the thymus is from numerous fine branches of the pericardiophrenic artery or the internal mammary artery. The upper portion of the gland may also be supplied by small branches from the inferior thyroid artery. The venous drainage is principally through a short vein of significant size that runs from the posterior surface of the gland directly into the left innominate vein. In two-thirds of patients, this vein is single, but in one-third, two veins exist. In a small percentage of patients, the venous drainage will be to a thyroid ima vein. Small veins also accompany the arteries from the lateral edges of the gland.

The technique used for thymectomy will vary depending on the surgeon's view of the necessity for removing all thymic tissue. Papatestas and colleagues (8) have advocated a transcervical approach, arguing that it results in a smoother postoperative course than does a transthoracic operation and that it produces an equally high percentage of remissions. At the other extreme, Jaretzki et al. (7) advocate the routine use of a complete median sternotomy plus an additional transverse cervical incision. They remove all thymic tissue and mediastinal fat above the diaphragm, extending the dissection posterior to each phrenic nerve in the thorax and above the thyroid in the neck. While no evidence exists that a total thymectomy is necessary for the treatment of myasthenia gravis, current understanding of the disease would suggest that it is desirable. Ectopic thymic tissue is reported in 20%–50% of patients; while some is found in the neck, it also occurs in small foci within mediastinal fat and along the pericardium or the mediastinal pleura over the hilus of the lung, areas that cannot be explored through a cervical incision. On the other hand, the potential morbidity of the extensive operation advocated by Jaretzki should be accepted only if convincing evidence of significantly superior results is presented. At the present, the following procedure seems to be an acceptable compromise.

A partial median sternotomy in which the sternum is divided from the manubrium to the third intercostal space, then angled off to the left (as described in Ch. 4) is used. This incision provides excellent exposure of the anterior–superior mediastinum from the root of the neck to just below the hilus of the lung, yet is limited enough in scope that it does not interfere significantly with ventilation. If the operation is done to remove a large or an invasive thymoma, the sternotomy may be extended into both the left

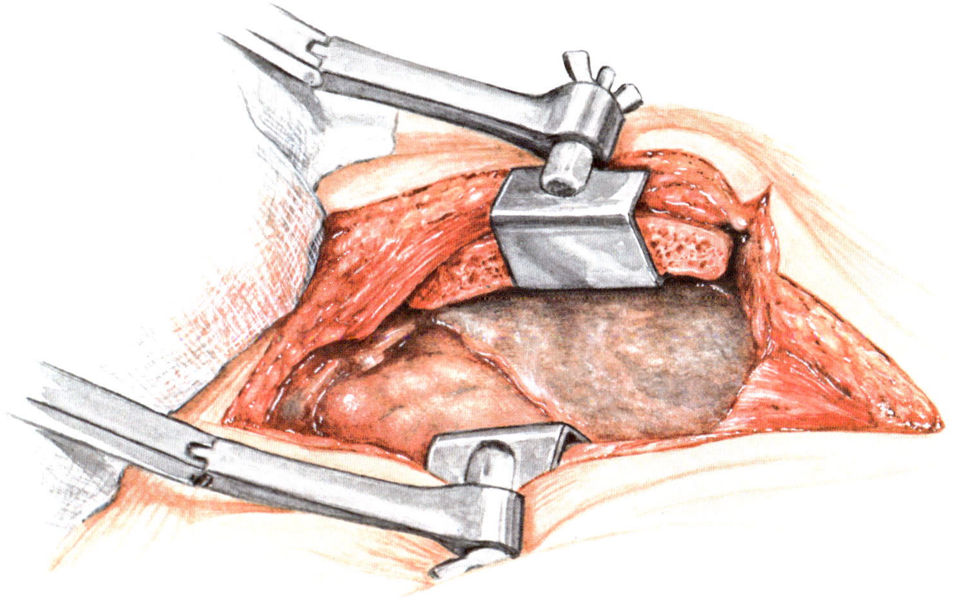

FIG. 8-2.

and right third interspaces. Usually the pleural cavity does not need to be entered, although the internal mammary vessels on the left should be divided. As the Himmelstein sternal spreader is gradually opened, the small vessels from the internal mammary artery can be controlled with hemostatic clips.

In the process of doing a thymectomy for myasthenia gravis, it is important that not only the obvious thymic tissue be removed, but also that the pericardial fat in the anterior–superior mediastinum be taken out to remove small regions of aberrant thymic tissue that are not detected by the surgeon. The reflection of the parietal pleura from each side should be identified; in Figure 8-2, notice the reflection of the left pleural cavity over the anterior surface of the thymus.

Using a Küttner dissector, bluntly sweep the pleura laterally from the thymus and the mediastinal fat as far as the phrenic nerve and pericardiophrenic vessels on the left and to the superior vena cava on the right. Beginning inferiorly, dissect the thymus and pericardial fat off the pericardium. The plane of dissection should be developed across the mediastinum from one pleuropericardial junction to the other. Usually, the thymus will be adherent to the mediastinal pleura at the pericardiophrenic vessels, where the small thymic arteries enter the gland. The lateral limits of the gland should be separated from the pleura and the thymic vessels controlled with clips. Figure 8-3 illustrates the operation after the inferior portion of the gland and the lower portion of the right lobe have been dissected free. Do not use cautery near the phrenic nerve, because a paralyzed diaphragm may mean the difference between a patient with myasthenia gravis developing or not developing respiratory distress.

Identify the innominate vein at the left superior extent of the dissection field and dissect the thymus and fat away until the thymic vein (or veins) is encountered. Because this vein is usually short, the use of hemostatic clips for control is convenient. Occasionally, the thymus extends posterior to the innominate vein rather than anterior, and unless the vein is identified early in the dissection, it is at risk of laceration. Continue the dissection superiorly as far as the inferior surface of the thyroid, which can be reached by retracting the strap muscles slightly. Ligate and divide the small arterial branches from

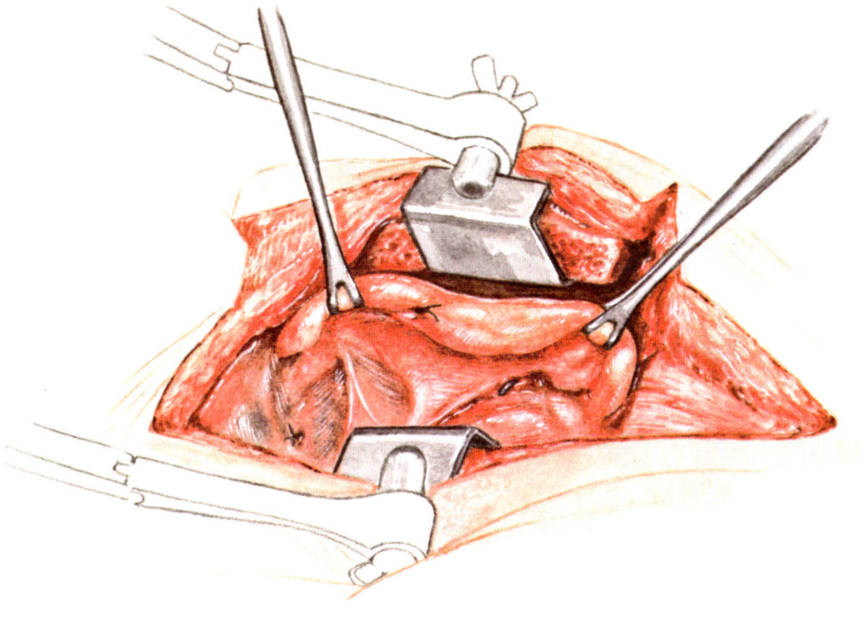

FIG. 8-3.

the inferior thyroid artery to the superior surface of the thymus and divide the fascia that connects the superior pole of each thymic lobe to the thyroid. It is important to visualize this region of dissection because the occurrence of thymic tissue slightly separated from the main lobes of the thymus is frequent. Figure 8-4 depicts the operative field of the superior mediastinum after the thymus and mediastinal fat have been removed.

Insert one 24 French catheter into the superior mediastinum and connect it to suction. Normally this catheter can be removed in 24 hours. If one or the other pleural cavities is entered and a pneumothorax is produced, an intrapleural catheter should also be placed. The criteria for discontinuing mechanical ventilator support and extubating the patient with myasthenia gravis are the same as those discussed in Chapter 9 for any other patient.

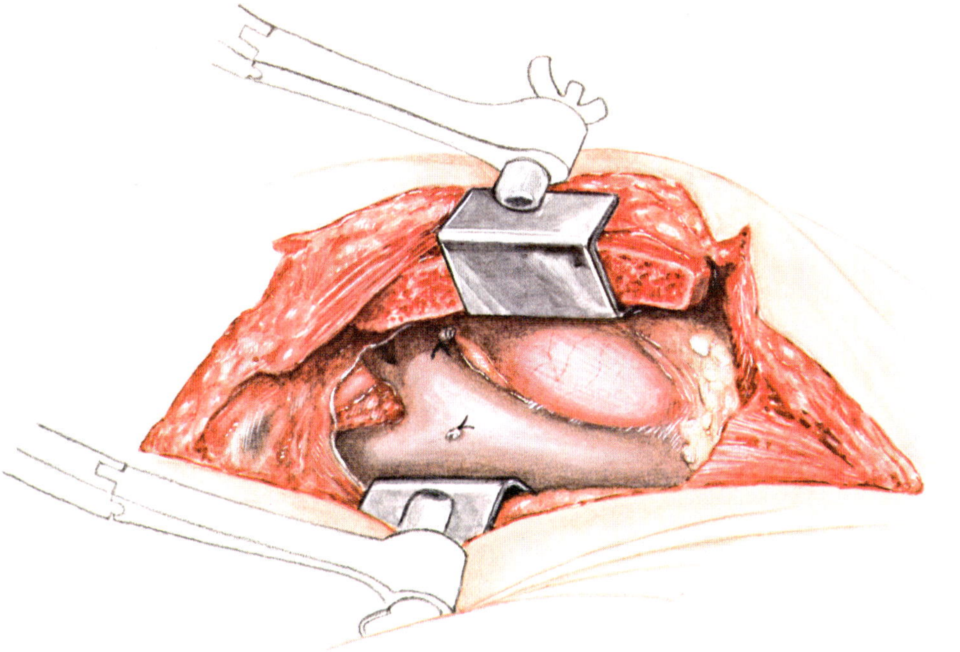

FIG. 8-4.

Thymoma

In adults, thymomas are the most common of the anterior–superior mediastinal tumors. A recent survey (1) reported that exclusive of lymphomas, thymomas made up 52% of the anterior–superior mediastinal tumors. Thymomas are very rare in childhood; when a thymoma has been diagnosed in childhood, it has usually been reclassified as a lymphoblastic lymphoma (9). The peak incidence occurs during the fifth and sixth decades. If patients with myasthenia gravis are excluded, most others with a thymoma are asymptomatic. However, a number of systemic syndromes do exist in association with thymoma; the more common ones are listed in Table 8-2. The results reported for a thymectomy in patients with myasthenia gravis have been discussed earlier in this chapter. Of the other syndromes, a thymectomy has been curative for some patients with erythroid hypoplasia, but it has not been helpful for patients with an immunoglobulin deficiency.

Although thymomas most commonly occur within the thymus in the anterior–superior mediastinum, they can be found any place in the mediastinum from the diaphragm to the neck, either anterior or posterior to the hilus of the lung. They vary in size from small tumors demonstrable only with computerized tomography to tumors that fill one hemithorax. About 10% of both invasive and noninvasive thymomas will show some areas of calcification, but they have no radiographic characteristics to distinguish them from any other mediastinal tumor or cyst.

Histologically, thymomas are characterized by the presence of both lymphocytes and epithelial cells; the tumor, however, is primarily one of thymic epithelial cells; the lymphocytes are probably not neoplastic (9). The histologic classification of thymomas by cellular type is often arbitrary and contributes little to the clinical management. With the exception of a few distinctive histologic types, such as squamous cell carcinoma, the histology cannot be used to differentiate benign from malignant tumors. The best criterion of a given thymoma's propensity for recurrence and spread is its gross appearance at surgery. If infiltration of surrounding structures is found, the tumor will probably behave as if malignant, while if the tumor is encapsulated, it will probably behave as if benign, but because of the difficulty in making a histologic diagnosis, many authors divide the tumors into the categories of invasive or noninvasive rather than malignant or benign. In the reported series, approximately 20% are invasive and 80% are noninvasive. The invasive tumors usually spread by direct extension and by implantation on the pleural surfaces; however, some will metastasize to sites outside of the thorax.

If the tumor is in the midline or is associated with myasthenia gravis, it should be resected through a median sternotomy using the technique described for thymectomy in the section on myasthenia gravis. However, the resection of a large thymoma that is predominantly within one hemithorax

TABLE 8-2 Syndromes Associated with Thymoma

Myasthenia gravis
Erythroid hypoplasia
Immunoglobulin deficiency
Myocarditis
Thyroid disease
Peripheral T-cell lymphocytosis
Collagen–autoimmune disease
Achylasia

is easiest through a standard posterior–lateral thoracotomy. The resection even for a noninvasive thymoma should include a total thymectomy. If a complete resection of an invasive thymoma is possible, it will require additionally the complete resection of all pericardial fat and may require the resection of a portion of the pericardium, the lung, or the left innominate vein. An effort should be made to resect the tumor intact in order to minimize the risk of implantation.

When the innominate vein must be resected, the left side of the superior vena cava and the right innominate vein should first be dissected free of the pericardial fat or tumor and the junction of the left innominate vein freed so a finger can be passed behind it (Fig. 8-4). Occlude the left innominate vein at its junction with the right innominate vein using two right-angled or curved vascular clamps; divide the vein between them. Oversew the stump of the vein on the superior vena cava with two running 5–0 Mersilene sutures. On the left side of the tumor, the vein can be ligated with two 2–0 nonabsorbable ligatures and a 3–0 suture ligature, then divided. Some edema of the left arm and left side of the neck may occur for a short time after the operation, but if the azygos vein is intact, this edema should disappear in one to two weeks.

Other Thymic Tumors and Cysts

Carcinoid tumors of the thymus are a relatively recently described entity (10). They arise in the thymus and have a natural history similar to that of other carcinoid tumors; they are malignant and have the potential to metastasize. Although an associated carcinoid syndrome has not been described, these tumors may be associated with Cushing's syndrome. The resection performed for this tumor should be the same as that for an invasive thymoma.

Thymolipomas are encapsulated benign tumors composed of a mixture of adipose tissue and normal thymic tissue. They usually cause no symptoms.

About 10% of masses that appear in the thymus are simple thymic cysts that have a squamous or columnar lining and some thymic tissue in the wall. These cysts may occur any place within the mediastinum or in the neck. Rosai (9) believes that many of the "nonspecific" cysts of the anterior–superior mediastinum are also of thymic origin. Thymic cysts may be of developmental origin or may arise from cystic dilatation of Hassall's corpuscles, but they must always be differentiated from a thymoma with cystic degeneration.

Germ Cell Tumors

Germ cell tumors are the second most common tumor of the anterior mediastinum. The varieties are similar to those found in the testes, teratoma–teratocarcinoma, seminoma, choriocarcinoma, and embryonal carcinoma. Because of this similarity, a possibility always exists that a mediastinal germ cell tumor is a metastasis, so the workup of these patients should include a careful examination of the testes or ovaries. Although these tumors have no histogenetic relationship to the thymus, they are often clinically difficult to distinguish from a thymoma, because they frequently occur anatomically close to, and even within, the thymus.

Teratomas and Teratocarcinomas

These tumors are the most frequent variety of mediastinal germ cell neoplasm; probably 10%–15% of them are malignant. Their greatest incidence is in the third and fourth decades of life. While mature teratomas affect both sexes equally, teratocarcinomas occur predominantly in men. Mature teratomas are composed of a variety of tissues foreign to the mediastinum, originating from all three germ cell layers. They are commonly cystic or partially cystic, and the cyst cavity frequently contains hair and sebaceous material. Either the cyst wall or the cyst contents may contain calcium. These tumors can grow to large size and become densely adherent to the surrounding structures. If they then become infected, the cyst may perforate into a bronchus, the pleural cavity, or the pericardial sac. If the perforation is into a bronchus, hair and sebaceous material may be expectorated; if into the pericardial sac, cardiac tamponade from the severe inflammatory response may occur. Teratocarcinomas are teratomas in which one histologic component, often squamous cell, has become malignant. They are rapidly growing tumors with areas of hemorrhage and necrosis that often invade the surrounding anatomic structures.

Under the influence of present intensive chemotherapy, some metastasis from teratocarcinoma or embryonal carcinoma of the testicle rather than disappear will evolve into adult teratomas (6). Occasionally, this phenomenon has occurred spontaneously, but the frequency with which it is encountered at present argues that it is related to the chemotherapy. Thoracic surgeons are now being asked to perform a thoracotomy on patients who are receiving chemotherapy for carcinoma of the testicle and who develop radiologic evidence of one or more mediastinal masses; the purpose of the thoracotomy is to determine whether these masses are malignant, therefore requiring further therapy, or are benign, in which case the chemotherapy may be discontinued. These masses, which are often cystic if they are teratomas, vary in size from 1 to 5 cm in diameter. They frequently lie posterior to the hilus of the lung along the anterior surface of the esophagus, and they probably represent lymph nodes that have been replaced completely by tumor tissue. They are usually not densely adherent to surrounding structures and can be dissected free of the lung and the esophagus without entering the cyst.

Seminoma

Mediastinal seminomas appear in young men usually as noncalcified, often lobulated tumors of the anterior mediastinum. They are not encapsulated and may attain large size, but they usually do not require a surgical resection because of their extreme radiosensitivity. The reported 5-year survival at present averages about 75%. The surgeon who performs a biopsy of a large mediastinal seminoma should be aware of the risk of tumor swelling that can occur from instrumentation of these tumors. If the biopsy is done by mediastinoscopy or through a mediastinotomy, this swelling may produce severe respiratory obstruction. Because of this, the surgeon should be prepared to perform an immediate median sternotomy and a subtotal resection of tumor, if necessary, to decompress the upper thorax.

Choriocarcinoma and Embryonal Carcinoma

Choriocarcinoma is a rare tumor of young men associated with gynecomastia and with high levels of chorionic gonadotropin. Embryonal carcinoma may produce elevated levels of α-fetoprotein or carcinoembryonic antigen. Both varieties of tumors should be totally excised if they are localized. If total excision is impossible, the response to intensive chemotherapy is still gratifying.

Malignant Lymphoma

Both Hodgkins and non-Hodgkins lymphoma may occur in the anterior–superior, the middle, or the posterior mediastinum, within the mediastinal and the hilar lymph nodes, or within the thymus. This is the most common neoplasm of the middle mediastinum and may represent either dissemination from other anatomic areas or, rarely, primary mediastinal disease. Hodgkins disease accounts for 55%–60% of the cases. Lymphoblastic lymphoma is a disease of T lymphocytes, commonly occurring in children, that often presents as a large anterior–superior mediastinal mass. It may produce respiratory symptoms, and an association with leukemia is common. Histocytic lymphoma is an aggressive tumor that commonly develops systemic spread, but may in certain patients have a very prolonged course.

These diseases do not require an extensive surgical resection; radiation therapy and chemotherapy are the treatments of choice, but adequate tissue must be obtained for a histologic diagnosis. Adequate tissue in many instances means one or more whole lymph nodes. Although the lymphomas that develop in the lymph nodes of the middle mediastinum may be characteristic enough to suggest the correct diagnosis from the chest radiograph, those that occur in the anterior–superior mediastinum, especially those within the thymus, may not be so characteristic. If a lymphoma is suspected on the basis of the radiograph, the diagnosis can often be made by mediastinoscopy or an anterior mediastinotomy, but in adults, if the abnormal mass is within the thymus and the possibility of a thymoma exists, a thoracotomy is usually the better choice. In children, however, a thymoma should never be the primary diagnosis for an anterior–superior mediastinal mass, because thymomas are a rarity in this age group.

Neurogenic Tumors

Neurogenic tumors are primarily tumors of the posterior mediastinum that arise from one of three sources: nerve sheath, the sympathetic nervous system, or the paraganglia. In adults, they are chiefly benign tumors of nerve-sheath origin (neurilemmoma or neurofibroma), but in children at least 50% are malignant tumors of sympathetic nervous system origin (neuroblastoma or ganglioneuroblastoma).

Tumors of Nerve Sheath Origin

Neurilemmoma, the most common of this group, is a benign, encapsulated tumor that can vary in size from 1 cm to more than 10 cm in diameter. Areas of hemorrhage and cystic degeneration are common; some may be completely cystic, and calcification within the tumor can sometimes be seen radiographically. Neurilemmomas almost never become malignant. These tumors, in common with neurofibromas, may occur anywhere along the course of the intercostal nerves, but most commonly they arise from segments of the nerves near the posterior mediastinum. In this location, the tumors rarely will grow through the intervertebral foramina and develop a dumbbell-shaped extension within the spinal canal. A search for this phenomenon by tomography of the intervertebral foramina should be made in any patient with a nerve sheath tumor near the spine. If an intraspinal extension of the tumor is demonstrated, the extension should be removed by a laminectomy at the same time or prior to the thoracotomy for removal of the intrathoracic tumor.

Neurofibromas are benign nerve-sheath tumors often associated with Recklinghausen's disease. Although they are often described as less well-encapsulated than neurilemmomas, most posterior mediastinal tumors of nerve-sheath origin are encapsulated. Neurofibromas may undergo malignant change to become malignant schwannomas, but this transformation occurs chiefly in patients with Recklinghausen's disease. The prognosis following the resection of this latter tumor is poor.

These tumors should be approached through a standard posterior–lateral thoracotomy. Because they are usually benign, the tumors do not require a radical resection. Incise the pleura overlying the tumor and isolate the intercostal nerve and blood vessels lateral to the tumor. When these structures have been ligated and divided, the tumor can be easily dissected free by staying just outside the capsule. As the medial portion of the tumor is freed, the intercostal nerve and blood vessels are ligated between the vertebra and the tumor, then divided. If the tumor is very large and located near the spine, the structures medial to the tumor may be controlled more easily by the application of stainless steel clips. Excess traction on the tumor should be avoided during this dissection because of the risk of producing long-term posterior rootlet pain.

Tumors of the Sympathetic Nervous System

Neuroblastoma, which may also occur in the retroperitoneum, is primarily a tumor of children. It is a nonencapsulated, poorly differentiated tumor that may infiltrate the surrounding tissue extensively. Many are associated with elevated levels of vanillylmandelic acid. These are highly malignant tumors that metastasize early and widely; yet the prognosis is better than for neuroblastomas that arise in the retroperitoneum, particularly for children less than 1 year of age. If the tumor cannot be totally resected, with the addition of irradiation and chemotherapy, long-term survival is still possible in a large percentage of patients.

Ganglioneuroblastoma, compared to neuroblastoma, shows an intermediate differentiation, but because each tumor of this type may show differing degrees of differentiation within itself, it is not always possible to make a sharp separation between the two classes. Ganglioneuroblastoma are often encapsulated and frequently have areas of calcification. They are, however, malignant and can metastasize widely. They should be completely resected if possible; if this cannot be done, the use of irradiation and chemotherapy can still produce long survivals.

Ganglioneuroma is a well-encapsulated benign tumor that arises from sympathetic ganglia, usually in adults or older children. These tumors may also be associated with elevated levels of vanillylmandelic acid. They should be completely excised.

Tumors of Paraganglia

Mediastinal paragangliomas may arise from the mediastinal aorticosympathetic paraganglia or from the aorticopulmonary chemoreceptor bodies around the aortic arch. Although most such tumors do not elaborate an active hormone, some secrete catecholamines at a level sufficient to cause hypertension. These active tumors have been termed extraadrenal pheochromocytomas by some authors, but Rosai (9) believes that the term pheochromocytoma should be reserved for tumors of the adrenal medulla, so he classifies even the actively secreting tumors as paraganglioma. From the surgeon's viewpoint, however, the preoperative preparation and the intraoperative management of a patient with an active mediastinal paraganglioma should be the same as that for a patient with a pheochromocytoma. Even though these tumors are histologically benign, they must be widely and totally resected because of their propensity for aggressive local spread and recurrence. The chance of long-term survival after resection of such a tumor is about 50%.

Mesenchymal Tumors

This is a heterogeneous group of tumors whose behavior resembles that of corresponding tumors in other anatomic sites. With the exception of lipomas, the identity of most such tumors cannot be determined without a thoracotomy.

Lipomas are the most common of this group. They are often large and located in the anterior–superior mediastinum or just above the diaphragm. They should not be confused with the mediastinal fat hypertrophy that occurs in patients on long-term steroid therapy. Lipomas may frequently be diagnosed from their characteristic low density exhibited by computerized tomography. Excision of these tumors is curative, but unless the diagnosis is in doubt, excision is usually not necessary in an asymptomatic patient. Liposarcomas may occur anywhere in the mediastinum, including within the pericardial sac. Total excision is usually not possible, but subtotal excision followed by radiation therapy may offer some palliation.

Other tumors in this group may occur within the thymus as well as in most regions of the mediastinum. Those reported are lymphangiomas, hemangiomas, leiomyomas, fibromas, and malignant mesenchymoma.

The treatment of these mediastinal tumors depends largely on their location. If an unknown tumor is found within the thymus, a total thymectomy with excision of the tumor should be done without a prior biopsy. If the tumor is located elsewhere in the mediastinum and is not invasive, a local resection with complete removal of the tumor is adequate. A biopsy of an invasive tumor should always be obtained if a complete resection is not possible.

Mediastinal Cysts

Pericardial Cysts

Pericardial cysts are solitary, soft, unilocular cysts that may occur any place along the pericardium, but are most commonly found in the cardiophrenic angle, usually on the right side. They are lined by thin mesothelium and contain a clear fluid. Usually they are very loosely connected to the pericardium and to the diaphragm, so they may be easily enucleated, but occasionally they may communicate with the pericardial cavity. They do not cause symptoms and are excised for diagnosis.

Bronchogenic Cysts

Bronchogenic cysts are unilocular, thin-walled cysts that are lined by ciliated columnar epithelium and contain a clear or gelatinous fluid. The wall may contain hyaline cartilage, smooth muscle, or bronchial glands. These cysts usually occur between the esophagus and the tracheobronchial tree, most commonly just posterior to the carina, but they can occur at any location down to the diaphragm and they may be embedded in the wall of the esophagus. In adults they are usually asymptomatic unless very large, but in children they may cause respiratory distress from airway compression. These cysts should be removed by simple enucleation. If they lie on the wall of the esophagus, the esophageal muscle should be reapproximated with 5–0 sutures after the excision.

Esophageal, Gastric, and Enteric Cysts

These are usually unilocular cysts lined by squamous, ciliated columnar, or gastric mucosa. Differentiation from a bronchogenic cyst is not always possible, because all may occur embedded in the wall of the esophagus. They infrequently communicate with the lumen of the esophagus. Approximately two-thirds of these cysts are discovered in infants and may be associated with esophageal or airway obstruction. The secretions from the cysts lined with gastric mucosa may cause life-threatening hemorrhage or perforation of a peptic ulcer. These cysts should be removed when diagnosed in infants. In adults they are usually resected to establish the diagnosis of an intrathoracic mass.

Other Cysts

Cystic hygromas are multiloculated, endothelial-lined cysts, often containing a thin, brown fluid, that occur in the anterior–superior mediastinum, often as an extension of a cervical hygroma. They are usually excised for diagnosis. A few thoracic duct cysts or cystic lymphangiomas in the superior portion of the mediastinum have been reported, as have nonspecific cysts that may have been thymic cysts.

References

1. Bergh NP, Gatzinsky P, Larsson S, Lunden P, Ridell B: Tumors of the thymus and thymic region: I, Clinicopathological studies on thymomas. Ann Thorac Surg 25:91–98, 1978.
2. Bolooki H, Schwartzman RJ: High-dose steroids for perioperative management of patients with myasthenia gravis undergoing thymectomy. J Thorac Cardiovasc Surg 75:754–757, 1978.
3. Buckingham JM, Howard SM Jr, Bernatz PE, Payne WS, Harrison EG Jr, O'Brien PC, Weiland LH: The value of thymectomy in myasthenia gravis. A computer-assisted matched study. Ann Surg 184:453–458, 1976.
4. Clark RE, Marbarger JP, West PN, Spratt JA, Florence JM, Roper CL, Ferguson TB, Weldon CS: Thymectomy for myasthenia gravis in the young adult. Long-term results. J Thorac Cardiovasc Surg 80:696–701, 1980.
5. Drachman DB: Myasthenia gravis, I and II. N Engl J Med 298:136–142; 186–193, 1978.
6. Hong WK, Wittes RE, Hajdu ST, Cvitkovic E, Whitmore WF, Golbey RB: The evolution of mature teratoma from malignant testicular tumors. Cancer 40:2987–2992, 1977.
7. Jaretzki A, Bethea M, Wolf M, Olarte MR, Lovelace RE, Penn AS, Rowland L: A rational approach to total thymectomy in the treatment of myasthenia gravis. Ann Thorac Surg 24:120–130, 1977.
8. Papatestas AE, Genkins G, Kornfeld P, Horowitz S, Kark AE: Transcervical thymectomy in myasthenia gravis. Surg Gynecol Obstet 140:535–540, 1975.
9. Rosai J: Ackerman's Surgical Pathology. St. Louis, Mosby, 1981.
10. Rosai J, Higa E: Mediastinal endocrine neoplasm of possible thymic origin, related to carcinoid tumor. Cancer 29:1061–1074, 1972.
11. Wechsler AS, Olanow CW: Myasthenia gravis. Surg Clin North Am 60:931–945, 1980.

Postoperative Care and Complications

9

Postoperative Care

This discussion will cover those aspects of postoperative care that are unique to pulmonary surgery, but it will not deal with those elements, such as wound dressing, fluid therapy, and pain medication, that are common to most major surgical procedures.

General Considerations

The endotracheal tube should not be removed after a pulmonary resection until the patient is fully awake, breathing spontaneously, and able to produce a tidal volume of at least 9 ml/kg body wt. Following operations on debilitated patients or on patients with a limited pulmonary reserve, it is frequently desirable to leave the endotracheal tube in place and to continue mechanical ventilation for the first 24 hours to prevent the patient from developing respiratory insufficiency through fatigue.

Patients should be encouraged to cough frequently and to breathe deeply. Most patients will breathe more easily in a Fowler's position than while horizontal; even so, the position of the patient should be changed frequently to prevent secretions from accumulating in one part of the lung.

Gastric distension will interfere with ventilation at any time, but it is especially dangerous after a right pneumonectomy. A distended stomach will elevate the left diaphragm and impair the function of the remaining lung. To prevent this complication, the nasogastric tube should not be removed until intestinal motility has returned to normal.

The frequency of respiratory and cardiovascular complications following a pulmonary resection requires that these systems be monitored closely. In addition to frequent measurement of the vital signs, the electrocardiogram should be monitored for the development of cardiac arrythmias, and the central venous pressure or pulmonary artery wedge pressure should be watched for evidence of excessive fluid administration. The adequacy of pulmonary function is monitored by frequent measurements of the Pa_{O_2}, the Pa_{CO_2}, and the tidal volume. The use of an indwelling arterial line facilitates drawing arterial blood samples, provides a continuous measurement of systemic arterial pressure, and if necessary, permits a measurement of cardiac output.

The lung usually becomes more susceptible to the development of edema after the handling that occurs during a thoracotomy. Of the factors controlling the movement of fluid across the microvascular endothelium into the interstitium, at the present only the luminal hydrostatic pressure can be altered, and this pressure is a function of the intravascular volume. It follows that to decrease the risk of pulmonary edema, the patient should be kept relatively dry. The change in body weight is generally a good guide to the precision of fluid replacement, except after a pneumonectomy, when a weight gain will occur because of intrathoracic fluid accumulation on the side of the pneumonectomy. A low central venous pressure or a low volume of urine output are not of themselves good criteria of the need for additional fluid administration.

Although the intrathoracic pressure should be adjusted at the end of a pneumonectomy to position the mediastinum 1–2 cm toward the side of the pneumonectomy, pressure changes in the postoperative period may displace the mediastinum toward or away from the remaining lung. If the mediastinum is shifted excessively toward the side of the pneumonectomy, the venous return to the heart may be impaired; if it is shifted toward the remaining lung, the vital capacity will be decreased. The chest radiogram should be examined each of the first three postoperative days for such a shift; if it occurs, air should either be removed from or injected into the hemithorax to return the mediastinum to the desired position. After the first three days, the mediastinum becomes so stiff that it cannot be readily moved.

Because a posterior–lateral thoracotomy involves the division of several muscles around the shoulder girdle, some pain is caused by motion of the shoulder, but if the shoulder is permitted to remain immobile during the postoperative period, it will become stiff. As soon as possible after surgery, active motion of the shoulder, with the goal of raising the elbow above shoulder level, should be started. The action of combing the hair on the back of the head is beneficial.

Pulmonary Care

In addition to auscultation of the chest, the daily evaluation of the patient's lungs should include a chest radiogram for the first three days or until the patient's pulmonary status has stabilized. If the radiogram shows areas of atelectasis or pneumonia, therapy should be initiated at once to improve the patient's bronchial toilet. The various therapeutic actions to cleanse the tracheobronchial tree should be instituted is a specific sequence.

First, the patient should be turned frequently and encouraged to cough effectively. This is easier if the patient has been taught how to cough before surgery. A patient in the sitting position can usually cough more effectively than when horizontal, and sometimes small doses of pain medication or an intercostal block around the incision are helpful in eliciting an effective cough.

When the cough is not effective in preventing or clearing the pulmonary infiltrate, the patient's trachea should be suctioned with a pliable 18 French catheter introduced through the nose. Grasp the patient's tongue with gauze and pull it forward. Using the other hand, pass the lubricated catheter, with the suction off, through one nostril until the tip is positioned just above the glottis. As the patient phonates or inspires deeply, quickly advance the catheter into the trachea and suction it out by moving the catheter up and down and rotating it. This action usually stimulates a violent cough that also helps to clear the trachea and bronchi of secretions.

If the secretions cannot be adequately removed by nasotracheal suctioning, the trachea and bronchi should be cleared with a bronchoscope. The wide-channel bronchofiberscope is adequate for most patients, but in some with very tenacious secretions, a rigid bronchoscope with a large suction cannula may be required. In the latter situation, the injection of small quantities of saline through the bronchoscope is helpful in removing the mucous.

Pleural Drainage Catheters

The occurrence or nonoccurrence of complications following a pulmonary resection often depends as much on the attention given to the intrapleural suction catheters, the associated tubing, and the chest drainage unit as it does on the operative procedure itself. Consequently, the surgeon should determine that all personnel involved with the patient's postoperative care are familiar with the functioning of the chest drainage unit to which the intrapleural catheters are coupled.

These units essentially consist of three connected compartments. The first compartment collects blood and fluid aspirated from the pleural cavity. The second compartment contains sterile water and provides an underwater seal to prevent air from entering the pleural cavity; it is also used to detect the presence of an air leak. The third compartment is connected to a source of suction and is filled with fluid to regulate the amount of negative pressure applied to the intrapleural catheters, usually a minus 20 cm H_2O. Valves are now included to prevent the aspiration of fluid from one compartment to another when large pressure changes occur from coughing or hyperventilation. When a patient is to be transported to another area of the hospital, the unit may be disconnected from the wall suction and sent with the patient, but the catheters or tubing between the patient and the water-seal unit should not be clamped for more than a few seconds.

Pain in the region of the catheters requires investigation; if the catheters were placed anterior to the posterior axillary line so that the patient does not lie on them, they should cause little pain.

The tubing that connects the intrapleural catheters to the chest drainage unit should be stripped ("milked") at hourly intervals to prevent obstruction of the catheters or tubing by clots. This tubing should not be permitted to sag or lie in a vertical loop, because fluid collecting in the dependent segment will decrease the negative pressure applied to the catheters. Intrapleural catheters that are part of a closed thoracostomy system should never be irrigated. Irrigation may wash in bacteria and produce an empyema. If catheters become obstructed, they should be removed or replaced as necessary.

Intrapleural catheters are usually removed when the fluid drainage has decreased to less than 100 ml in 24 hours and the surgeon is certain that any pulmonary air leak has stopped. Removal is most easily performed by two persons. Place a large clamp on each catheter and disconnect the catheters from the tubing. Cut the skin suture, and use a large syringe with a connector that fits tightly into the catheter to maintain a negative pressure after the clamp has been removed. Gradually withdraw the catheter until the most proximal side hole is even with the pleura, then remove the catheter rapidly while the assistant occludes the skin opening with petrolatum gauze or some similar dressing. If a pocket containing more than 30 ml of fluid is encountered during the removal, the catheter should be left in that pocket and reconnected to suction for another 24 hours. After the catheters have been removed and the skin openings occluded with petrolatum gauze and a tight dressing, a chest radiogram should be obtained to determine if a pneumothorax has developed.

Oxygen Therapy

The mismatch of blood flow with ventilation is the most common cause of hypoxia in the postoperative period. Among the many causes associated with a pulmonary resection that may contribute to such ventilation–perfusion ($\dot{V}A/\dot{Q}$) abnormalities are advanced age of the patient, a general anesthetic, handling of the lung, poor bronchial toilet, inaccuracies in fluid administration, chronic pulmonary disease, and a recumbent position. Some of these factors significantly decrease the ventilation to areas of the lung by producing intraalveolar hemorrhage and patchy atelectasis and by increasing fluid in the airways and in the pulmonary interstitium. An abnormal $\dot{V}A/\dot{Q}$ results in the lung's becoming a less efficient gas exchanger. This necessitates an increase in ventilation, thereby increasing respiratory work. Carried to an extreme degree, this abnormality can cause death from repiratory insufficiency.

The arterial oxygen tension (Pa_{O_2}) is the most useful and readily available measure of the degree of $\dot{V}A/\dot{Q}$ abnormality. The Pa_{O_2}, however, is a complex function of $\dot{V}A/\dot{Q}$, oxygen concentration in the inspired air (FI_{O_2}), cardiac output, alveolar ventilation, mixed venous oxygen tension ($P\bar{V}_{O_2}$), pulmonary shunts, and additional minor factors, so an increase or decrease in the Pa_{O_2} cannot be translated directly to a change in $\dot{V}A/\dot{Q}$ without knowledge of these other variables. The Pa_{CO_2} is such a sensitive function of alveolar ventilation that it is of little help in detecting $\dot{V}A/\dot{Q}$ inequalities.

The frequency of postoperative $\dot{V}A/\dot{Q}$ inequalities and the finding that the hypoxia resulting from these abnormalities can often be corrected by small increases in the concentration of oxygen has resulted in the routine administration of supplemental oxygen at low concentration to all postthoracotomy patients for the first 24–48 hours. As explained by West (15), alveolar units with a low $\dot{V}A/\dot{Q}$ in the range of 0.01–0.1 will increase their oxygen content rapidly with small increases in the inspired PO_2. Small increases in the FI_{O_2} are commonly delivered by the use of nasal cannulae. In a normal subject during quiet normal breathing, 100% oxygen from nasal cannulae at a flow rate of 2 liters/min. will produce an FI_{O_2} of between 0.25 and 0.30, while at a flow rate of 4 liters/min., the FI_{O_2} will be 0.35–0.40 (7); however, the actual FI_{O_2} of the patient will depend upon both the tidal volume and the ventilatory pattern. The oxygen supplied will be more comfortable for the patient to breathe if it has increased humidity, but unless strict sterile conditions are maintained, the humidifier can be the source of a nosocomial Gram-negative pneumonia. Sterile water must be used in the humidifier, and all tubing and equipment should be changed at least daily.

Pulmonary units with a $\dot{V}A/\dot{Q}$ below 0.01 will show little change until the FI_{O_2} exceeds 0.5 (15). If the required FI_{O_2} cannot be obtained by nasal cannulae, a mask or an endotracheal tube must be used. However, it is not necessary to increase the FI_{O_2} above the level necessary to maintain the Pa_{O_2} at 60–70 torr. The results of increasing the FI_{O_2} are not all beneficial, and the higher the concentration of oxygen, the greater the deleterious effects may be. Alveoli with significantly decreased ventilation are kept open by the relatively fixed volume of nitrogen within the alveolus. When a higher concentration of oxygen develops in these poorly ventilated alveoli, a greater fraction of the total gas volume will be absorbed and the alveoli may become unstable and collapse, thus converting poorly ventilated regions to unventilated regions and increasing the areas of atelectasis. Other kinds of toxicity from high concentrations of oxygen have been described periodically, and although the impression of many clinicians is that an F_{IO_2} greater than 0.5 for prolonged periods is harmful, the objective evidence supporting such toxicity in adult humans is not strong.

Mechanical Ventilation

The most common indication for the use of mechanical ventilators is to provide adequate oxygenation and carbon dioxide elimination for patients with established respiratory failure, but they are also used prophylactically after surgery in patients who might not be able to perform the work of breathing or in whom the performance of that work might cause a deterioration in cardiac status.

In determining the need for a mechanical ventilator, arterial blood gas tensions are the most important tests. In general, if the Pa_{CO_2} rises above 55 torr or if the Pa_{O_2} cannot be maintained above 55 torr with the highest inspiratory oxygen concentration that can be delivered by mask, the patient should have an endotracheal tube inserted and should be placed on a ventilator. A continuing trend of deterioration in the arterial blood gases and in the patient's clinical course, however, should signal to the clinician that mechanical ventilator support ought to be instituted or a severe blood gas derangement could develop.

At the present, the mechanical ventilators used for surgical patients produce lung inflation by applying a positive pressure to the airway. Two types of positive pressure ventilators are available: pressure-cycled ventilators, which terminate the inspiratory phase when a preset airway pressure is reached, and volume-cycled ventilators, which terminate the inspiratory phase when a preset volume of gas has been delivered.

Pressure-cycled ventilators have a disadvantage that limits their usefulness: any increase in airway resistance or decrease in lung compliance can significantly decrease the tidal volume that they deliver; therefore they cannot be used for patients with a low compliance, such as those with ARDS. Volume-cycled ventilators, such as the Siemens–Elema Servo ventilator, can deliver the set minute volume of gas to the lungs with better than a 90% accuracy, independent of resistance, if the predetermined pressure limits are not exceeded. This feature has made volume-cycled ventilators the most widely used, but this same feature may result in high airway pressures that can cause considerable barotrauma to the lung and that can significantly decrease the cardiac output.

A ventilator should be able to deliver a wide range of inspiratory oxygen concentration. The minimum concentration that will maintain the patient's Pa_{O_2} between 60 and 70 torr should be employed. A higher arterial oxygen tension serves little useful purpose, and the higher inspiratory oxygen concentration needed to maintain it increases the risk of pulmonary damage. The ability of the current available ventilators to deliver accurately the set concentration of oxygen is improved greatly over past models; nevertheless the clinician should not rely on the oxygen concentration setting, but should measure the concentration in the inspiratory gas daily.

Although the normal tidal volume averages about 7 ml/kg body wt., when a patient is placed on a ventilator, the tidal volume is usually set initially at 10–12 ml/kg body wt. in order to compensate for the increased dead space of the apparatus and of a patient in respiratory failure. If the patient can exert an inspiratory effort strong enough to trip the ventilator and if the frequency of the patient's spontaneous respiration while on the ventilator is

10–20 breaths/min., the ventilator can be used in the assist mode. If machine-controlled ventilation is necessary, use a beginning respiratory rate of 12–14 breaths/min.

Arterial blood gas tensions should be measured 15–20 min after putting the patient on a ventilator. If the Pa_{CO_2} is not within the normal range, the tidal volume may be increased up to 15 ml/kg body wt., unless this results in an excessive airway pressure. Any further increase in minute volume should be obtained by increasing the respiratory rate. If the Pa_{CO_2} has fallen below 30 torr, the respiratory rate should be decreased.

The configuration of the inspiratory pressure flow pattern probably is not of major clinical importance; however, if the patient fights the ventilator, better synchrony between the patient and the machine can often be obtained by adjusting the inspiratory flow rate (the inspiratory time). If the Pa_{O_2} is not at an adequate level, a short inspiratory pause of 0.5–1.0 sec will sometimes improve the lung's ventilation–perfusion ratios and will often decrease atelectasis. The likelihood of atelectasis is also decreased by periodic, single, large tidal volumes, called sighs. Any time the duration of positive intrathoracic pressure is increased, the cardiac output must be closely monitored.

Positive End-Expiratory Pressure (PEEP)

PEEP has been an extremely useful technique for improving arterial oxygenation in patients with pulmonary failure; it may often succeed when ventilation with increased inspiratory oxygen concentrations alone fails. PEEP does not decrease pulmonary edema. Rather, it decreases the ventilation–perfusion inequality by increasing the functional residual capacity and maintaining small airways open that otherwise might close during expiration.

As a corollary to the increase in functional residual capacity, however, PEEP increases the pulmonary vascular resistance, and this increase in resistance is greatest in those segments of the lung that are well ventilated. Because of this change in vascular resistance, it is possible that the use of PEEP will decrease the Pa_{O_2} in certain clinical conditions in which one lung is relatively normal and the other is poorly ventilated. The lung usually reacts to such a situation by shunting the blood flow from the poorly ventilated lung to the normal lung, but the use of PEEP increases the vascular resistance in the normal lung with the result that the poorly ventilated lung becomes well perfused and the ventilation–perfusion inequality increases.

Usually PEEP is started at 5 cm H_2O and is then increased as necessary to maintain the Pa_{O_2} above 60 torr with an inspiratory oxygen concentration of 50% or less. However, as PEEP increases, so does the chance of adverse consequences. Because there is a proportional decrease in venous return to the heart as the mean intrathoracic pressure increases from the PEEP, the cardiac output must be monitored closely. The mixed venous Po_2 can be used as an index of tissue perfusion and oxygenation if the possible errors in this use are understood. The decrease in cardiac output caused by PEEP can often be corrected by increasing the intravascular volume. In determining the need for an infusion of fluid to increase the cardiac output, one cannot rely on the central venous pressure and the pulmonary artery wedge pressure, because during the use of PEEP, these two measurements may be spuriously increased.

Complications of Mechanical Ventilation

If the complications resulting from tracheal intubation and from mechanical failure of the ventilator are excluded, the important complications of positive-pressure ventilation are 1) a decrease in the cardiac output, 2) barotrauma, 3) cardiac arrhythmias, and 4) nosocomial pulmonary infections. Except for the last, these complications are all intensified by PEEP.

The decrease in cardiac output is caused by a decrease in the transmural right ventricular filling pressure and by an increase in the right ventricular afterload. The magnitude of these changes was shown by Cournand et al. (3) to be functions of the mean airway pressure elevation and of the inspiratory–expiratory time ratio. Cournand recommended a ventilation pattern of a short inspiratory phase of less than half of the total ventilatory cycle, followed by a rapid drop to atmospheric pressure, but this pattern increases the risk of atelectasis. Peak airway pressures above 35 cm H_2O are frequently associated with some decrease in cardiac output, but this decrease can often be corrected by an infusion of fluid.

A pneumothorax can result from high inspiratory pressures alone, but the occurrence seems to be more common with PEEP values above 12 cm H_2O. Recall that the value of PEEP is added to both end-expiration and to peak inspiration pressures. Some physicians advocate the prophylactic insertion of bilateral intrapleural catheters if the peak inspiratory pressure with PEEP exceeds 55 cm H_2O.

When a patient is acidotic from a high Pa_{CO_2} and is suddenly hyperventilated, serious ventricular arrhythmias may occur, probably from a change in the ratio of potassium to ionized calcium (1). These patients should have mechanical ventilation started slowly and the Pa_{CO_2} brought back to a normal value over a period of 12 hours to allow the necessary electrolyte equilibration to occur.

Pulmonary infections are a common complication of mechanical ventilation. Within a few hours of institution of ventilation bacteria can be cultured from the tubing of most patients on mechanical ventilators. Infections may be minimized by changing all tubing and humidifiers for sterile ones every 24 hours, by filtering the inspired air, and by maintaining a strict aseptic technique for suctioning and other procedures on the airway.

High-Frequency Ventilation

Many of the problems encountered with postive-pressure ventilators relate to the high inspiratory pressures necessary to ventilate patients with low lung compliance: 1) Patients with a large bronchopleural or bronchoesophageal fistula often cannot be adequately ventilated because they lose a large part of each tidal volume through the fistula during the time of high inspiratory pressure. 2) The high inspiratory pressure often causes a pneumothorax. 3) The high inspiratory pressure and the prolonged inspiratory–expiratory ratio decreases venous return and so decreases cardiac output.

One recent approach to these problems is the use of high-frequency ventilation (HFV). HFV is defined by Slutsky et al. (14) as ventilation with a frequency at least four times greater than normal. Many methods of delivering HFV have been described, but no completely satisfactory high-frequency ventilator is available yet. HFV utilizes frequencies from 60–100 breaths/min. using very high tracheal flows, and tidal volumes that may be less than the pulmonary dead space. Such frequencies and flow rates require a ventilator with a negligible compressible volume; consequently the current commercially available positive-pressure ventilators cannot be used. Sjöstrand, one of the early workers in the field, uses a pneumatic valve (13); most systems deliver the inspiratory gases through a cannula within the endotracheal tube.

During HFV, high peak inspiratory pressures are not generated; consequently the incidence of barotrauma should be less. Of even greater importance for those patients with bronchial fistulas, the pressure difference between the airway and the pleural space or esophagus should change less; therefore, the loss of a large portion of the minute volume through the fistula should be reduced. With the lower peak pressures, less circulatory interference should occur than with conventional ventilators.

The clinical experience with this method has not been great. Sjöstrand (13) and his colleagues have utilized HFV during laryngoscopy and bronchoscopy when endotracheal intubation and conventional high volume positive-pressure ventilation would have interfered with the procedure. Carlon et al. (12) reported their use of HFV in 17 patients who could not be supported with conventional ventilators. Eleven of these patients had large fistulas between the airway and the pleural cavity or the esophagus, and five had large airleaks as a result of barotrauma from conventional ventilators. In all cases, even in those patients who ultimately died, adequate alveolar ventilation could be maintained with HFV. The cardiac output improved in 10 of the 17 patients.

Weaning from the Ventilator

The use of the many published criteria for predicting successful weaning from a ventilator (4,9) may have value in a population of patients without severe underlying chronic lung disease, but such patients rarely present difficult problems in weaning. In many surgical intensive care units, postoperative patients on ventilators may be found who could not meet most of these criteria prior to the onset of their acute surgical illness at a time when they were not on a ventilator. It is with these patients that most of the difficulties with weaning are encountered, and for these patients, few methods other than "trial and fail" are available to predict whether the patient can sustain unassisted breathing at an adequate level.

A few guidelines do exist for weaning these difficult patients. Short periods of unassisted ventilation should be interspersed during the day as soon as the patient's clinical condition permits. As the patient's tolerance for these periods improves, an early attempt should be made to wean the patient, because the longer such a patient is kept on a ventilator, the more difficult is the weaning process. Although this statement may impress some as a tautology, many physicians agree that a cause and effect relationship does exist between the duration of ventilation and the difficulty in weaning.

A definable trend of general clinical improvement is of vital importance. The problem that originally precipitated respiratory failure should be controlled. The patient should be out of heart failure, with no life-threatening arrythmias, and without the need for pressor drugs. The patient should be mentally alert and able to attempt a cough.

It has been my experience that if the patients cannot meet the following three ventilatory criteria, they usually cannot be weaned permanently from a ventilator. First they should be able to sustain a tidal volume of at least 6 ml/kg body wt. and should have a vital capacity of not less than 9 ml/kg body wt. These measurements can be made easily in the intubated patient with a Wright respirometer. Second, they should be able to maintain a Pa_{O_2} of greater than 60 torr on an inspiratory oxygen concentration that can be attained with a mask, generally 35%–40% oxygen. Third, they should not require PEEP to maintain the above stated Pa_{O_2}.

The use of intermittent mandatory ventilation (IMV) is recommended by some authors as an improved method of weaning. This technique provides periodic inspiratory positive pressure ventilation, while permitting the patient to breath spontaneously between controlled breaths. The chosen tidal volume is delivered at intervals that can be varied from a few seconds to several minutes. Pontoppidan et al. (9) believe that the use of IMV permits weaning to be initiated at an earlier stage in the patient's course and lessens the demand for close observation of the patient. On the other hand, Schachter et al. (11) concluded that the use of IMV did not reduce the length of ventilator management when compared to a group of patients who were treated with conventional mechanical ventilation.

When the IMV on commercially available mechanical ventilators is used, the inspiratory gas mixture must be pulled through the tubing and humidifier of the ventilator, thus increasing the resistance that the patient must inspire against when the ventilator is not controlling respiration. I have had the experience of being able to wean a debilitated patient with severe lung disease only when he was taken off the ventilator and put on a T-piece; he could not be weaned using the IMV of the ventilator.

It is essential that the patient be monitored closely after discontinuing ventilator support and that mechanical ventilation be reinstituted at any sign of inadequate ventilation. The signs that should be watched for are 1) a change in mental status, such as depression of the sensorium or apprehension; 2) evidence of fatigue, such as sweating or increased use of the accessory muscles of respiration; 3) a significant increase in the pulse rate or the respiratory rate; 4) a decrease in the systemic blood pressure; and 5) most important, an increase in the Pa_{CO_2} or a decrease in the Pa_{O_2}. The personnel responsible for the patient must not wait for the above signs to become well established. Many poor risk patients may develop a respiratory or cardiac arrest within minutes of showing the first clinical sign of inadequate ventilation. Never extubate a patient until the patient has demonstrated an ability to remain off the ventilator. In some patients, 24–48 hours may be required to establish this.

Complications

Hemothorax

If a patient has no clotting abnormality and if the residual lung completely fills the pleural cavity, any significant bleeding that occurs after a pulmonary resection will usually be from a systemic blood vessel. Frequent sites are intercostal arteries that were lacerated during closure of the incision, or adhesions from the diaphragm or the region of the pulmonary ligament that were divided during the resection and retracted to an area not readily observed. Bleeding from adhesions is more common in patients with a chronic inflammatory disease of the lungs because of the ingrowth of larger systemic vessels. Bleeding from the lung itself after surgery is frequent only if lobar atelectasis has occurred or if an unresectable carcinoma of the lung is encountered. Although it is rare for clotting abnormalities not present before surgery to develop following a thoracotomy that did not involve cardiopulmonary bypass, an assessment of clotting factors should still be made if bleeding continues.

The indication for reoperation because of postthoracotomy bleeding will obviously vary from patient to patient, but as a guide, I have used the following criteria: 1) after the initial irrigation fluid has been evacuated, if the bleeding continues at greater than 200 ml/hour for 4 or more hours; 2) if the volume of blood clot that accumulates in the pleural cavity exceeds 25% of the volume of one hemithorax; and 3) massive bleeding that causes hypotension. At the reoperation, all clots should be evacuated and a search made for a site of bleeding. If the site cannot be located, the rib retractor should be removed and the area of the chest wall near the incision examined. Even when no bleeding site can be identified, the evacuation of the pleural clot is sometimes enough to stop the bleeding.

Subcutaneous Emphysema

Lesser degrees of subcutaneous emphysema are common after a pneumonectomy, particularly if an extensive mediastinal lymph node dissection has been done or a wide area of pleura has been removed. Because it is not common practice to leave an intrapleural catheter after a pneumonectomy, the accumulation of fluid in the pleural cavity, along with a vigorous cough, can elevate the intrapleural pressure enough to force some air out of the chest. However, the volume of air present in one hemithorax is limited, so the degree of subcutaneous emphysema that can develop after a pneumonectomy is also limited unless a bronchopleural fistula develops.

Massive subcutaneous emphysema can develop following any pulmonary resection of a magnitude less than a pneumonectomy, but it will occur only if an air leak from the lung is coupled with intrapleural catheters that are nonfunctional or that have one catheter hole positioned outside the pleural cavity. Although subcutaneous emphysema may result in a grotesque appearance, it is not a threat to the patient's life and it requires no specific therapy other than the removal of its cause. If the chest radiogram shows one catheter hole to be outside of the pleural cavity, the catheter should be removed or repositioned. If the catheters are clogged and cannot be reopened by stripping the tubing, they should be removed and new catheters inserted. When the lung fills the pleural cavity completely, there is no reason to increase the negative pressure applied to the intrapleural catheters in an attempt to evacuate more air.

Air Leaks and Intrapleural Pockets

If the remaining lung after a pulmonary resection fills the pleural cavity, most air leaks from the pulmonary parenchyma will stop within 24–48 hours by being sealed against the parietal pleura. The process by which the remaining lung and its associated pleural cavity conform and so permit air leaks to seal includes both expansion of the two lungs and a decrease in the size of the associated pleural cavity resulting from an elevation of the diaphragm and a shift of the mediastinum toward the side operated on. Factors which interfere with this process are atelectasis or pneumonia, pulmonary fibrosis, rigidity of the mediastinum or diaphragm, and poorly functioning intrapleural catheters.

In the event of a large or a prolonged air leak, the first action should be to examine for an air leak the tubing and connections between the intrapleural catheters and the chest drainage unit. An easy method is to clamp the catheters at the skin level for a few seconds. If the air leak persists, it is from some place in the drainage system, not from the lung. To determine if air is leaking into the chest around the intrapleural catheters, find out if the air leak will stop with the application of sterile ointment and pressure to the skin entrances for the catheters.

When a patient with an air leak has an area of atelectasis or an inadequate bronchial toilet, efforts should be made to improve the patient's cough; if necessary, suction out the tracheobronchial tree with a bronchoscope so the lung can expand completely and fill the pleural cavity. If the intrapleural catheters are occluded, attempt to open them by vigorous stripping. When this is impossible, remove them and insert new ones. If an intrapleural pocket does not communicate with the catheters in place, an additional catheter should be inserted into the pocket. Within the first 24 hours, if the air leak is not massive, but the lung does not fill the pleural cavity completely, it is sometimes helpful to increase the negative pressure applied to the catheters to 45 cm H_2O for a period of no longer than 8 hours. This increased negative pressure may assist in pulling the diaphragm up and shifting the mediastinum toward the side operated on, thus decreasing the size of the pleural cavity and permitting the lung to fill it completely. This action does little good after 24–36 hours due to the increased rigidity of the mediastinum. If it is not successful within 8 hours, it will usually not be successful if continued for longer periods. The use of greater negative pressure than 45 cm H_2O or a longer period of time than 8 hours increases the risk of producing pulmonary edema.

If a patient has a continuous maximal bubbling in the water seal compartment of the chest drainage unit, unchanged throughout both inspiration and expiration, that continues for more than 30 min after the chest incision has been tightly closed, the patient should be reexplored at once and the bronchial fistula sutured closed. If such a fistula is suspected later in the postoperative period after a lobectomy, the bronchial closure should be examined by bronchoscopy to determine if a significant bronchopleural fistula exists. If one is found, the patient should be reexplored and the fistula closed by reamputating the bronchial stump if it is long enough or by suturing an intercostal muscle bundle into it if the stump is short.

Most troublesome air leaks are not massive, but rather are small leaks that persist for long periods. When an air leak is still present after the seventh postoperative day, each of the intrapleural catheters should be connected to a separate chest drainage unit so that the catheter evacuating the air leak can be identified. The catheters that do not show a leak can then be removed. The management of the remaining catheter depends on the presence or absence of an associated intrapleural air space, i.e., it depends on whether or not the lung completely fills the pleural cavity. If no intrapleural air space is present, withdraw the remaining catheter 1–2 cm each day, until the most proximal side hole in the catheter is just inside the pleural cavity. This permits the lung to seal the tube track behind the catheter and so stop any parenchymal air leaks kept open by the presence of the catheter. If the air leak is still present when the tube has been withdrawn as much as possible, discontinue the use of suction to the catheter, but let it remain connected to a water seal for 24 hours. If the lung does not collapse away from the chest wall during that period, the intrapleural catheter should be opened to the atmosphere for an additional 24 hours, after which it may be removed if an intrapleural air pocket has not developed.

When an intrapleural air pocket continues to exist after 14 or more days, but no air leak can be discovered on careful and prolonged examination, and no evidence of an infection in the intrapleural pocket is found, the catheter draining the air pocket should be clamped and the other catheters removed. If after 24 hours the air pocket has not enlarged, the remaining catheter can also be removed.

In the presence of a small air leak, but no intrapleural pocket, and also in the presence of an intrapleural pocket, but no air leak, all intrapleural catheters can be removed if the lung is adherent to the parietal pleura; however, an intrapleural pocket with an associated air leak cannot be left undrained, because if it were, an infection in the pocket would surely develop. Commonly such a pocket forms in the apex of the chest. When a persistent air pocket with a persistent parenchymal air leak is encountered, the intrapleural catheters not primarily involved in evacuating the pocket may be removed, but the catheter that drains the pocket most directly must be left in place. After 2 weeks, when the lung is firmly adherent to the parietal pleura, the remaining catheter may be cut off a few centimeters from the skin and left open to the atmosphere until the pocket is obliterated and the air leak ceases. This procedure entails a small risk of an empyema developing in the residual pocket;

the risk is probably not much greater than if the catheter remained on suction, yet the procedure permits the patient to be fully ambulant. If a pocket such as this is not obliterated, sooner or later an infection will develop in it. Such an apical empyema is most effectively and expeditiously treated by an apical thoracoplasty (discussed in Ch. 6).

Empyema and Bronchopleural Fistula After Pneumonectomy

After a pneumonectomy, the hemithorax decreases in size, and the pleural cavity becomes layered with fibrous tissue, but a residual pocket of serum, often 200–400 ml, will continue to exist within the hemithorax for the rest of the patient's life. Fortunately, the development of an empyema after a pneumonectomy is rare. If it occurs, it is usually within the first month of surgery and is secondary to a small bronchopleural fistula, a wound infection, or a contamination at the time of surgery; the residual pocket of serum, however, can become infected from a transient bacteremia at any time following surgery. I have seen patients develop an empyema eight years after a pneumonectomy. Those empyemas that develop years after a pneumonectomy performed for cancer of the lung are particularly treacherous, because such a patient who presents with malaise, weight loss, and an unexplained fever is often assumed to have a recurrence of the cancer. At any time after a pneumonectomy, early or late, a patient with an unexplained fever, or any of the other signs mentioned previously, should have a diagnostic thoracentesis, using fluoroscopy if necessary, and a microscopic smear and a culture made of the fluid.

A bronchopleural fistula that develops after a pneumonectomy commonly occurs within the first 2 weeks, but it may occur up to several months after surgery. Such fistulas are commonly heralded by two signs: an increase in the volume of air in the pleural cavity of the resected lung or the production of serosanguinous sputum, often in large amounts. Occasionally, however, the first sign will be evidence of sepsis from an infection in the pleural cavity. The fistula may be small, such as a laceration of the membranous portion of the bronchus from tying a suture too tightly, or it may be so large that the whole bronchial stump is open. Large or small, any bronchopleural fistula that develops after a pneumonectomy poses a serious threat to the patient's life. If the fistula is sizable, the patient may drown from aspirating a massive volume of intrapleural fluid into the remaining lung or may die of asphyxiation because the large bronchial opening makes adequate ventilation of the remaining lung impossible. If the fistula is small, pneumonia in the remaining lung with pulmonary insufficiency may develop from repeated small volume aspiration, or the patient may become septic from an empyema on the side of the pneumonectomy.

The treatment of a patient with an empyema following a pneumonectomy requires the complete evacuation of all infected fluid and clot and the elimination of the infecting organism. If the empyema develops within the first week, a closed thoracostomy using an intercostal catheter connected to a chest drainage unit should be employed to empty the hemithorax as much as possible. After the seventh day following a pneumonectomy, the mediastinum will have become sufficiently stiff and immobile to perform an open thoracostomy over the most dependent portion of the residual space (described in Ch. 7). In all such patients, bronchoscopy should be performed and the bronchial stump examined for the presence of a bronchopleural fistula. The detection of small fistulas by bronchoscopy is not always easy. A strategy that I have used after the hemithorax has been emptied of fluid is to drop enough saline on the bronchial stump to form a small pool and then to examine the pool for the formation of air bubbles. The presence of air movement out of an open thoracostomy cannot be used to diagnose a bronchopleural fistula; such air flow can occur from diaphragmatic motion alone in the absence of a fistula.

If no bronchopleural fistula can be identified, the pleural cavity should be irrigated through the open thoracostomy twice a day with a saline solution containing an antibiotic appropriate for the resident organism. When that organism can no longer be cultured from the pleural cavity, the cavity should be filled with a dilute antibiotic solution and the thoracostomy opening closed tightly. The total dose of the antibiotic placed in the pleural cavity should not exceed the maximum recommended single dose because an antibiotic such as neomycin can cause eighth nerve or renal damage. Using this method, 85%–90% of patients that do not have a bronchopleural fistula will have no further difficulty with an infection in the residual cavity. The alternative to this procedure is the performance of an extensive thoracoplasty to obliterate completely the residual cavity.

A large bronchopleural fistula from the stump of the right or left main bronchus shortly after a pneumonectomy is an immediate threat to the patient's life. Any patient who displays evidence of such a fistula by coughing up serosanguinous fluid should be considered a surgical emergency. The first action is to empty the hemithorax of fluid by an intercostal catheter attached to suction or, if the postoperative period has been more than 7–10 days, by an open thoracostomy. If the size of the fistula is contributing to inadequate ventilation of the remaining lung as evidence by an elevated Pa_{CO_2}, the fistula should be surgically closed at once. In order to maintain adequate ventilation until the fistula is closed, an endobronchial tube should be positioned so the fistula is occluded by the cuff of the tube. Such placement is not difficult if the fistula is into the right pleural cavity, but positioning a tube in the right main bronchus to occlude a fistula to the left pleural cavity can easily obstruct the right upper lobe bronchus.

It is rare that an attempt to suture close such a fistula by reapproximating the walls of the bronchial stump will be successful. The fistula often appears as a hole with friable edges in a stiff and fibrotic mediastinum. The most successful method is to plug the fistula with an intercostal muscle bundle. Choose the muscle bundle that will lie with its center on the fistula after the muscle has been dissected free of the adjacent ribs and is suspended from both ends. Usually this will be the third intercostal muscle. From the inside of the chest, incise the pleura and periosteum along the center of both the rib above and the rib below the selected muscle bundle, from the anterior to the posterior end of each rib. Reflect the periosteum off the upper half of the rib below and the lower half of the rib above, being careful not to damage the intercostal artery and vein. Incise the outer leaf of the periosteum and dissect free the intercostal muscle bundle with its artery and vein, but leave it attached at both ends to ensure an adequate blood supply. The portion of the muscle that overlies the bronchial opening should be stuffed into the bronchus and carefully sutured to the bronchial wall around the whole circumference. Recall, while placing the sutures, that the stump of the pulmonary artery lies immediately adjacent to the bronchial stump after a pneumonectomy. The chest cavity must be left with an open thoracostomy for 2–3 months. After that period, if the fistula is closed and if cultures taken from the chest cavity do not show a significant bacterial content, the hemithorax is filled with an appropriate antibiotic solution, as previously described, and the thoracostomy is closed. The alternative to this method is the use of a 7–8 rib thoracoplasty to collapse the hemithorax completely, in addition to the use of an intercostal muscle bundle to plug the bronchus. A prolonged period of open drainage of the thorax is still required after a thoracoplasty.

Rarely, a bronchopleural fistula after a pneumonectomy may be so small that the only sign is a slight increase in the volume of air within the hemithorax. If no evidence of sepsis is found and if the pleural fluid is sterile on culture, some of these fistulas will heal with prolonged antibiotic treatment. Patients treated in this manner must be followed closely and their pleural cavity drained if any evidence of an infection is found.

Respiratory Failure

Respiratory failure is the inability of the respiratory system (lungs, thoracic cage, and respiratory muscles) to provide an adequate level of gas exchange for the support of the body's metabolism. It differs only in degree from respiratory insufficiency, which is often defined as the inability to maintain blood gas tensions at a normal value.

The etiologies of pulmonary insufficiency in the postthoracotomy patient are diverse. A partial list of causes is given in Table 9-1. Only the first three causes listed are peculiar to thoracic surgery, and these three are of a nature different than the others because they do not represent an acute process affecting the lung parenchyma. This does not imply that they are of lesser importance. At the present, respiratory muscle fatigue is probably the leading cause of respiratory failure and death following a pulmonary resection.

Pulmonary failure due to any of the first three causes is more easily prevented than treated. An excessive pulmonary resection should be largely prevented by setting an absolute limit to the extent of the resection, a limit based on the preoperative evaluation of pulmonary function. An unstable chest wall can be prevented by an adequate reconstruction. If pulmonary failure from an unstable chest wall does occur in the postoperative period, the patient should be managed with a mechanical ventilator until the chest wall and mediastinum become rigid enough to permit weaning from the ventilator, usually 1–2 weeks. During this period an attempt should be made to keep the patient relatively dry so that an increase in pulmonary interstitial water does not also occur.

No routinely successful therapy is available for respiratory muscle fatigue in debilitated patients who require increased ventilatory work. They must

TABLE 9-1 Causes of Pulmonary Insufficiency.

1. Excessive pulmonary resection
2. Unstable chest wall
3. Respiratory muscle fatigue
4. Pulmonary thromboembolism
5. Poor bronchial toilet and atelectasis
6. Aspiration
7. Pneumonia
8. Excessive infusion of fluid
9. Allergic drug alveolitis
10. Pulmonary contusion
11. Oxygen toxicity
12. Remote sepsis
13. Hemorrhagic shock
14. Fat embolism
15. Diffuse intravascular coagulation
16. Pancreatitis
17. Head injury

be managed with a mechanical ventilator until they can continue spontaneous respiration without tiring excessively. Any associated bronchitis, pneumonia, or atelectasis should be vigorously treated, and the patients should be encouraged to change position and to get out of bed frequently. An attempt should be made to improve muscle strength by better nutrition and by supervised exercise. Improved nutrition often requires parenteral alimentation; however, the volume of fluid that can be utilized must be limited in order to prevent an increase in lung water.

The remaining causes listed in Table 9-1 may be divided into two groups: those that produce transient pulmonary insufficiency, such as an excessive infusion of fluid during surgery, and those that may lead to progressive pulmonary failure and death, a condition often termed the adult respiratory distress syndrome (ARDS). This syndrome is a part of the multiple organ failure associated with severe illness or injury that also includes failure of the kidneys, the liver, the immune system, and the gastric mucosa. By far the most common cause of ARDS is sepsis. However, in only half of the cases of sepsis is the lung itself clinically infected; in the rest, the infection is remote from the lung.

The pathogenesis of ARDS is generally believed to involve an increase in the permeability of the pulmonary microvasculature to macromolecules with a resultant increase in pulmonary extravascular water, but the mechanism by which a remote infection can cause an increase in the permeability of the pulmonary microvasculature is unknown. Three theories are currently held: 1) The change is mediated by the extrinsic or intrinsic nerve supply of the lung, possibly by causing pulmonary venospasm and subsequent capillary disruption. 2) Either increased concentrations of normally occurring substances or novel biologically active material in the blood may damage the pulmonary microvascular endothelium. 3) The pulmonary microvascular endothelium is damaged by some of the formed elements of the blood, such as blood clots resulting from diffuse intravascular coagulation or by granulocytes stimulated by activated compliment (10). Possibly several of these postulated mechanisms may play a role.

Pathology

Because the lung has limited means of reacting to injury, ARDS caused by any of the listed etiologies results in similar pathologic changes. Early in the course, petechial hemorrhages occur on the pleural surface, and scattered areas of atelectasis can be seen. Histologic examination shows capillary and venous engorgement, some interstitial edema, and areas of alveolar collapse.

As the syndrome develops, the alveolar lining shows damage. The type I alveolar cells are replaced by hyaline membranes; interstitial and alveolar edema increase. A marked infiltrate of polymorphonuclear leukocytes develops, and peribronchial, perivascular, and intraalveolar hemorrhage occurs. In the fully developed syndrome, the lungs become solid, and they grossly resemble liver. If the patient survives, beginning at about the second week interstitial fibrosis progressively increases for several months, after which it may or may not regress.

Clinical Course

The early course of the adult respiratory distress syndrome varies with the etiology. If the syndrome is caused by aspiration, the onset will be abrupt; if it is caused by a pulmonary or an abdominal infection, it will develop gradually; if it follows resuscitation from trauma and shock, the onset usually develops gradually after a latent period of 12–24 hours. The initial sign is usually tachypnea with a greater than normal minute volume. The Pa_{CO_2} is low, and because of persisting ventilation–perfusion inequalities, the alveolar–arterial gradient for oxygen is larger than normal, even on an increased concentration of inspired oxygen. Usually such inequalities are partially corrected by the lung's ability to decrease the blood flow to poorly ventilated areas, but after shock the high levels of catecholamines cause a generalized tensing of the pulmonary vasculature that prevents development of regional increases in resistance (5).

As the condition progresses, the chest radiograph will show patchy infiltrates quite characteristic of pulmonary edema, at a time when the left atrial pressure is normal. Areas of atelectasis develop, perhaps due to the decrease in the functional residual capacity and to an inactivation of surfactant by alveolar edema fluid and fibrin. Progressive hypoxemia occurs, and even for the patient on a ventilator, very high concentrations of oxygen may be required to maintain the Pa_{O_2} at 50–60 torr. There is a decrease in lung compliance, i.e., the resistance of the lung to inflation increases. The decrease in compliance may be due to pulmonary vascular engorgement. It is probably not due to the increase in lung water, because the compliance of a lung filled with water and ventilated with water is little different from the compliance of a lung ventilated with air. Compliance can be measured in patients on a ventilator by dividing the tidal volume by the change in the airway pressure used to produce that volume.

A fatal outcome for patients with ARDS is often signalled by an increasing pulmonary vascular resistance, a rising Pa_{CO_2} with a consequent increase in calculated dead space ventilation, and an increasing alveolar–arterial gradient for oxygen while being ventilated with 100% oxygen.

Therapy

Treatment of a patient with ARDS has two major aspects: first, the removal of the initiating mechanism, and second, the support of respiration as the lung recovers. In addition, an attempt should be made to protect the other organ systems that are at risk. If the pulmonary failure is due to pneumonia, the infecting organism should be isolated and intensively treated. If an intraabdominal abscess or fistula is suspected, the patient's abdomen should be explored and the abscess promptly and adequately drained. To prevent upper gastrointestinal bleeding, the patient should receive both cimetidine and frequent antacids to maintain the gastric pH above 3.5.

The principal support of respiration in most patients with ARDS will come from the use of a mechanical ventilator. The patient's tracheobronchial tree should be kept clean, and supplemental oxygen should be given first by nasal cannulae or mask, but when the Pa_{O_2} cannot be maintained above 60 torr with oxygen delivered by mask, the trachea should be intubated and the patient placed on a volume-cycled respirator. If an inspiratory oxygen concentration of 50% does not maintain the Pa_{O_2} at 60 torr or above, positive end-expiration pressure should be utilized to improve oxygenation. If the Pa_{O_2} is below 60 torr with 50% oxygen and 15 cm H_2O PEEP, the oxygen concentration should be increased to 100% before the PEEP is raised further.

The only treatment presently available to improve lung function is to decrease the lung water content. Diuretics should be used, and the fluid volume infused should be limited to the smallest amount that is still compatible with an adequate cardiac output. The administration of albumin in an attempt to decrease lung water by increasing plasma oncotic pressure is *not* advisable. A significant increase in the permeability of the lung microvasculature to albumin is associated with ARDS (8). Because of this increase in permeability, an increase in the concentration of albumin within the vascular system cannot significantly change the oncotic pressure of the plasma within the lung microvasculature. However, the albumin infusion will increase the vascular volume and consequently increase the capillary hydrostatic pressure. This increased pressure can amplify the transudation of water into the interstitium of the lung.

The use of corticosteroids to treat patients with ARDS is of probable value only for patients with pulmonary failure caused by fat embolism. High doses of corticosteroids in experimental animals decreases the lungs' ability to correct ventilation–perfusion inequalities (12), and Lucas and Ledgerwood (6) have reported that seriously injured patients who received massive doses of steroids had a Pa_{O_2} decrease compared to patients who did not receive steroids. They concluded that massive steroids neither prevent nor ameliorate pulmonary failure after shock.

References

1. Brown EB, Goot B: Intracellular hydrogen ion changes and potassium movement. Am J Physiol 204:765–770, 1963.
2. Carlon GC, Kahn RC, Howland WS, Ray C, Turnbull AD: Clinical experience with high frequency jet ventilation. Crit Care Med 9:1–6, 1981.
3. Cournand A, Motley HL, Werko L, Richards DW: Physiological studies of the effects of intermittent positive pressure breathing on cardiac output in man. Am J Physiol 152:162–174, 1948.
4. Geer RT: Mechanical ventilation. *In* Fishman AP (Ed): Pulmonary Diseases and Disorders. New York, McGraw-Hill, 1980.
5. Kersten TE, Mayer JE, Varco RL, Humphrey EW: The nature of failure of pulmonary adaptation to atelectasis. Surgery 82:90–98, 1977.
6. Lucas CE, Ledgerwood AM: Pulmonary response of massive steroids in seriously injured patients. Ann Surg 194:256–261, 1981.
7. Mithoefer JC: Oxygen therapy. *In* Fishman AP (Ed): Pulmonary Diseases and Disorders. New York, McGraw-Hill, 1980.
8. Northrup WF, Humphrey EW: The effect of hemorrhagic shock on pulmonary vascular permeability to plasma proteins. Surgery 83:264–273, 1978.
9. Pontoppidan H, Wilson RS, Rie MA, Schneider RC: Respiratory intensive care. Anesthesiology 47:96–116, 1977.
10. Sachs T, Moldow CF, Craddock PR, Bowers TK, Jacob HS: Oxygen radicals mediate endothelial cell damage by complement-stimulated granulocytes. J Clin Invest 61:1161–1167, 1978.
11. Schachter EN, Tucker D, Beck GJ: Does intermittent mandatory ventilation accelerate weaning. JAMA 246:1210–1214, 1981.
12. Schwartz ML, Northrup WF, Nicoloff DM, Humphrey EW: The effect of steroids on adaptation to atelectatic shunting. J Thorac Cardiovasc Surg 68:822–829, 1974.
13. Sjöstrand U: High-frequency positive-pressure ventilation (HEPPV): A review. Crit Care Med 8:345–364, 1980.
14. Slutsky AS, Brown R, Lehr J, Rossing T, Drazen JM: High-frequency ventilation: A promising new approach to mechanical ventilation. Med Instrum 15:229–233, 1981.
15. West JB: Ventilation–perfusion relationships. Am Rev Respir Dis 116:919–943, 1977.

Index

Q

R